Laboratory Diagnosis of
Inherited Metabolic Diseases

Laboratory Diagnosis of Inherited Metabolic Diseases

Edited by
Uttam Garg, PhD
Laurie D. Smith, MD, PhD
Bryce A. Heese, MD

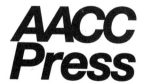

1850 K Street, NW, Suite 625
Washington, DC 20006

Cover design by Janet Harward

1 2 3 4 5 6 7 8 9 0   VGI   14 13 12

Printed in the United States of America

Library of Congress Cataloging-in-Publication Data

Laboratory diagnosis : inherited metabolic diseases / edited by Uttam Garg, Laurie D. Smith, Bryce A. Heese.
    p. cm.
  Title from table of contents: Laboratory diagnosis of inherited metabolic diseases
  Includes bibliographical references and index.
  ISBN 978-1-59425-140-5 (alk. paper)
  1. Metabolism, Inborn errors of—Diagnosis. 2. Diagnosis, Laboratory. I. Garg, Uttam.
II. Smith, Laurie D. III. Heese, Bryce A. IV. Title: Inherited metabolic diseases. V. Title:
Laboratory diagnosis of inherited metabolic diseases.
  RC627.8.L315 2012
  616.07´56—dc23
                                                    2012012727

This book is dedicated to—
My daughters, Megha and Mohini, and wife, Jyotsna (UG);
My children who inspired me to go to medical school,
my husband who continually encourages me,
and the patients who inspire me daily (LDS); and
My children and my wife, Jennifer (BAH).

Contents

Preface

With increased recognition, the expansion of newborn screening, and continued successes in treatment, patients with inherited metabolic diseases are experiencing better outcomes and longer survival. Thus, an increasing number of laboratory and clinical professionals are encountering patients with inherited metabolic diseases and are challenged with the diagnosis and initial management of individuals with these conditions. However, these diseases are still rare and infrequently encountered, and the laboratory workup can often be complex, especially because the information about laboratory test selection and interpretation is not readily available. The laboratory plays a vital role in the diagnosis and monitoring of patients with inherited metabolic diseases; therefore, knowledge about laboratory testing is extremely important for patient management and better outcome. *Laboratory Diagnosis of Inherited Metabolic Diseases* is intended to provide information about laboratory test selection; sample collection, processing, and handling; and interpretation of results in patients with suspected inherited metabolic diseases. Laboratory tests are generally categorized into initial tests, which are typically available in a routine hospital laboratory, and specialized tests. Specialized follow-up and confirmatory tests generally include amino acid, organic acid, acylcarnitine, enzyme assay, and DNA analyses that are not available in most hospital laboratories and require special attention to sample collection and handling as well as result interpretation. This book, written by practicing laboratorians and healthcare providers, provides information about these important aspects along with interpretation of laboratory data. Several illustrative chromatograms generated from patients with inherited metabolic disorders are provided. Laboratorians will find enough information on most laboratory tests to identify necessary resources to set up a particular method. Although the main emphasis of the book is on the laboratory diagnosis of metabolic disorders, basic information on clinical presentation, genetics, pathogenesis, treatment, and prognosis on selected inherited metabolic diseases is also provided.

We are indebted to our authors and colleagues who made this book possible. Also, we whole-heartedly acknowledge the support of Joanna Grimes at AACC Press.

Uttam Garg
Laurie D. Smith
Bryce A. Heese

Editors

Uttam Garg, PhD, DABCC, FACB
Professor of Pathology
University of Missouri School of Medicine
Director of Clinical Chemistry Laboratories
Department of Pathology and Laboratory Medicine
Children's Mercy Hospitals and Clinics
Kansas City, Missouri

Laurie D. Smith, MD, PhD
Associate Professor of Pediatrics
University of Missouri School of Medicine
Clinical and Biochemical Geneticist
Section of Genetics
Department of Pediatrics
Department of Pathology and Laboratory Medicine
Children's Mercy Hospitals and Clinics
Kansas City, Missouri

Bryce A. Heese, MD
Assistant Professor of Pediatrics
University of Missouri School of Medicine
Clinical and Biochemical Geneticist
Section of Genetics
Department of Pediatrics
Department of Pathology and Laboratory Medicine
Children's Mercy Hospitals and Clinics
Kansas City, Missouri

Contributors

Andrea M. Atherton, MS, CGC
Genetic Counselor
Section of Genetics
Children's Mercy Hospitals and Clinics
Kansas City, Missouri
Chapters 7 and 8

Michael J. Bennett, PhD, FRCPath, FACB, DABCC
Professor of Pathology and Laboratory
  Medicine
University of Pennsylvania
Evelyn Willing Bromley Endowed Chair in
  Clinical Laboratories and Pathology
Director, Metabolic Disease Laboratory
The Children's Hospital of Philadelphia
Philadelphia, Pennsylvania
Chapter 5

Dennis J. Dietzen, PhD, DABCC, FACB
Associate Professor of Pediatrics
Washington University School of Medicine
Director, Core Laboratory and Metabolic
  Genetics Laboratory
St. Louis Children's Hospital
St. Louis, Missouri
Chapter 2

Angela M. Ferguson, PhD, DABCC, FACB
Assistant Professor
University of Missouri School of Medicine
Assistant Director, Clinical Chemistry
  Laboratory
Department of Pathology and
  Laboratory Medicine
Children's Mercy Hospitals and Clinics
Kansas City, Missouri
Chapter 6

Uttam Garg, PhD, DABCC, FACB
Professor of Pathology
University of Missouri School of Medicine
Director of Clinical Chemistry Laboratories
Department of Pathology and
  Laboratory Medicine
Children's Mercy Hospitals and Clinics
Kansas City, Missouri
Chapters 1, 4, 6–9, 15, and 16

Miao He, PhD, FACMG
Assistant Professor
Director, Emory Biochemical Genetics
  Laboratory
Department of Human Genetics
Emory University
Atlanta, Georgia
Chapter 13

Bryce A. Heese, MD
Assistant Professor of Pediatrics
University of Missouri School of Medicine
Clinical and Biochemical Geneticist
Section of Genetics
Department of Pediatrics
Department of Pathology and
  Laboratory Medicine
Children's Mercy Hospitals and Clinics
Kansas City, Missouri
Chapters 1, 7, 8, 10, 14, and 15

Keith Hyland, PhD
Vice President
Director, Department of Neurochemistry
Medical Neurogenetics
Atlanta, Georgia
Chapter 11

Lauren A. Hyland, MS
Department of Neurochemistry
Medical Neurogenetics
Atlanta, Georgia
Chapter 11

Patricia M. Jones, PhD, DABCC, FACB
Professor
Pathology and Medical Laboratory Sciences
University of Texas Southwestern
    Medical Center
Clinical Director of Chemistry
Children's Medical Center Dallas
Dallas, Texas
Chapter 5

Van Leung-Pineda, PhD, DABCC
Director of Clinical Chemistry
Department of Pathology and Laboratory
Cook Children's Medical Center
Fort Worth, Texas
Chapter 2

Stanley F. Lo, PhD, DABCC
Associate Professor of Pathology
Department of Pathology
Medical College of Wisconsin
Milwaukee, Wisconsin
Chapter 3

Dietrich Matern, MD, FACMG
Professor of Laboratory Medicine, Medical
    Genetics, and Pediatrics
Department of Laboratory Medicine
    and Pathology
Mayo Clinic
Rochester, Minnesota
Chapter 13

William E. O'Brien, PhD
Professor
Department of Molecular and Human Genetics
Baylor College of Medicine
Houston, Texas
Chapter 12

Devin Oglesbee, PhD, FACMG
Assistant Professor
Department of Laboratory Medicine
    and Pathology, and Department of
    Medical Genetics
Mayo Clinic
Rochester, Minnesota
Chapter 14

Kimiyo M. Raymond, MD
Assistant Professor of Laboratory Medicine
    and Medical Genetics
Department of Laboratory Medicine
    and Pathology
Mayo Clinic
Rochester, Minnesota
Chapter 13

William J. Rhead, MD, PhD
Professor of Pediatrics and Pathology
Department of Pediatrics
Medical College of Wisconsin
Milwaukee, Wisconsin
Chapter 3

Jessica A. Scott-Schwoerer, MD
Assistant Professor
Department of Pediatrics
University of Wisconsin Hospital and Clinics
Madison, Wisconsin
Chapter 3

Laurie D. Smith, MD, PhD
Associate Professor of Pediatrics
University of Missouri School of Medicine
Clinical and Biochemical Geneticist
Section of Genetics
Department of Pediatrics
Department of Pathology and
    Laboratory Medicine
Children's Mercy Hospitals and Clinics
Kansas City, Missouri
Chapters 1, 4, 6–9, 15, and 16

Qin Sun, PhD, FACMG
Assistant Professor
Department of Molecular and Human Genetics
Baylor College of Medicine
Houston, Texas
Chapter 12

V. Reid Sutton, MD, FACMG
Associate Professor
Department of Molecular and Human Genetics
Baylor College of Medicine
Houston, Texas
Chapter 12

Lynne Wolfe, MS, CRNP, BC
Nurse Practitioner
Undiagnosed Diseases Program
National Institutes of Health/National Human
    Genome Research Institute
Bethesda, Maryland
Chapter 13

Zhen Zhao, PhD
Clinical Chemistry Fellow
Department of Pathology/Immunology
Washington University School of Medicine
St. Louis, Missouri
Chapter 2

Chapter 1

Introduction to the Laboratory Diagnosis of Inherited Metabolic Diseases

Uttam Garg, Laurie D. Smith, and Bryce A. Heese

Inherited metabolic diseases, "inborn errors of metabolism," are genetic disorders that involve defects in intermediary metabolism. Individually rare, inherited metabolic diseases are collectively common. According to some estimates the frequency of inherited metabolic diseases is as high as 1:500. Most of these diseases are due to defects in single genes that code for enzymes or membrane transporters. The defects lead to accumulation of substrates before the metabolic block, formation of toxic intermediates by metabolism of substrates by alternative metabolic pathways, and/or lack of essential products. These metabolic changes can interrupt normal metabolism.

The clinical presentations of inherited metabolic disorders can be quite variable. Saudubray et al. *(1)* have presented a classification scheme that groups inherited metabolic disorders into different categories: those that involve complex molecules, those that lead to intoxication, and those that affect energy metabolism. Several clinical scenarios might suggest the diagnosis of an inborn error of metabolism. The acutely ill neonate who might appear to have sepsis but does not respond to the appropriate interventions suggests a metabolic disorder that results from intoxication. The child or adult with later-onset or recurrent symptoms such as vomiting, metabolic acidosis, ataxia, or coma might suggest an intermittent disorder of intoxication or energy metabolism. Any of these disorders may present with chronic and progressive symptoms that involve the muscles, gastrointestinal tract, or central nervous system. The disorders involving the accumulation of complex molecules may also present with behavioral changes, coarsening of facial features, or joint contractures. Acute behavioral disturbances and psychoses can also be associated with some of these disorders, ranging from lysosomal disorders such as Niemann-Pick C to disorders of metal transport such as Wilson disease. The inborn errors of metabolism can also present with specific organ involvement such as a cardiomyopathy or hepatic dysfunction. An inborn error of metabolism should generally be considered in any patient without a clear diagnosis for their clinical findings. Several excellent resources are available on the clinical aspects of inherited metabolic diseases *(2–8)*.

Laboratory tests are often required in the diagnosis and confirmation of suspected inherited metabolic diseases. In recent years, in developed countries, newborn screening programs have expanded significantly and are capable of making laboratory diagnoses of many inherited metabolic disorders at birth *(9–11)*. Laboratory tests are used in the confirmation of screen positive results *(11)*. Laboratory tests can broadly be divided into two categories: routine and specialized tests. Routine laboratory tests such as glucose, electrolytes, ammonia, lactate, renal function tests, liver function tests, urinalysis, and basic hematological tests are available in a routine hospital laboratory and can provide important clues in the diagnosis and initial management of a patient with suspected inherited metabolic disorders. More specialized tests such as amino acids, organic acids, acylcarnitines, enzyme assays, and DNA tests are generally not available in a local hospital and are sent out to specialized laboratories. It is important that the samples be collected, processed, and transported carefully according to the instructions provided by the specialized laboratory.

LABORATORY DIAGNOSIS

The clinical laboratory plays a vital role in the diagnosis of inherited metabolic diseases. Body fluids, most commonly blood and urine, and less commonly cerebrospinal and amniotic fluids, are analyzed for the diagnosis and confirmation of metabolic disorders *(5, 12)*. Enzyme assays and DNA analyses are also frequently used in the diagnosis and confirmation of inherited metabolic diseases. In postmortem investigations, additional samples may include bile acids and vitreous fluids. In general, metabolites are less variable in blood and cerebrospinal fluid (CSF) as compared with urine. However, many metabolic disorders cause accumulation of metabolites in urine to much higher concentrations than blood, making urine the specimen of choice. When testing is performed on urine, expressing results relative to creatinine concentration to account for sample dilution generally provides more diagnostic value.

For patient management, in general, laboratory tests can be divided into screening spot tests, routine tests, and specialized tests. Although spot tests are now less frequently used, they may be helpful in quick screening when other tests are not available. These tests suffer from lack of sensitivity and specificity. Some simple metabolic screening tests are listed in Table 1-1.

The routine tests are generally available in most hospital laboratories and are helpful in the initial management of a patient with a suspected inherited metabolic disorder. These tests include pH, arterial blood gases, electrolytes, glucose, renal function tests, liver function tests, ammonia, lactate, urinalysis and routine hematological tests. Changes in these tests in various metabolic disorders are given in Table 1-2.

The specialized tests are generally not available in a routine hospital laboratory but are needed for the establishment and confirmation of a suspected disorder. Commonly used specialized laboratory tests include plasma and urine amino acid profiles, urine organic acid profiles, and plasma acylcarnitine profiles *(13)*. The other specialized tests include plasma pyruvate, acetoacetate, 3-hydroxybutyrate, mucopolysaccharides, oligosaccharides, enzyme assays, and mutational analyses.

Although with the availability of better tests the need for functional tests has decreased in recent years, it may be necessary to perform a functional test to uncover a metabolic disorder. In general, functional tests expose the patient to high concentrations of a specific substrate. This may cause dangerously high concentrations of toxic metabolites causing serious complications. Therefore, it is important to strictly follow the established protocols to perform functional tests. Some functional tests and the associated metabolic disorders are listed in Table 1-3.

Sample Collection and Processing

The importance of correct sample collection and processing cannot be overemphasized. Many laboratory tests used in the diagnosis of metabolic disorders need special attention. For example, samples for lactate and ammonia need to be collected and transported to the laboratory on ice, and plasma must be separated immediately. Samples for plasma amino acid profiles should be collected after fasting. Table 1-4 provides the list of commonly used tests along with sample requirements and handling.

Sample Analysis

Sample analysis in a biochemical genetics laboratory is quite different as compared to a routine chemistry laboratory. The common differences from the routine analyses include manual assays, in-house preparation of reagents, unavailability of commercial controls, calibrators and internal standards, lack of external proficiency testing materials for most assays, multicomponent analysis, and less defined reference intervals. Because of these differences, methods evaluations in a biochemical genetics laboratory pose unique challenges and may not follow the typical methods evaluations in a routine laboratory. However, the basic components of methods evaluation and implementation are the same and discussed in the following subsection.

Table 1-1 Metabolic Screening Tests

Test	Analyte	Common disorder	Comment
Cyanide nitroprusside (sodium nitroprusside and sodium cyanide)	Cystine	Cystinuria Generalized aminoaciduria	Cyanide nitroprusside reacts with disulfide-containing compounds to form pink to purple color. Other substances it reacts with include cysteine-homocysteine, glutathione, 2-mercapto-lactate-cysteine, dithiodiglycol, dithiodiglycolic acid, diethyl disulfide, drugs (sulfur-containing drugs such as *N*-acetylcysteine, captopril, penicillamine), and aceto-acetate.
	Homocysteine	Homocystinuria Severe B12/cobalamin deficiency	
Dinitrophenyl-hydrazine (DNPH)	Branched chain 2-ketoacids (2-keto-isovaleric, 2-keto-isocaproic, 2-keto-3-methylvaleric acids)	Maple syrup urine disease (MSUD)	DNPH reacts with 2-ketoacids to form hydrazones, which form precipitates. DNPH causes positive test with imidazolepyruvic acid (histidinemia), acetone, 2-ketobutyric acid (methionine malabsorption), and acetone.
	Phenylpyruvic acid 4-Hydroxyphenyl-pyruvic acid	Phenylketonuria Liver disease, tyrosinemia types 1 and 2	
Reducing substances	Fructose Galactose Homogentisic acid 4-Hydroxyphenyl-pyruvic acid Xylose	Fructose intolerance Galactosemia Alkaptonuria Tyrosinemia type 1 and 2 Pentosuria	Reducing substances reduce copper (cupric ions) to form green to orange color. Many other substances including glucose, lactose, maltose, arabinose, ribose, uric acid, ascorbic acid, cysteine, ketones, sulfanilamide, oxalic acid, hippuric acid, glucuronic acid, formaldehyde, isoniazid, salicylates, cinchophen, and salicyluric acid cause positive test.
Sulfite	Sulfite	Sulfite oxidase deficiency Molybdenum cofactor deficiency	The sample should be tested fresh.

Method Evaluation

Before starting the method evaluation, it is important to select the right method. Method selection is generally achieved through literature search and consultation with colleagues. Method selection involves evaluating clinical needs and other logistics such as instrumentation, reagents, staffing, employee competency, number of samples being analyzed, and sample requirements/collection/transportation/processing, etc.

Table 1-2   Routine Laboratory Tests/Investigations and Commonly Associated Diseases

Test	Disorders
Ammonia, high	Urea cycle disorders
	Dibasic amino aciduria
	Hyperinsulinism-hyperammonemia
	Lysinuric protein intolerance
	Carnitine uptake defect
	Carnitine palmitoyltransferase-1 deficiency
	Acylcarnitine translocase deficiency
	Maple syrup urine disease (maybe)
	Branched chain amino acids organic acidurias (maybe)
	Severe liver disease
AST/ALT/bilirubin—	Tyrosinemia type 1
abnormal liver function tests	Fatty acid oxidation defects:
	Carnitine uptake defect
	Carnitine palmitoyltransferase-1 deficiency
	Carnitine palmitoyltransferase-2 deficiency
	Very-long-chain acyl-CoA dehydrogenase deficiency
	Medium-chain acyl-CoA dehydrogenase deficiency
	Short-chain acyl-CoA dehydrogenase deficiency
	Long-chain 3-hydroxyacyl-CoA dehydrogenase deficiency
	Multiple acyl-CoA dehydrogenase deficiency
	Carbohydrate metabolism defects:
	Glycogen storage disease types 1, 3, 6, 9
	Glycogen synthase deficiency
	Pyruvate carboxylase deficiency
	Galactose-1-phosphate uridyltransferase deficiency
	Hereditary fructose intolerance
	Fructose-1,6-diphosphatase deficiency
	Glycogen storage disorders 3–7
	Lipid metabolism defects:
	Cholesterol-7-hydroxylase deficiency
	3-Hydroxy-Δ^5-C27-steroid dehydrogenase deficiency
	3-Oxo-Δ^4-5β-reductase deficiency
	3-Hydroxy-3-methylglutaryl-CoA synthase deficiency
	Cholesteryl ester storage disease
	Gaucher disease, type 1
	Niemann-Pick disease, types A and B
	Acid lipase deficiency/Wolman disease
	Hyperammonemias
	Ornithine transcarbamylase
	Argininosuccinic aciduria
	Arginase deficiency
	Lysinuric protein intolerance
	Hemochromatosis
	α1-Antitrypsin deficiency
	Wilson disease
	Zellweger syndrome
	CDG-1e
Cholesterol, high	Lipoprotein lipase deficiency
	Dysbetalipoproteinemia
	Defective apoB-100
	Hepatic lipase deficiency
	Lecithin cholesterol acyltransferase deficiency
	Sterol 27-hydroxylase deficiency

Table 1-2   Routine Laboratory Tests/Investigations and Commonly Associated Diseases *(Continued)*

Test	Disorders
Cholesterol, low	Mevalonic aciduria
	Abetalipoproteinemia
	Hypobetalipoproteinemia
	Smith-Lemli-Opitz syndrome
	Other cholesterol biosynthesis disorders
	Barth syndrome
	Glucosyltransferase I deficiency
	CDG-Ic
Creatine kinase, high	Fatty acid oxidation defects:
	Carnitine palmitoyltransferase-2 deficiency
	Very-long-chain acyl-CoA dehydrogenase deficiency
	Long-chain 3-hydroxyacyl-CoA dehydrogenase deficiency
	Multiple acyl-CoA dehydrogenase deficiency
	Glycogen storage disorders 2, 3, 5
	CDG-Ic
	Myoadenylate deaminase deficiency
Creatinine, low	Creatine synthetic defects
Creatinine/urea, high	Lysosomal cystine transport
	Hyperoxaluria type 1
Glucose, low	Fatty acid oxidation disorders
	Glycogen storage disorders
	Galactosemia
	Fructose-1,6-diphosphatase deficiency
	Pyruvate carboxylase deficiency
	Multiple acyl-CoA dehydrogenase deficiency
	Hereditary fructose intolerance
Hemoglobin, low	B12 metabolism deficiency
	Folate metabolism disorders
	Glucose-6-phosphate dehydrogenase deficiency
	5-Oxoprolinuria
	Glutathione synthesis defects
	Glycolysis defects
Iron/transferrin saturation, high	Hemochromatosis
Lactate, high	Glycogen metabolism disorders:
	Amylo-1,6-glucosidase deficiency
	Glucose-6-phosphatase deficiency
	Glucose-6-phosphate translocase deficiency
	Glycogen synthetase deficiency
	Liver phosphorylase deficiency
	Lactate/pyruvate disorders:
	Pyruvate dehydrogenase deficiency
	Pyruvate carboxylase deficiency
	Krebs cycle/respiratory chain/mitochondrial defects:
	Ketoglutarate dehydrogenase defect
	Fumarase defect
	Respiratory chain complexes I–V
	Hyperammonemias
	Fatty acid oxidation defects
	Fructose-1,6-diphosphatase deficiency

(Continued)

Table 1-2   Routine Laboratory Tests/Investigations and Commonly Associated Diseases (*Continued*)

Test	Disorders
Lactate, high *(continued)*	Organic aciduria:
	Methylmalonic aciduria
	Propionic aciduria
	Isovaleric aciduria
	Biotinidase deficiency
	Holocarboxylase synthetase deficiency
	L-2-Hydroxyglutaric aciduria
	Acquired causes:
	Hypoxia
	Drug intoxications—salicylate, cyanide
pH, low, acidosis	Organic acidurias:
	Methylmalonic aciduria
	Propionic aciduria
	Isovaleric aciduria
	3-Methylcrotonylglycinuria
	3-Methylglutaconic aciduria
	3-Hydroxy-3-methylglutaryl-CoA lyase deficiency
	Biotinidase deficiency
	Holocarboxylase synthetase deficiency
	3-Oxothiolase deficiency
	2-Ketoglutarate dehydrogenase complex deficiency
	3-Hydroxyisobutyric aciduria
	Maple syrup urine disease
	Mitochondrial disorders
	Fatty acid oxidation defects:
	Carnitine uptake defect
	Carnitine palmitoyltransferase-1 deficiency
	Very-long-chain acyl-CoA dehydrogenase deficiency
	Medium-chain acyl-CoA dehydrogenase deficiency
	Short-chain acyl-CoA dehydrogenase deficiency
	Long-chain 3-hydroxyacyl-CoA dehydrogenase deficiency
	Multiple acyl-CoA dehydrogenase deficiency
	Carbohydrate metabolism defects:
	Glycogen storage disease types 1, 3, 6, 9
	Glycogen synthase deficiency
	Pyruvate carboxylase deficiency
	Galactosemia
	Fructose-1,6-diphosphatase deficiency
	Glycerol kinase deficiency
Phosphate, low	Fanconi syndrome
	X-linked hypophosphatemic rickets
Triglycerides, high	Glycogen storage disease type 1
	Lipoprotein lipase deficiency
	Dysbetalipoproteinemia
	Hepatic lipase deficiency
	Lecithin cholesterol acyltransferase deficiency
Uric acid, high	Hypoxanthine phosphorybosyl transferase deficiency
	Phosphorybosylpyrophosphate synthetase deficiency
	Glycogen storage disease type 1
Uric acid, low	Purine nucleoside phosphorylase deficiency
	Molybdenum cofactor deficiency
	Xanthine oxidase/dehydrogenase

Table 1-3   Functional Tests and Associated Disorders

Test	Indication
Allopurinol test	Diagnosis of heterozygous or mild cases of ornithine transcarbamylase deficiency. There will be an increase in urinary orotic acid excretion. Urinary orotic acid will also increase in phosphoribosylpyrophosphate deficiency.
Glucagon stimulation test	Diagnosis of glycogen storage disease type 1 (von Gierke disease)
Oral galactose loading test	Diagnosis of glycogen storage disease types 0, 1, 3, 6, 9. Lactate increases in these disorders.
Tetrahydrobiopterin (BH_4)	Identify BH_4-responsive phenylketonuric patients.

Once the method is selected, it should undergo rigorous validation before patient testing is started and results are used for diagnostic purposes. Validation is defined as confirmation, through evidence, that the method meets the intended use. Common components of a method validation include evaluation of accuracy, precision/imprecision, reportable range, analytical measurement range/linearity, clinical reportable range, analytical sensitivity/limit of quantitation, and analytical selectivity/specificity *(14)*. Other components may include method comparison, carryover monitoring, recovery, and sample stability. Establishment or verification of reference ranges is required for most quantitative methods.

Accuracy, which is defined as closeness of the test result to the true value, is evaluated by preparing matrix matched samples containing known amounts of the analyte. It can be achieved by acquiring samples with known concentrations from a reputable source. A minimum of three, but generally five to six, concentrations covering the range of expected concentrations should be used. These samples are analyzed several times, generally 3–5 times, and the mean is calculated and compared with the target value. Accuracy is considered acceptable if the deviation of the results is within acceptable limits. If reportable lower and upper concentrations are covered with these samples, analytical measurement range/linearity can be evaluated with these data. Any sample with the concentration above the highest tested concentration should be diluted and rerun. In many cases this may not be needed for the diagnosis of a specific disease and the results may be reported as more than the upper limit of linearity.

The precision of an analytical method describes the closeness of individual results. The measure of precision is generally evaluated by measuring imprecision and is expressed as the standard deviation (SD) or more commonly as the coefficient of variation (CV) that is defined as relative standard deviation (RSD) and is calculated as $SD \times 100/Mean$. Two types of imprecision should be evaluated: within-run or within-day (short-term) imprecision and between-run or between-day (long-term) imprecision. Two to three concentrations in the expected range are generally used. A commonly used method for evaluating short-term imprecision is to run quality-control samples approximately 20 times within a run or within a day. For evaluation of long-term imprecision, quality-control samples are run approximately 20 times within different runs at different days. Imprecision is considered acceptable if the experimental CVs are less than the established goals.

In evaluating analytical sensitivity, generally two parameters—limit of detection and limit of quantitation—are evaluated. Limit of detection is defined as the lowest concentration a method can detect. There are several methods for establishing limit of detection. One way of calculating the limit of detection is to run a blank sample (containing no analyte of interest) several times and calculate the mean and SD. The limit of detection is calculated as the mean plus 2 or 3 SD. In chromatographic techniques, the lowest concentration that gives a clear peak can be considered as the lower limit of detection. The limit of quantitation is defined as the concentration that can be measured with defined accuracy. Limit of quantitation can be calculated by running several samples containing low analyte concentrations and calculating the CV at each concentration. The lower limit of quantitation is defined as the lowest concentration at which an acceptable CV is obtained.

Table 1-4   Sample Collection and Storage[a]

Analyte	Sample type	Storage/shipping/comment
Acylcarnitines	Plasma (ethylenediaminetetra-acetic acid [EDTA] or heparin)	Freeze.
Alkaline phosphatase	Serum or plasma (heparin)	Refrigerate if sample cannot be analyzed in 4 h.
Amino acids	Plasma (heparin) or urine (random)	Refrigerate if done in-house. Freeze for shipping. Fasting blood sample is preferred.
Ammonia	Plasma (heparin)	Send immediately on ice. Postprandial sample is preferred. Recollect if sample is hemolyzed. Freeze plasma if analysis cannot be done in 4 h.
Complete blood count (CBC)	Blood (EDTA)	Refrigerate if sample cannot be analyzed the same day.
Creatine kinase	Serum or plasma (heparin)	Hemolysis will falsely increase creatine kinase. Refrigerate if sample cannot be analyzed in 4 h.
Creatinine/urea	Serum or plasma (heparin)	Stable at room temperature for 3 days.
Electrolytes	Serum or plasma (heparin)	Hemolysis will cause increase in potassium.
Glucose	Plasma (fluoride)	Send as soon as possible. Heparin plasma is acceptable if sample can be processed and analyzed within 30 min. Fasting sample when possible.
Lactate	Plasma (heparin or fluoride)	Send immediately on ice. Separate plasma immediately. Freeze if sample cannot be analyzed in 4 h.
Lactate dehydro-genase	Serum or plasma (heparin)	Hemolysis will cause false increase in lactate dehydrogenase.
Lipids	Serum or plasma (heparin)	Refrigerate.
Liver enzymes	Serum or plasma (heparin)	Hemolysis will increase aspartate amino-transferase (AST).
Organic acids	Urine (random)	Refrigerate if done in-house. Freeze for shipping. Scope of testing varies among laboratories.
pH and blood gases	Whole blood (heparin)	Send immediately on ice.
Pyruvate	Whole blood (heparin)	Add sample to prechilled tube containing perchloric acid.
Uric acid	Serum, plasma (heparin), or urine (random or timed collection)	Many drugs interfere in uric acid methods. Consult laboratory.
Urinalysis	Urine (random or timed)	Tests generally include pH, specific gravity, protein, glucose, bilirubin, urobilinogen, leukocyte esterase, and cell count.

[a]For long-term storage, freeze serum or plasma.

It is important to keep in mind that the method evaluation described above works well with routine methods. In fact, routine laboratory tests, for the last several decades, have become very well established. Reagents and instruments have become robust, and it is a common practice that manufacturers of the instruments will do the methods evaluation and the laboratory will have to just validate the manufacturers' claims. However, it may be more challenging to validate all of the components of method evaluation as described above in a more complex multiple component analysis. For example, it is very difficult to validate very high concentrations of individual amino acids by an amino acid analyzer in which the analytical runs are very long, and there are an unlimited number of combinations for amino acid concentrations that can exist in a particular sample. In addition, it is not known how a very high concentration of one amino acid can affect the quantitation of another amino acid. Therefore, it is not practical to perform detailed linearity studies for all possible combinations. Reporting a value that is roughly close to the actual value may be enough for diagnosis and serve the clinical purpose of interpretation of patient data. Furthermore, the laboratory data are interpreted along with the patient's clinical information.

Whenever possible, the results of a new method should be compared with the results from another established laboratory. This is particularly important when interpretation of results is involved. Any major discrepancy should be evaluated before putting the method into a clinical use.

Quality Control and Quality Assurance

Quality control and quality assurance are integral parts of a clinical laboratory. Because of frequently available quality-control materials and external proficiency schemes, the quality control and quality assurance are well maintained and established for common laboratory tests. However, quality control and quality assurance are more challenging for rare metabolic tests. For many important diagnostic metabolites, quality-control materials are not available. Furthermore, it is not uncommon to not have standard materials for many metabolites of interest. For example, many organic acids and acylcarnitines of clinical interest are not available as pure compounds; their estimation is at best semiquantitative. These limitations make laboratory diagnosis of metabolic disorders challenging and complicated. For adequate interpretation, it is important that the laboratory results are interpreted in context with patient clinical information. It is not uncommon, particularly for commercial laboratories, to not have adequate patient information during interpretation of laboratory data. Also, it is important to keep in mind that many inherited metabolic disorders are rare and are not frequently encountered, making quality control and assurance for these disorders challenging.

Quality control is generally maintained by running two to three quality-control samples with each batch of patients' samples. For qualitative assays the inclusion of a normal and an abnormal quality-control sample is recommended. For quantitative assays, the inclusion of two to three samples with known values (normal and abnormal) is recommended. Generally, when the results of quality-control samples are within acceptable limits, the patients' results are considered acceptable. One frequently used criterion for establishing an acceptable quality-control range is the use of the mean ± 2 or 3 SDs. This method of quality control works well for the methods measuring single analytes, but it may not work well when multicomponent analysis is done, such as amino acid, acylcarnitine, and organic acid profiles. For example, if the 2 SD rule is used, the chances of having the value of one quality-control sample within quality-control range is 95%, and the probability of two controls within quality-control ranges is $0.95 \times 0.95 = 0.9025$ or 90.25%. If it is a 20-component analysis, with two controls for each component, the probability of all controls within quality-control ranges is only $(0.95)^{20 \times 2} = 0.128$ or 12.8%. Although, this may be an overestimation of failure rate because the quality-control measurements in multicomponent analysis may not be completely independent, it is certain that multicomponent quality control will have a much greater rate of at least one quality-control failure strictly because of random variation than will occur for a single component quality control using the 2 SD rule. Using wider quality-control ranges such as the mean ± 3 SD will lead to higher acceptance of analytical runs but may miss subtle changes in patient values. Sometimes the mean plus/minus a certain percentage, such as the mean $\pm 20\%$, may be used for establishing quality-control ranges. It is important to keep in mind the pros and cons of different approaches of quality control. It is also important to interpret the data in context with specific analytes. For example, detection of succinylacetone on a urine organic acid profile may be clinically significant despite the lack of a succinylacetone control. The analyst should be knowledgeable in the interpretation of minor deviations from the established quality-control rules and be able to objectively judge the performance of a method to be acceptable for clinical use.

In addition to internal quality-control and quality-assurance practices, it is important that the laboratory involved in metabolic testing participate in external proficiency testing programs such as those offered by the College of American Pathologists (CAP) in the United States *(15)* and the European Research Network for evaluation and improvement of screening, Diagnosis and treatment of Inherited disorders of Metabolism (ERNDIM) in Europe *(16)*.

Reference Intervals

Reference intervals, sometimes referred to as "reference values," "normal values," and "expected values," are needed for clinical decision-making because they are used for comparing patients' results to the results from an apparently healthy population. Therefore, it is important that reliable reference intervals are established and provided along with the patients' results. Reference intervals are customarily defined as limits covering the central 95% of the values or the mean ±2 SD (if the data have a Gaussian distribution) and theoretically encompass 95% of healthy individuals. Although not an easy task, reference intervals must be established systematically using well-defined approaches *(17)*. Many factors including age, sex, race, geographic location, fasting, specimen type, etc., can influence reference intervals. If significant differences occur among these factors, partitioning may be required to establish different reference intervals to account for these factors. In general, reference intervals are relatively well defined for the routine laboratory tests. However, this is not the case for many specialized tests, particularly those for which quality-control and standard materials are not available. Approximate reference intervals for common analytes are provided in Table 1-5.

Table 1-5   Approximate Reference Ranges for Common Chemistry Tests

Tests	Age	Conventional units	SI units
Alanine amino-transferase[a]	All ages	5–50 U/L	0.08–0.83 µkat/L
Alkaline phosphatase	0–3 years	110–320 U/L	1.8–5.3 µkat/L
	3–19 years	140–400 U/L	2.3–6.7 µkat/L
	10–12 years	140–560 U/L	2.3–8.3 µkat/L
	12–14 years	105–420 U/L	1.7–7.0 µkat/L
	14–16 years	70–230 U/L	1.2–3.8 µkat/L
	>16 years	50–130 U/L	0.8–2.2 µkat/L
Ammonia	0–2 weeks	15–92 µmol/L	15–92 µmol/L
	2 weeks–2 years	10–62 µmol/L	10–62 µmol/L
	>2 years	4–33 µmol/L	4–33 µmol/L
Aspartate amino-transferase[a]	0–1 week	10–100 U/L	0.16–1.67 µkat/L
	1 week–2 years	20–77 U/L	0.33–1.28 µkat/L
	>2 years	12–50 U/L	0.20–0.83 µkat/L
Bicarbonate	All ages	20–28 meq/L	20–28 mmol/L
Chloride	All ages	98–108 mmol/L	98–108 mmol/L
Cholesterol	0–3 days	45–167 mg/dL	1.2–4.3 mmol/L
	3 days–1 year	65–175 mg/dL	1.7–4.5 mmol/L
	1–4 years	45–182 mg/dL	1.2–4.7 mmol/L
	>4 years	107–200 mg/dL	2.8–5.2 mmol/L
Creatine kinase[a]	0–3 years	60–305 U/L	1.0–5.1 µkat/L
	3–6 years	75–230 U/L	1.3–3.8 µkat/L
	6–9 years	60–365 U/L	1.0–6.1 µkat/L
	9–11 years	60–220 U/L	1.0–3.7 µkat/L
	11–13 years	55–315 U/L	0.9–5.3 µkat/L
	13–15 years, male	60–335 U/L	1.0–5.6 µkat/L
	13–15 years, female	50–240 U/L	0.8–4.0 µkat/L
	>15 years, male	55–370 U/L	0.9–6.2 µkat/L
	>15 years, female	45–230 U/L	0.8–3.8 µkat/L

Table 1-5   Approximate Reference Ranges for Common Chemistry Tests *(Continued)*

Tests	Age	Conventional units	SI units
Creatinine	0–2 weeks	0.06 to 0.64 mg/dL	5.3 to 56.7 µmol/L
	2 weeks–2 years	0.06–0.45 mg/dL	5.3 to 39.9 µmol/L
	2–10 years	0.26–0.64 mg/dL	23.1–56.7 µmol/L
	10–12 years	0.35–0.84 mg/dL	31.0–74.5 µmol/L
	>12 years, male	0.35–1.13 mg/dL	31.0–100.2 µmol/L
	>12 years, female	0.35–0.84 mg/dL	31.0–74.5 µmol/L
Glucose	0–30 days	45–100 mg/dL	2.5–5.6 mmol/L
	>30 days	65 to 110 mg/dL	3.6–6.1 mmol/L
	All ages	50–80 mg/dL (CSF)	2.8–4.4 mmol/L (CSF)
Lactate	All ages	0.6–2.1 mmol/L	0.6–2.1 mmol/L
		0.5–3.2 mmol/L (CSF)	0.5–3.2 mmol/L (CSF)
Lactate dehydrogenase[a]	0–14 days	616–2040 U/L	103–34.0 µkat/L
	14 days–5 years	425–975 U/L	7.1–16.3 µkat/L
	5–12 years	370–840 U/L	6.2–14.0 µkat/L
	12–14 years	370–785 U/L	6.2–13.1 µkat/L
	14–18 years	370–645 U/L	6.2–10.8 µkat/L
	>18 years	313–618 U/L	5.2–10.3 µkat/L
pCO_2, arterial	All ages	35 to 45 mm Hg	4.7 to 6.0 kPa
pH, arterial	All ages	7.35 to 7.45	7.35 to 7.45
Phosphate	0–1 day	4.2–9.0 mg/dL	1.4–2.9 mmol/L
	1 day–2 years	4.2–7.0 mg/dL	1.4–2.3 mmol/L
	2–4 years	3.5–6.8 mg/dL	1.1–2.2 mmol/L
	4–6 years	3.1–6.3 mg/dL	1.0–2.0 mmol/L
	6–12 years	3.0–6.0 mg/dL	1.0–1.9 mmol/L
	12–14 years	2.5–5.0 mg/dL	0.8–1.6 mmol/L
	>14 years	2.3–4.8 mg/dL	0.7–1.5 mmol/L
pO_2, arterial	All ages	80–100 mmHg	10.7 to 13.3 kPa
Potassium	0–3 months	3.5–6.2 mmol/L	3.5–6.2 mmol/L
	>3 months	3.5–5.2 mmol/L	3.5–5.2 mmol/L
Sodium	All ages	135–145 mmol/L	135–145 mmol/L
Triglycerides	All ages	40–150 mg/dL	0.45–1.69 mmol/L
Urea nitrogen	All ages	8–20 mg/dL	2.9–7.1 mmol/L
Uric acid	0–12 years	2.0–7.0 mg/dL	119–417 µmol/L
	>14 years, male	3.0–8.0 mg/dL	179–476 µmol/L
	>14 years, female	2.0–7.0 mg/dL	119–417 µmol/L

[a]Varies significantly with methodology. Reference ranges provided are from the editors' laboratory using Ortho-Clinical Diagnostics Chemistry System (Raritan, NJ).

Whenever possible, each laboratory should establish its own reference intervals. However, most inherited metabolic tests are performed on children, the values change significantly with age, and a large enough number of samples are often not available from apparently healthy individuals, so it may not be possible to establish reference intervals in the laboratory. If the reference intervals cannot be established, the laboratory should verify reference intervals taken from another laboratory or the literature. This can be achieved by comparing the results among different laboratories. Detailed guidelines on establishing and verifying the reference intervals have been published *(17)*.

TREATMENT AND PROGNOSIS

Treatment and prognosis of these disorders are also quite variable. Considerable research has resulted in the development of new treatments for disorders that originally depended solely on dietary restriction of precursor molecules to the development of enzyme replacement therapies and bone marrow transplantation for several of the lysosomal storage diseases. These disorders and developing possible therapeutic interventions remain active areas of clinical research and development. The prognoses for these disorders obviously rely on the underlying diagnosis and the availability of more than just supportive interventions for each of the disorders. Both patient morbidity and mortality are affected by some interventions; however, for some patients, palliation remains the only available intervention, with little effect on final outcomes.

REFERENCES

1. Saudubray JM, Desguerre I, Sedel F, Charpentier C. A clinical approach to inherited metabolic diseases. In: Fernandes J, Saudubray JM, van den Berghe G, Walter JH, eds. Inborn Metabolic Diseases: Diagnosis and Treatment, 4th, Rev. ed. Heidelberg, Germany: Springer, 2006:3–48.
2. Saudubray JM, van den Berghe G, Walter JH, eds. Inborn Metabolic Diseases: Diagnosis and Treatment, 5th ed. New York: Springer-Verlag, 2011.
3. Hoffmann GF, Zschocke J, Nyhan WL, eds. Inherited Metabolic Diseases: A Clinical Approach. Heidelberg, Germany: Springer, 2010.
4. Clarke JTR. A Clinical Guide to Inherited Metabolic Diseases, 3rd ed. Cambridge, UK, New York: Cambridge University Press, 2006.
5. Blau N, Duran M, Blaskovics MD, Gibson KM, eds. Physician's Guide to the Laboratory Diagnosis of Metabolic Diseases, 2nd ed. Berlin: Springer, 2003.
6. GeneTests. http://www.genetests.org (Accessed February 2012).
7. Nyhan WL, Barshop BA, Ozand PT. Atlas of Metabolic Diseases, 2nd ed. London: Hodder Arnold, 2005.
8. Scriver CR, Sly WS, Childs B, Beaudet AL, Valle D, Kinzler KW, Vogelstein B. The Metabolic & Molecular Bases of Inherited Disease, 8th ed. New York: McGraw-Hill, 2001.
9. Rinaldo P, Lim JS, Tortorelli S, Gavrilov D, Matern D. Newborn screening of metabolic disorders: recent progress and future developments. Nestle Nutr Workshop Ser Pediatr Program 2008;62:81–93; discussion 93–6.
10. Yu CL, Gu XF. Newborn screening of inherited metabolic diseases by tandem mass spectrometry. Beijing Da Xue Xue Bao 2006;38:103–6.
11. Dietzen DJ, Rinaldo P, Whitley RJ, Rhead WJ, Hannon WH, Garg UC, et al. National Academy of Clinical Biochemistry laboratory medicine practice guidelines: Follow-up testing for metabolic disease identified by expanded newborn screening using tandem mass spectrometry; executive summary. Clin Chem 2009;55:1615–26.
12. Blau N, Duran M, Gibson KM. Laboratory Guide to the Methods in Biochemical Genetics. Berlin: Springer, 2008.
13. Rinaldo P, Hahn S, Matern D. Inborn errors of amino acid, organic acid and fatty acid metabolism. In: Burtis CA, Ashwood ER, Bruns DE, eds. Tietz Textbook of Clinical Chemistry and Molecular Diagnostics, 4th ed. St. Louis, MO: Saunders, 2006:2207–47.
14. Linnet K, Boyd JC. Selection and analytical evaluation of methods with statistical techniques. In: Burtis CA, Ashwood ER, Bruns DE, eds. Tietz Textbook of Clinical Chemistry and Molecular Diagnostics, 4th ed. St. Louis, MO: Saunders, 2006:353–407.
15. College of American Pathologists. http://www.cap.org/apps/cap.portal (Accessed February 2012).
16. European Research Network for Evaluation and Improvement of Screening, Diagnosis and Treatment of Inherited Disorders of Metabolism. http://www.erndim.unibas.ch/ (Accessed February 2012).
17. Horowitz GL, Altaie S, Boyd JC, Ceriotti F, Garg U, Horn P, et al. Defining, establishing, and verifying reference intervals in the clinical laboratory: Approved guideline—3rd ed. Document C24-A3. Wayne, PA: Clinical and Laboratory Standards Institute, 2008.

Chapter 2

Amino Acid Disorders

Zhen Zhao, Van Leung-Pineda, and Dennis J. Dietzen

Amino acids are best known as the building blocks of proteins. These 20 protein-forming amino acids, as well as others not found in polypeptides, play key roles in the detoxification of ammonia (NH_3), neurotransmission, the generation of vasoactive molecules (e.g., nitric oxide), and the production of precursors of respiratory fuels (e.g., glucose and ketones). Amino acid disorders are by and large autosomally inherited and include not only those conditions in which the transformation of the carbon skeleton is disrupted but also heritable defects in amino acid transport. The clinical phenotype of these disorders is highly variable and nonspecific, but many are effectively detected by comprehensive amino acid profiling of blood, urine, and/or cerebrospinal fluid (CSF). Many are detectable in the neonatal period by biochemical analysis in dried blood spots before the onset of symptoms and development of lifetime physical and neurologic deficits. Amino acid profiles have historically been performed by anion-exchange chromatography with photometric detection of ninhydrin conjugates, but tandem mass spectrometry (MS/MS) is now also being used in newborn screening programs and hospital laboratories. Dietary protein restriction and selective amino acid supplementation are mainstays in the management of these disorders. Combined with early detection, such treatment allows infants affected with many of these disorders to develop normally and live long, healthy lives. In other disorders, despite deep understanding of their biochemical and genetic basis, treatment options are limited and lead to early death or lifelong physical and cognitive impairment. This chapter will detail the laboratory investigation necessary for the diagnosis of amino acidopathies.

PREANALYTIC, ANALYTIC, AND POSTANALYTIC CONSIDERATIONS IN THE DIAGNOSIS OF AMINO ACIDOPATHIES

The concentration of amino acids in blood reflects a balance among dietary intake, enteral extraction, utilization, and excretion. Fasting specimens better reflect metabolic utilization of amino acids than those obtained shortly after feeding. Specimens obtained shortly after feeding will necessarily portray the amino acid content and extraction of dietary protein. In general, amino acid profiles obtained after feeding are dominated by arginine, lysine, serine, threonine, and branched-chain amino acids that are overrepresented in dietary protein *(1, 2)*. Pediatric populations present a particular challenge to obtaining a "fasting" blood specimen because even healthy children are fed frequently. In addition, the parenteral feeding of critically ill children is administered via lengthy infusion, and blood content may reflect the underlying disease process or the content of the amino acid supplement more than the metabolic processes of the child *(3)*.

Blood amino acids may be assessed in plasma or serum samples by chromatographic and, increasingly, by mass spectrometric techniques. In general, plasma is preferred because some artifacts may be introduced by proteolysis during clotting. Amino acids are in general stable for 48–72 h at 4 °C and for months to years when stored at −20 °C or lower. The most labile molecules are cystine, which tends to precipitate with storage, and glutamine, which slowly metabolizes to glutamate via loss of the epsilon

Table 2-1   Common Physiologic, Dietary, and Iatrogenic Effects on Amino Acid Concentrations in Biologic Fluids

Amino acid(s)	Effect	Mechanism
Arginine, lysine, serine, threonine, isoleucine, leucine, valine	↑ Blood	Diet (animal protein)
Alanine	↑ Blood	Lactic acidosis
Arginine	↓ Blood	Hemolysis (erythrocyte arginase), storage artifact
Ornithine	↑ Blood	Hemolysis (erythrocyte arginase), storage artifact
Glutamine	↑ Blood	Hyperammonemia
Glutamine	↓ Blood	Storage artifact (deamidation)
Glutamine	↑ CSF	Anticonvulsant therapy
Glutamate	↑ Blood	Storage artifact (via glutamine deamidation)
Isoleucine, leucine, valine	↑ Blood	Catabolism (starvation, ketogenesis)
Glycine	↑ Blood	Starvation, ketogenesis, valproate therapy, carbamazepine therapy
Methionine, tyrosine	↑ Blood	Hepatic disease
Homocyst(e)ine	↑ Blood	Vitamin B12/folate deficiency
Cystine	↓ Blood	Storage artifact (precipitation)
β-Aminoisobutyric	↑ Blood	Tissue destruction, chemotherapy
γ-Aminobutyrate	↑ Urine	Bacterial contamination (via glutamate)

amino group. Common storage artifacts, dietary effects, as well as physiologic and iatrogenic factors that alter amino acid concentrations in biologic fluids are summarized in Table 2-1.

For decades, amino acid profiles have been generated via time-consuming (hours) ion-exchange chromatography profiles that rely on amino acid-ninhydrin conjugates for detection and quantitation *(4)*. These systems typically use cation-exchange resins (e.g., those containing sulfonate, carboxylate functional groups) with a lithium-citrate gradient to achieve elution. Primary amine-ninhydrin conjugates are formed after chromatography and are detected by absorbance using a primary wavelength of 570 nm. A second wavelength such as 440 nm is also commonly monitored to detect the unusual ninhydrin conjugate with proline, a secondary amine. Amino acid-ninhydrin conjugates have characteristic absorptivity at 570 and 440 nm, so these wavelengths are also useful to assess peak purity. Common coeluents in these systems are phenylalanine and aminoglycosides, histidine and gabapentin, as well as methionine and homocitrulline.

MS/MS has become the standard for newborn screening programs and is being adopted by an increasing number of clinical laboratories. Most of the example analyses cited in this chapter were obtained using a 20-min liquid chromatography (LC)-MS/MS profile *(5)*. This technique uses butylation of a methanol-extracted sample followed by C8 reversed-phase chromatography with an isocratic mobile phase containing 20% acetonitrile and 0.1% formic acid. Each butylated amino acid is identified as a positive ion using unique combinations of precursor and fragment ions. Isobaric amino acids (e.g., leucine, isoleucine, alloisoleucine or alanine, β-alanine) are distinguished by chromatographic separation or unique fragmentation patterns. Quantitation is achieved using a mixture of internal standards and multipoint external calibration curves. The use of mass spectrometric detection of amino acids enables more definitive molecular identification, a broader dynamic analytic range, and higher throughput.

HYPERPHENYLALANINEMIAS

Hyperphenylalaninemia (HPA) is the most common inborn error of amino acid metabolism affecting approximately 1:20,000 infants in the United States. HPA results from abnormal accumulation of the essential amino acid phenylalanine (PHE), which is detrimental to central nervous system (CNS) development and function. Most HPAs are due to autosomal-recessive mutations in the phenylalanine hydroxylase gene (phenylketonuria [PKU]), but some are due to defects in the synthesis or regeneration of tetrahydrobiopterin (BH_4). BH_4 is an essential cofactor for phenylalanine hydroxylase (PAH). Mutations in genes that code for enzymes involved in the synthesis and degradation of BH_4 alter flux through PAH. The end result of BH_4 deficiency is similar to classic PKU: abnormally elevated PHE. These patients exhibit similar clinical signs as those exhibited by individuals with PAH mutations.

Clinical Presentation

Infants with HPA can appear normal before the onset of symptoms. The primary phenotype of untreated HPA is mental retardation. However, this may not be evident until 6 months to 1 year of age. Mental retardation can be accompanied by seizures, dystonia, abnormal movements, recurrent hyperthermia, hypersalivation, convulsions, swallowing difficulties, and irritability. Poorly controlled maternal PKU increases the risk of miscarriage whereas surviving embryos exhibit intrauterine growth retardation, microcephaly, cardiac malformations, and impaired cognitive development.

Genetics and Pathogenesis

The mode of inheritance for mutations that cause HPA (classic PKU and BH_4 deficiency) is autosomal recessive. Most cases of HPA are caused by *PAH* gene mutations (at least 90%) as observed in classic PKU. In the remainder of patients, HPA is caused by mutations that affect BH_4 metabolism. PAH is primarily expressed in the liver, but the major pathological effect is alteration of brain development. The main toxin appears to be PHE itself because other PHE metabolites have not been observed at concentrations considered toxic. Pathogenesis may be related to competitive inhibition of neutral amino acid transport across the blood-brain barrier resulting in CNS tyrosine deficiency or deficiency of neurotransmitters derived from tyrosine (e.g., dopamine) *(6)*.

BH_4 [2-amino-4-hydroxy-6(L-erythro-1′,2′-dihydroxypropyl)-tetrahydropteridine] facilitates splitting of molecular oxygen in the hydroxylation of PHE (Figure 2-1). This enzyme cofactor also plays a role in the hydroxylation of tyrosine and tryptophan to form dopamine and serotonin, respectively. Defects in enzymes responsible for biopterin synthesis and regeneration cause HPA and may lead to

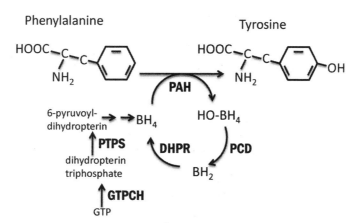

Figure 2-1 Tetrahydrobiopterin (BH_4) synthesis, reclamation, and conversion of phenylalanine to tyrosine by phenylalanine hydroxylase (PAH). 4-Hydroxytetrahydropterin(OH-BH_4) is converted back to BH_4 via successive activities of pterin-4α-carbinolamine dehydratase (PCD) and dihydropteridine reductase (DHPR). The initial steps of BH_4 synthesis are catalyzed by GTP cyclohydrolase (GTPCH) and 6-pyruvoyl-tetrahydrobiopterin synthase (PTPS). Hydrogens in the carbon backbone not involved in key reactions are omitted for simplicity.

deficiencies of dopamine and serotonin derived from tyrosine and tryptophan, respectively. Biosynthetic BH$_4$ enzymes include GTP cyclohydrolase I (GTPCH) and 6-pyruvoyl-tetrahydrobiopterin synthase (PTPS). Regenerating enzymes include dihydropteridine reductase (DHPR) and pterin-4α-carbinolamine dehydratase (PCD). GTPCH is the first enzyme in the biosynthesis of BH$_4$. Approximately 42 mutations have been described in GTPCH and they are associated with normal to mildly elevated plasma PHE concentrations and dopa-responsive dystonia *(7)*. PTPS deficiency is the most prevalent BH$_4$-linked form of HPA. Patients with PTPS deficiency have high urinary concentrations of neopterin and high neopterin:biopterin ratios. DHPR mutations are widespread and random. Most are missense, but there have also been insertions, deletions, and splicing mutations reported. Most patients experience almost complete or complete lack of DHPR function. The clinical presentation is similar to severe forms of GTPCH and PTPS deficiencies. Additional features of DHPR deficiency include abnormalities in vascular proliferation in the CNS and neuronal loss. Most mutations that affect PCD activity are targeted to exon 4 of the gene, which affects PCD's dehydratase activity. These mutations affect the solubility of the protein. Clinical symptoms of PCD deficiency in the neonatal period of some patients include transient electroencephalography (EEG) abnormalities, delayed motor development, and progressive hypotonia. Alterations in tone are generally transient and no other significant clinical signs are observed.

Laboratory Diagnosis

Newborn screening detects abnormally high concentrations of PHE in blood (Figure 2-2). Laboratory diagnosis of HPA is based on elevated plasma PHE (>120 µmol/L) and elevation of the PHE/tyrosine ratio (>3). In general, plasma concentrations of PHE at diagnosis reflect residual hepatic PAH activity. Concentrations >1,200 µmol/L typically reflect <1% residual PAH activity. PHE concentrations of 600–1,200 µmol/L indicate 1–3% residual PAH activity. Plasma PHE of 360–600 µmol/L are consistent with >3% residual PAH activity. HPA can be manifested in urine by increased excretion of phenylpyruvic, phenyllactic, and phenylacetic acids.

Measurement of PHE in newborn screening programs relies on MS/MS. This technique has largely replaced previous microbiological and enzymatic tests because of its superior sensitivity, precision, sample throughput, turnaround time, precision, and accuracy. In addition, MS/MS allows for simultaneous measurement of PHE and tyrosine. Confirmatory plasma analyses still largely rely on amino acid profiles using ion-exchange chromatography and postcolumn photometric detection of ninhydrin-amino acid conjugates. In some ninhydrin systems, ampicillin coelutes with PHE, causing falsely elevated concentrations. Typical reference intervals for PHE are 40–140 µmol/L up to 1 month of age, 30–75 µmol/L from 1 to 24 months of age, and 25–90 µmol/L from 2 to 18 years of age.

Authentic cases of PAH deficiency must be distinguished from those mediated by mutations in genes responsible for biosynthesis or regeneration of BH$_4$ to determine if BH$_4$ supplementation is indicated. Plasma PHE concentrations in BH$_4$ deficiency typically decrease within 8 h after BH$_4$ challenge but up to one third of PAH defects also respond to BH$_4$. In these situations urinary pterin analysis may be informative. Classic PKU cases (deficient PAH) have high total pterin concentrations with normal neopterin:biopterin ratios. In DHPR deficiency, total pterin is elevated, but there is low BH$_4$ concentration. In 6-pyruvoyltetrahydropterin synthase (6-PTS) deficiency, elevated neopterin and neopterin:biopterin ratios are expected, whereas in GTPCH deficiency, there are low pterin values and normal ratios.

Tests of enzymatic activity can also aid in pinpointing the specific enzymatic defect. Enzymatic activity can be measured from liver biopsy specimens or cultured cells from the patient, depending on the enzyme. Tests are available for PAH, DHPR, PCD, PTS, and GTPCH. Affected individuals will show lower enzymatic activities than normal. Molecular genetic testing can be useful for confirming the diagnosis of HPA. However, it is not recommended that they take the place of phenotypic testing because there are several mutations and no clear genotype:phenotype correlation. Lack of a mutation does not preclude the presence of disease. Identification of the PAH mutation can be useful for predicting the degree of enzymatic defect and influence treatment.

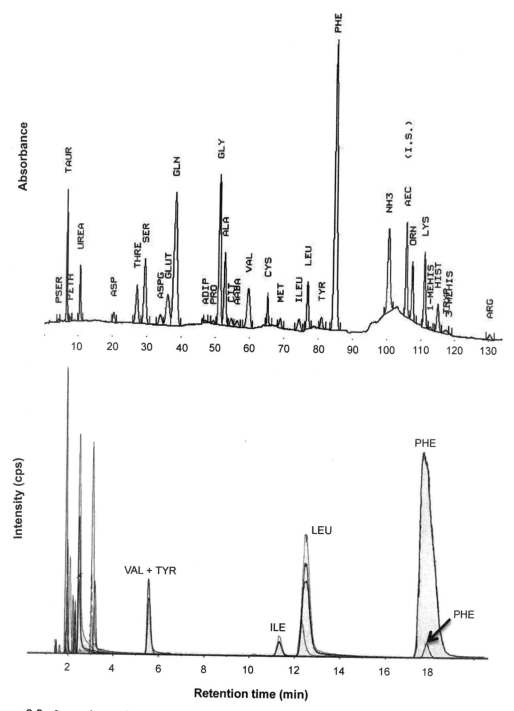

Figure 2-2 Ion-exchange chromatogram (upper) using aminoethylcysteine (AEC) as internal standard and LC-MS/MS total ion chromatogram (lower) of plasma from patient with PKU. Phenylalanine peak (arrow) from normal patient is superimposed on lower chromatogram to indicate extent of phenylalanine elevation in disease.

Treatment and Prognosis

Early initiation (before 1 month of age) and strict maintenance of dietary restriction of PHE is required to avoid damage to the developing nervous system. This dietary regimen requires constant monitoring of PHE concentrations in the patient, not just to prevent toxic accumulation but also to ensure adequate nutritional amounts of tyrosine, which becomes an essential amino acid in PKU. Treatment termination has adverse outcomes, including neurologic deficits that can manifest later in life. This is because HPA can be toxic to the brain throughout life, even if the effects in adulthood are less prominent than in childhood. Some patients with PKU, but no deficiency in BH_4, have responded well to treatment with BH_4 (8). Most newly diagnosed patients receive a trial of BH_4 supplementation to assess the utility of this approach. When BH_4 metabolism is disrupted, the objective is to control PHE concentrations and supplement potential deficiencies of dopamine and serotonin. PHE restriction actually has to be more strictly regulated than in classic PAH deficiency because PHE elevation can impede neurotransmitter transport and metabolism. L-Dopa and 5-hydroxytryptophan are commonly used dopamine and serotonin precursors, respectively, that cross the blood-brain barrier. CSF concentrations of neurotransmitter metabolites (homovanillic acid and 5-hydroxyindoleacetic acid) may be monitored to assess adequacy of replacement therapy.

TYROSINEMIAS AND ALKAPTONURIA

Tyrosinemia is an elevation of blood tyrosine concentration caused by an inherited defect in tyrosine catabolism (Figure 2-3). Diagnosis of tyrosinemia in the neonatal period is commonly confounded by the transient elevation of blood tyrosine due to delayed expression of p-hydroxyphenylpyruvate dioxygenase. Tyrosine is made from PHE by PAH. The catabolism of tyrosine starts like that of many other amino acids with transamination. Subsequent steps of the pathway decarboxylate the side chain and open the phenyl ring, ultimately yielding acetoacetate and fumarate. Four types of tyrosinemia have been described. In type I, there is a deficiency of the enzyme fumarylacetoacetate hydrolase (FAH), which mediates the final step in tyrosine degradation. Tyrosine aminotransferase is deficient in type II disease. Type III is due to deficiency of p-hydroxyphenylpyruvate dioxygenase, and in alkaptonuria, the enzymatic defect resides at the level of homogentisate-1,2-dioxygenase.

Clinical Presentation

Type I tyrosinemia is also known as hepatorenal tyrosinemia. Acute liver failure indicated by a severely prolonged prothrombin time and renal failure characterized by generalized aminoaciduria is the hallmark of this disorder (9). Phenotypic variation is considerable in type I disease, ranging from acute, irreversible liver failure in the neonatal period to later-onset presentations characterized by the development of hepatocellular carcinoma. Neurological, eye, and skin symptoms are characteristic of type II tyrosinemia. Eye symptoms include photophobia, irritation, pain, and lacrimation. Skin lesions are painful and present on soles, palms, and plantar surfaces of the digits. About half of patients with this disorder present with severely delayed cognitive development and aggressive behavior. Only a few cases of type III tyrosinemia have been reported. Of those described, symptoms are primarily neurologic and include ataxia and seizures. The main finding in children with alkaptonuria is the presence of dark urine, a consequence of the formation of melanin-like polymers in a process termed ochronosis (dark tissue pigmentation). Later in life the darkening of cartilage can occur along with bone and connective tissue disease leading to painful arthritic complications. Also later in life, patients can exhibit cardiac symptoms and development of kidney stones related to pigment crystallization (10).

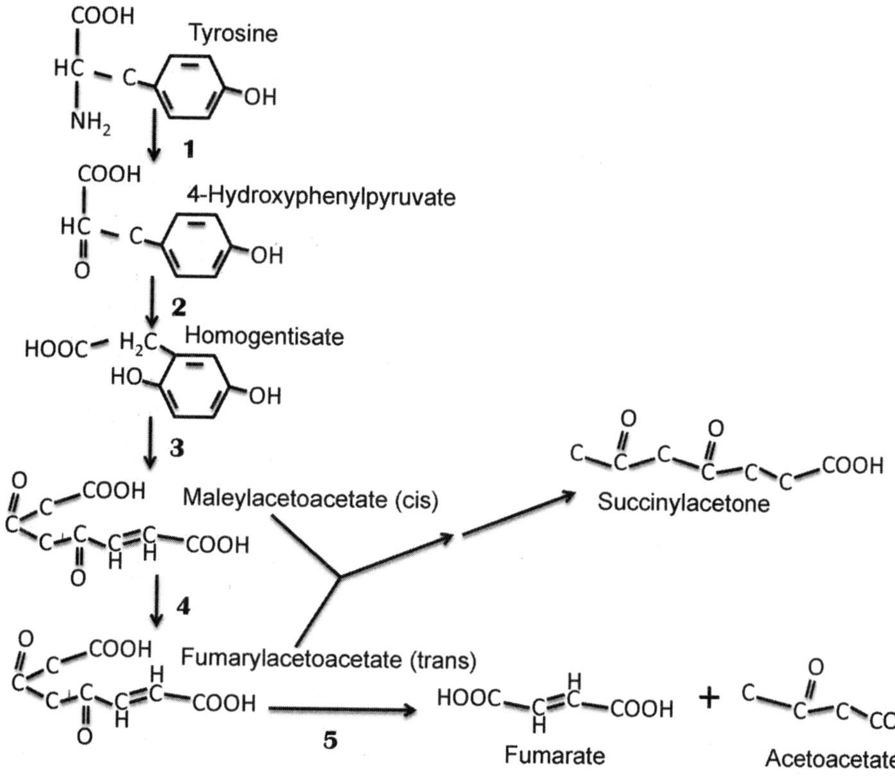

Figure 2-3 Tyrosine catabolism. Enzymes indicated are (1) tyrosine aminotransferase, (2) 4-hydroxyphenyl-pyruvate dioxygenase, (3) homogentisate-1,2-dioxygenase, (4) maleylacetoacetate isomerase, and (5) fumarylace-toacetate hydrolase. Succinylacetone is formed from accumulating maleylacetoacetate and fumarylacetoacetate in deficiency of fumarylacetoacetate hydrolase. Hydrogen atoms in the carbon backbone are omitted unless involved in key enzymatic reactions.

Genetics and Pathogenesis

Type I tyrosinemia is caused by a defect in the gene encoding the most distal step of tyrosine catabolism, *FAH* on chromosome 15. At least 34 mutations in this gene have been documented. Liver and renal pathogenesis is related to the accumulation of maleylacetoacetate, fumarylacetoacetate, and succinylacetone. These metabolites lead to accumulation of the heme precursor, δ-aminolevulinic acid, causing neuropathy similar to that observed in porphyrias. Tyrosinemia type II is characterized by a deficient tyrosine aminotransferase encoded on chromosome 16. The pathogenesis of type II disease is believed to result from tyrosine accumulation and crystallization in corneal epithelial cells that trigger inflammation. Skin abnormalities are also thought to be a result of tyrosine accumulation leading to hyperkeratotic skin lesions. 4-Hydroxyphenylpyruvate dioxygenase encoded on chromosome 12 is deficient in tyrosinemia type III. There have been only a few individuals identified with type III tyrosinemia. Affected patients show no liver abnormalities, but neurologic impairment has been observed.

Mutations that cause alkaptonuria affect the gene that encodes homogentisic acid oxidase on chromosome 3. This is another autosomal-recessive inherited disease in which mutations are spread throughout the gene. Approximately 65 mutations have been identified that include missense, nonsense, splice/intronic, and frameshift mutations. Pathogenesis results from the conversion of excess homogentisic acid to benzoquinone acetic acid. Benzoquinone acetic acid forms the melanin-like polymers that cause ochronosis. Polymer deposition disrupts the normal structure of connective tissue, causing damage that leads to arthritic symptoms.

Laboratory Diagnosis

The tyrosinemias display distinctive biochemical features in blood (Figure 2-4) and urine. Normal concentrations of tyrosine in blood range from 50 to 150 µmol/L in term newborns and from 20 to 100 µmol/L thereafter through adolescence. The highest blood tyrosine concentrations (1,000–3,000 µmol/L) are associated with deficient transamination (type II). More distal catabolic defects generally produce lower tyrosine concentrations (300–1,000 µmol/L). In many cases, blood tyrosine concentrations in affected infants overlap significantly with those from unaffected infants that have hepatic dysfunction secondary to premature birth, viral infection, galactosemia, toxins, or medications.

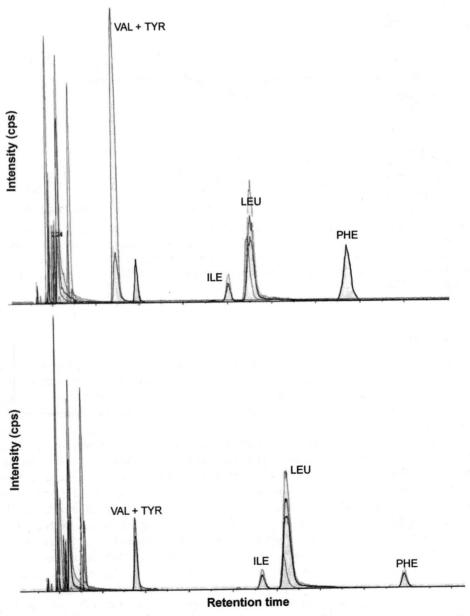

Figure 2-4   LC-MS/MS total ion chromatogram (C8) of plasma from patient with type 1 tyrosinemia (upper) and normal patient (lower).

Urine from patients with tyrosinemia contains some metabolites common to all forms of tyrosinemia and others that pinpoint the metabolic defect. The transaminated metabolites of tyrosine, 4-hydroxyphenyllactate, and 4-hydoxyphenylpyruvate are common features of inhibited tyrosine catabolism even in tyrosine aminotransferase deficiency (type II disease). In these cases, transamination is thought to occur via an alternative enzyme such as aspartate aminotransferase. In all forms of tyrosinemia, urine may also contain 4-hydroxyphenylacetic acid, which is formed by decarboxylation of tyrosine by enteric bacteria. The presence of succinylacetone and homogentisic acid is pathognomonic for type I disease and alkaptonuria, respectively. In rare cases, urine from individuals with type III disease contains pyroglutamic acid (5-oxoproline) and an unusual amino acid, Hawkinsin, formed via conjugation of glutathione with hydroxyphenylpyruvate *(11)*.

Treatment and Prognosis

Historically, tyrosinemia type I was treated with dietary restriction of PHE and tyrosine. Such treatment did not generally prevent hepatic crises, renal tubular failure, or development of hepatocellular carcinoma. As a last resort, liver transplantation was used to prevent hepatic complications but did not impede progression of renal disease. Treatment of type I tyrosinemia has been revolutionized by the introduction of 2-[2-nitro-4-(trifluoromethyl)benzoyl]cyclohexane-1,4-dione, known as nitisinone (Orfadin®, NTBC). Nitisinone is a potent ($IC_{50} \approx 40$ nmol/L) competitive inhibitor of 4-hydroxyphenylpyruvate dioxygenase, a step upstream of FAH. Nitisinone prevents accumulation of succinylacetone and prevents acute liver and neurologic disease *(12)*. The long-term effects of NTBC treatment have not yet been comprehensively documented.

Dietary restriction of PHE and tyrosine remains the mainstay of treatment in type II and type III tyrosinemia as well as alkaptonuria. Maintenance of blood tyrosine concentrations <500 µmol/L is associated with improvement of ophthalmic, cutaneous, and neurologic symptoms in type II disease. Dietary treatment alone does not effectively limit accumulation of homogentisic acid in alkaptonuria. Ascorbic acid may reduce oxidation of homogentisic acid to benzoquinone acetic acid, and nitisinone has been shown to blunt accumulation of homogentisic acid, but the long-term benefits of these approaches remain unclear.

MAPLE SYRUP URINE DISEASE

Branched-chain amino acids are important sources of energy in catabolic states. Glucose can be produced from the carbon skeleton of valine and isoleucine, and ketone bodies can be generated from leucine and isoleucine. The transformation of branched-chain amino acid carbon begins with transamination to an α-keto derivative, which is subsequently metabolized by the branched-chain α-keto acid dehydrogenase complex (BCKDH). Deficiency of the BCKDH complex is responsible for maple syrup urine disease (MSUD; Figure 2-5).

Clinical Presentation

The clinical symptoms of MSUD are predominantly neurologic. Symptoms include poor feeding, lethargy, ataxia, seizures, and coma. MSUD patients can be divided into five clinical subtypes on the basis of age of onset, clinical presentation, tolerance to dietary protein, enzyme activity levels, growth rate, and response to thiamine treatment. Classic MSUD is the most common and most severe form of the disease, accounting for 75% of MSUD patients and typically presenting during the neonatal period. Residual BCKDH enzyme activity is generally <2% of normal in classic MSUD. In untreated neonates, classic MSUD is characterized by a maple syrup or burnt sugar odor of urine, feeding problems, and alternating irritability and lethargy progressing to coma. The other subtypes may have 2–30% of normal enzyme activity with variable age of onset and clinical signs *(13)*.

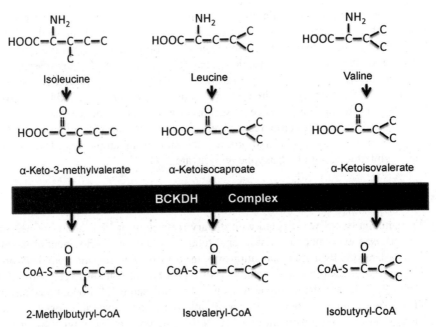

Figure 2-5   Proximal branched-chain amino acid catabolism via transamination and branched-chain ketoacid dehydrogenase complex (BCKDH). Hydrogen atoms in the carbon backbone are omitted unless involved in key enzymatic reactions.

Genetics and Pathogenesis

MSUD is inherited in an autosomal-recessive pattern. It occurs in the general population at a frequency of approximately 1 in 185,000 live births on the basis of newborn screening data. The highest frequency of MSUD is observed in Old Order Mennonites of Pennsylvania, with an estimated prevalence of 1 in 176 live births. The BCKDH complex is composed of three catalytic components (E1, E2, and E3) *(14)*. The E1 subunit has decarboxylase and dehydrogenase activities and requires thiamine as a cofactor. The E2 subunit is responsible for coenzyme A (CoA) esterification through a dihydrolipoyl group. The E3 subunit is common to other α-ketoacid dehydrogenase complexes (pyruvate and α-ketoglutarate dehydrogenase) and reoxidizes the lipoate moiety. Hundreds of disease-causing mutations have been documented covering four genes: *BCKDHA* (chromosome 19), *BCKDHB* (chromosome 6), *DBT* (chromosome 1), and *DLD* (chromosome 7) encoding the E1α, E1β, E2, and E3 subunits, respectively, of the BCKDH complex. Correlation of genotype with phenotype is typically poor. The pathology of MSUD is likely mediated by accumulation of branched-chain amino (primarily leucine) and α-keto acids (primarily α-ketoisocaproate) that disrupt transport at the blood-brain barrier leading to deficient protein and neurotransmitter synthesis. α-Ketoisocaproate may also have direct toxic effects on cellular respiration, leading to glial and neuronal apoptosis.

Laboratory Diagnosis

MSUD is biochemically characterized by elevated blood concentrations of isoleucine, leucine, and valine as well as increased urinary excretion of corresponding α-keto acids—α-keto-3-methylvaleric, α-ketoisocaproate, and α-ketoisovaleric, respectively. Diagnosis is most commonly achieved by analysis of blood amino acids (Figure 2-6) because the transamination step before BCKDH is reversible. Normal plasma concentrations of isoleucine, leucine, and valine are typically <75, 150, and 300 μmol/L, respectively. Sample acquisition during catabolic stress or after natural protein

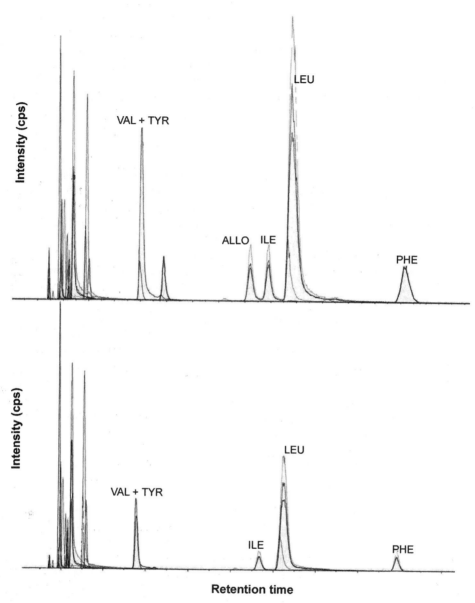

Figure 2-6 LC-MS/MS total ion chromatogram (C8) of plasma from patient with MSUD (upper) and normal patient (lower).

ingestion increases plasma concentrations of the branched-chain amino acids two- to threefold, but the isoleucine:leucine:valine ratio typically remains 1:2:4. In untreated MSUD, leucine concentrations are increased disproportionately, reaching 500–5,000 μmol/L, whereas isoleucine and valine concentrations range from 200 to 1,300 and 500 to 1,800 μmol/L, respectively. Isomerization of α-keto-3-methylvaleric acid at the 3 carbon followed by transamination leads to formation of alloisoleucine *(15)*. Alloisoleucine concentrations of up to 5 μmol/L have been observed in catabolic states, but concentrations >5 μmol/L are pathognomonic for MSUD. Significant concentrations of alloisoleucine persist even in treated, well-controlled MSUD patients.

Analysis of branched-chain amino acids in body fluids presents some unique challenges. In amino acid analyses performed by ion-exchange chromatography, alloisoleucine typically elutes very close to methionine, making small concentrations difficult to appreciate. MS/MS techniques such as those performed in newborn screening programs are unable to distinguish isoleucine, leucine, alloisoleucine, and hydroxyproline because these are isobaric (precursor ion $m/z = 132$). Therefore, newborn screening programs report the sum of these isomers along with the valine concentration. Confirmatory testing performed by MS/MS must include chromatographic separation and separate quantitation of these isomers to exclude false-positive findings due to increased hydroxyproline and to allow individual adjustment of isoleucine, leucine, and valine in the diet.

Treatment and Prognosis

The treatment of MSUD has two goals. The first is to promote anabolism, thereby decreasing carbon flux through BCKDH. This is achieved by persistent high caloric intake with particular attention paid during periods of intercurrent illness. The second goal is correct high concentrations of branched-chain amino and ketoacids. This is achieved by lifelong dietary restriction of the branched-chain amino acids, sometimes accompanied by thiamine supplementation. Thiamine is an obligatory catalytic constituent of BCKDH involved in ketoacid decarboxylation. Some patients with mutations in the E2 subunit have a significant response to thiamine, but dietary therapy is not precluded in this circumstance. Monitoring is performed every 1–2 weeks in infancy and less frequently as the patient ages. In extreme circumstances, liver transplantation has been used to correct BCKDH deficiency.

Severely affected patients die within the first few months of life if not treated. Patients with the milder variant types of MSUD may show normal early development without neurological manifestations, but without appropriate recognition and treatment they are at risk of acute metabolic decompensation and death. With early diagnosis and treatment, patients with MSUD are able to survive and a favorable neurologic outcome is possible. Patients receiving liver transplants often have a dramatic reversal of branched-chain amino acidemia and their protein intake can be liberalized. However, such patients must still cope with the risks of lifelong immunosuppression and the eventual need for retransplantation.

HOMOCYSTINURIA

Homocysteine is a metabolite of the essential amino acid methionine. Methionine in the form of *S*-adenosyl methionine is an important methyl donor in the formation of creatine, choline, and several other biomolecules *(16)*. Homocystinuria is a rare autosomal-recessive disorder caused by a defect in the remethylation of homocysteine. The disorder is biochemically characterized by an abnormal accumulation of homocysteine in plasma and urine. Multiple systems are affected, including connective tissue, muscles, brain, and the cardiovascular system, leading to developmental delay, osteoporosis, ocular impairment, thromboembolic disorders, and severe premature atherosclerosis *(17)*.

Clinical Presentation

Homocystinuria caused by cystathionine β-synthase (CBS) deficiency is a multisystem disease characterized by a normal presentation at birth followed by clinical manifestations in the ocular, skeletal, vascular, and central nervous systems. The deficiency is characterized by ectopia lentis, myopia, osteoporosis, thromboembolism, mental retardation, developmental delay, and a Marfanoid appearance. Thromboses may be arterial or venous and most commonly involve the cerebrovasculature. Expressivity is variable for all of the clinical findings. For example, in mildly affected patients, dislocation of the optic lenses may be the only sign. Two clinical phenotypic types have been recognized based on changes in the biochemical abnormalities after pyridoxine (vitamin B6) administration: pyridoxine responsive and pyridoxine nonresponsive. The former is in general, but not always, milder than the latter form.

Genetics and Pathogenesis

Homocysteine may be remethylated to form methionine or metabolized through cystathionine to form cysteine (Figure 2-7). Homocysteine concentrations are normally very low (<15 μmol/L). Homocysteine may accumulate secondary to dietary vitamin B12 (cobalamin) deficiency and various genetic defects involving methionine adenosyltransferase, glycine-*N*-methyltransferase, adenosylhomocysteine hydrolase, methylenetetrahydrofolate reductase (MTHFR), CBS, and a host of enzymes involved in cobalamin metabolism and transport *(18)*. The most common of these disorders, and the one referred to commonly as "homocystinuria," is CBS deficiency. The disorder is inherited in an autosomal-recessive manner with a worldwide frequency of approximately 1 in 300,000. CBS activity requires pyridoxine (vitamin B6) as a cofactor. Methionine formation from homocysteine is catalyzed by methionine synthase using methylcobalamin as a cofactor. Methylcobalamin is in turn regenerated by a methyl group derived from 5,10-methylenetetrahydrofalate. An alternative remethylation reaction catalyzed by betaine-homocysteine *S*-methyltransferase using betaine as a methyl donor is also expressed in liver and kidney tissue.

Homocysteine circulates predominantly (70%) linked via disulfide bonds to cysteine residues in protein. Most of the remaining 30% circulates as homocysteine-cysteine disulfides or homocysteine-homocysteine disulfides (termed homocystine). Only 1–2% of circulating homocysteine circulates as a free thiol. In CBS deficiency, as total homocysteine concentrations increase to 150–400 μmol/L, the free thiol fraction may increase to 10–25% of the total. Small quantities of homocysteine may also form an intramolecular thiolactone. Much of the disease burden is attributed to altered protein disulfide formation mediated by free thiol and by modification of lysine residues by homocysteine thiolactone. Disruption of intramolecular disulfide bonds in fibrillin and tropoelastin may account for the similar skeletal features of Marfan syndrome and CBS deficiency *(19)*. However, thrombosis is unique to homocystinuria. Increased homocysteine has been associated with endothelial dysfunction, enhanced platelet activation, and prothrombotic changes mediated through factor V, fibrinogen, thrombomodulin, and plasminogen. A direct mechanistic link between increased homocysteine and the hyperthrombotic state has yet to be demonstrated.

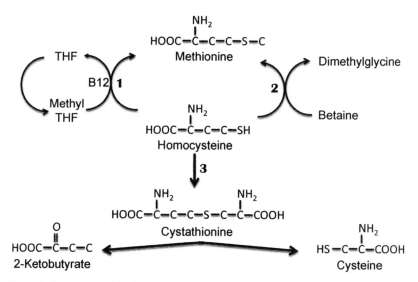

Figure 2-7 Remethylation of methionine. Homocysteine may be remethylated via methionine synthase (1), by the action of betaine:homocysteine methyltransferase (2), or metabolized to cystathionine via cystathionine-β-synthetase (3). Homocysteine accumulates in deficiency of cystathionine-β-synthase and in disruption of normal tetrahydrofolate (THF) and vitamin B12 metabolism. Hydrogen atoms in the carbon backbone are omitted unless involved in key reactions.

Laboratory Diagnosis

Analysis of plasma amino acids, carnitine esters, and urine organic acids all provide data relevant to confirm and refine the diagnosis of CBS deficiency. The most direct evidence for CBS deficiency is an increased blood concentration of total homocysteine. Highly automated competitive immunoassays are available that detect homocysteine after reduction of disulfide-linked thiols. Fasting blood amino acid profiles from CBS-deficient individuals show elevated concentrations of methionine, and the oxidized homocysteine-homocysteine homodimer is often referred to as homocystine (Figure 2-8). In ion-exchange methods that detect amino acid-ninhydrin conjugates, methionine and

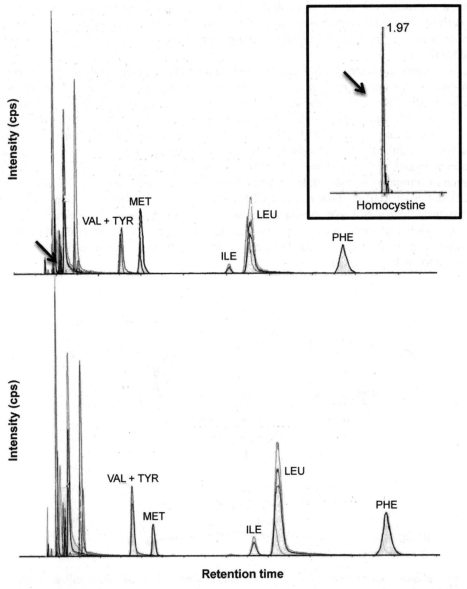

Figure 2-8   LC-MS/MS total ion chromatogram (C8) of plasma from patient with homocystinuria (upper) and normal patient (lower) showing elevated methionine concentration. Inset: Extracted ion chromatogram of the m/z 325→190 precursor-to-product transition for monobutyl homocystine at retention time indicated by arrow in total ion chromatogram.

homocitrulline often coelute and may lead to overestimation of methionine concentrations. Homocystine accumulation is typically more exaggerated in urine specimens. Total plasma homocysteine concentrations are typically >200 μmol/L, and methionine concentrations range from 100 to 2,000 μmol/L. Normal concentrations of total plasma homocysteine and methionine are 5–15 and 10–50 μmol/L, respectively. Homocystine is not normally detected (<1 μmol/L) in blood or urine. Urine organic acid and plasma acylcarnitine profiles are useful to distinguish elevation of homocysteine due to CBS deficiency from defects in cobalamin metabolism that also cause isolated homocystinuria (*cblE*, *cblG*) or combined homocystinuria with methylmalonic aciduria (*cblC*, *cblD*, *cblF*), which require a distinct therapeutic approach.

Treatment and Prognosis

CBS deficiency is usually asymptomatic for the first few months of life. If untreated, patients eventually develop mental retardation, developmental delay, ectopia lentis, osteoporosis, and other complications. The detection and immediate treatment of homocystinuria during the neonatal period is critical because many of these complications are irreversible. Once the diagnosis is established, it is critical to determine if the patient is responsive or nonresponsive to pyridoxine. Pyridoxine mitigates the biochemical abnormalities and improves IQ, reduces frequency of lens dislocation, and decreases the risk of thromboembolism. However, half of CBS-deficient patients do not respond to pyridoxine. These patients are treated with methionine-restricted diets. Early dietary treatment has been reported to effectively delay and prevent several serious problems in some patients, including mental retardation, ophthalmic and skeletal abnormalities, seizures, osteoporosis, and thromboembolism. However, dietary treatment is difficult and satisfactory compliance is hard to achieve, especially in older children or adults. Another treatment option in these patients is the use of the methyl donor, betaine, to remethylate homocysteine to methionine. Methionine concentrations may rise excessively in betaine therapy. Hypermethioninemia does not appear to modulate the pathophysiology of CBS, but cerebral edema has been reported in betaine-treated patients.

NONKETOTIC HYPERGLYCINEMIA

Nonketotic hyperglycinemia (NKH) is a hereditary metabolic disease inherited in an autosomal-recessive manner. Its incidence is unknown except in a few countries. The highest incidence of NKH has been documented in Finland (1 in 55,000) and in British Columbia, Canada (1 in 63,000). Glycine is structurally the simplest amino acid and a component of almost all animal protein. An average adult U.S. diet contains 3–5 g of glycine per day. NKH, also known as glycine encephalopathy, is an inborn error of glycine catabolism characterized by abnormal accumulation of large quantities of glycine in all body tissues, particularly the brain, most often leading to intractable neonatal seizures, although milder cases have been described. There is no specific treatment available. Patients with neonatal onset of the disease often die in the first few months of life, and survivors have severe neurologic impairment. The metabolic defect of the disease is in the glycine cleavage system (GCS), a mitochondrial enzyme complex *(20)*.

Clinical Presentation

A broad spectrum of clinical phenotypes of NKH has been documented and is usually classified based on the age of onset and severity of symptoms. The vast majority of NKH patients present in the neonatal period with lethargy, profound hypotonia, feeding problems, myoclonic jerks, and coma progressing to apnea. Even with assisted ventilation, approximately 30% of patients do not survive the neonatal period. Those patients who survive usually regain spontaneous respiration by the second to third week of age. However, they may live for several years with intractable seizures and severe neurologic disability. Phenotypically mild and late-onset cases of NKH termed "atypical" have also been described (21). Infantile NKH is the most common atypical presentation of the disease. Patients have normal growth and development until at least 6 months of age followed by the development of seizures, hypotonia, and developmental delay/regression. Patients with a mild-episodic form have the age of onset in childhood with mild intellectual disability and episodes of delirium, chorea, and vertical gaze palsy associated with febrile illness. A late-onset form with onset from childhood to late adulthood has been described in a few individuals who develop nonspecific neurological symptoms with or without cognitive impairment. Patients who develop clinical and biochemical features of neonatal NKH that then resolve have also been described. This "transient" NKH has been putatively ascribed to slow maturation of the GCS. Neurologic deficits may persist throughout life or resolve at 2–4 months of age.

Genetics and Pathogenesis

Glycine functions as an inhibitory neurotransmitter via specific receptors in the spinal cord by enhancing postsynaptic chloride flux, which leads to hyperpolarized membranes (22). In the cortex, glycine potentiates excitatory sodium flux mediated by glutamate at the N-methyl D-aspartate (NMDA) receptor (23). Glycine carbon is incorporated in various biomolecules (phospholipids, ceramides, purines) via cytoplasmic transformation to serine. Glycine is also catabolized to carbon dioxide (CO_2), NH_3, and a methyl group (as 5,10-methylene tetrahydrofolate) primarily in liver mitochondria via the GCS (Figure 2-9).

The biochemical defect in NKH is in GCS. The GCS consists of P-protein (glycine decarboxylase) encoded by *GLDC* on chromosome 9, T-protein encoded by *GCST* on chromosome 3, H-protein encoded by *GCSH* on chromosome 16, and L-protein (dihydrolipoamide dehydrogenase) encoded by *DLD* on chromosome 7. Of the 136 mutations reported to cause NKH, 109 are in the *GLDC*, 25 in *GCST*, and 2 in *GCSH*. Approximately 5% of patients with clinical disease do not have a mutation identified in any of the genes known to cause NKH. The product of the *DLD* gene is also a

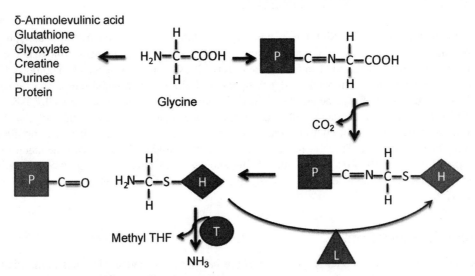

Figure 2-9   Glycine cleavage system (GCS). Glycine carbon not required for other synthetic functions is disposed of by the GCS. The concerted actions of P- and H-proteins liberate CO_2 using pyridoxal phosphate and lipoic acid, respectively. T-protein catalyzes transfer of the α-carbon to THF while releasing NH_3. The L-protein reoxidizes the lipoic acid moiety of the H protein using NAD^+ to prepare for another reaction cycle.

component of multiple α-ketoacid dehydrogenase complexes (BCKDH, pyruvate dehydrogenase, and α-ketoglutarate dehydrogenase) that use lipoic acid as a cofactor. Therefore, *DLD* mutations cause a spectrum of clinical and biochemical abnormalities because of impaired branched-chain amino acid catabolism and defective function of the citric acid cycle.

Laboratory Diagnosis

Amino acid analysis of glycine in plasma and CSF is required to establish the diagnosis of NKH. Plasma and CSF specimens should be collected on the same day. CSF glycine is more markedly elevated than plasma glycine in NKH, reaching concentrations 8–10 times normal (normal <10 μmol/L). Elevated plasma concentrations may be difficult to appreciate in the immediate newborn period because normal glycine concentrations may reach 800 μmol/L. This makes pathologic hyperglycinemia particularly difficult to appreciate in newborn screening. After the first year of life, glycine concentrations in unaffected children typically do not exceed 400 μmol/L. In addition to NKH, common causes of hyperglycinemia include ketosis, propionic and methylmalonic acidemias, and valproate therapy. Therefore, distinction of children with NKH is best assessed using the ratio of glycine concentrations in CSF to those in plasma. A ratio >0.08 is considered diagnostic of NKH (normal <0.04). GCS activity measurement is generally not available, but molecular analysis of the gene products involved may provide further support for the presence of NKH.

Treatment and Prognosis

There are few effective strategies to prevent primary manifestations of NKH. Anticonvulsant therapy, dietary glycine restriction, and sodium benzoate treatment are commonly used to control seizures and reduce plasma concentration of glycine. Amidation of benzoic acid with glycine leads to excretion of glycine in the form of hippuric acid. NMDA receptor antagonists such as dextromethorphan, ketamine, and felabamate have also been used in an effort to minimize the effect of elevated glycine concentrations in neural synapses. These therapeutic approaches have had limited benefit to the neurological and developmental outcomes of NKH patients. The prognosis of severely affected NKH patients remains poor.

SULFITE OXIDASE AND MOLYBDENUM COFACTOR DEFICIENCY

Isolated sulfite oxidase deficiency and molybdenum cofactor deficiency are rare genetic disorders affecting the catabolism of the sulfur-containing amino acids methionine and cysteine. Both disorders are panethnic and inherited as autosomal-recessive traits with nearly equal numbers of males and females affected. To date, more than 100 patients with one of these two deficiencies have been described. Both disorders are characterized by severe neonatal seizures and progressive neurological deterioration. No effective therapy has been developed. Although the general clinical presentation is similar, the two disorders can be differentiated by their biochemical findings. Given their similar clinical phenotype, it is reasonable to assume that most of the signs and symptoms of molybdenum cofactor deficiency may be attributed to the deficiency of sulfite oxidase activity *(24)*.

Clinical Presentation

Affected patients are usually the products of uncomplicated pregnancies and appear normal during the immediate neonatal period. Symptoms present shortly after birth with severe feeding difficulties, convulsions, axial hypotonia, peripheral hypertonicity, and progressive neurological damage. Most of the known patients died at an early age, and survivors are severely developmentally impaired. A subset of patients have dysmorphic features and dislocated ocular lenses.

Genetics and Pathogenesis

Sulfite oxidase plays a role in the distal steps of catabolism of the sulfur-containing amino acids methionine and cysteine. Methionine is a precursor for the formation of cysteine, which is normally catabolized to pyruvate and sulfite, which is then oxidized to sulfate by sulfite oxidase in the mitochondrial intermembrane space. Taurine and sulfocysteine (Figure 2-10) accumulate as a result of increased sulfite concentrations. The pathogenesis of the neurological damage in sulfite oxidase deficiency is not fully understood, but it may be a direct consequence of elevated concentrations of neurotoxic sulfite, the deficit of sulfate, or the combination of both. Sulfite may disrupt disulfide bonds, which disrupts protein folding. S-Sulfocysteine may also be an agonist for the NMDA receptor, leading to neonatal seizures similar to those observed in NKH. More than 16 pathogenic mutations have been described for the sulfite oxidase (*SUOX*) gene, and most of the mutations are private. A missense mutation R160Q has been identified in more than one patient *(25)*.

Sulfite oxidase requires molybdenum cofactor, in which the metal is complexed to pterin as molybdopterin *(26)*. Like other transition metals involved in electron transfer, molybdenum undergoes a reversible two-electron reduction mediating the transfer of oxygen to substrate. In addition to sulfite oxidase, molybdenum cofactor is also required by xanthine dehydrogenase and aldehyde oxidase. These two enzymes share many physicochemical properties and show some overlap in substrate specificity. Xanthine dehydrogenase catalyzes the conversion of hypoxanthine and xanthine to uric acid whereas aldehyde oxidase only catalyzes the hydroxylation of hypoxanthine to xanthine. In patients with molybdenum cofactor deficiency, all three enzymes are defective because of a lack of functional molybdenum cofactor. The gene products of four genes *MOCS1, MOCS2, MOCS3,* and *GEPH* are required for molybdenum cofactor biosynthesis. Mutations have been identified in *MOCS1, MOCS2,* and *GEPH* genes. All are inherited in an autosomal-recessive fashion. Most disease-causing mutations were identified in *MOCS1* and *MOCS2* genes *(27)* with only one case reported in the *GEPH* gene. No mutation in *MOCS3* has yet been described.

Molybdenum cofactor deficiencies and isolated sulfite oxidase deficiency are indistinguishable with the exception that xanthinuria is present in molybdenum cofactor deficiency. An isolated deficiency

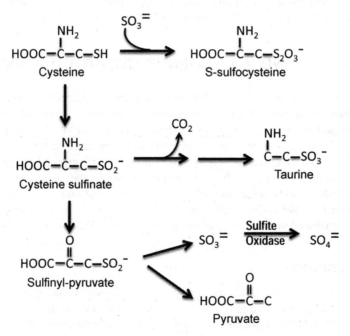

Figure 2-10 Metabolism of cysteine secondary to sulfite oxidase/molybdenum cofactor deficiency. Hydrogen atoms in the carbon backbone are omitted unless involved in key reactions.

of aldehyde oxidase has never been reported. The individuals with isolated xanthine dehydrogenase deficiency or combined xanthine dehydrogenase and aldehyde oxidase deficiencies present with xanthinuria, which does not cause apparent serious clinical consequences. The absence of encephalopathy in isolated xanthine dehydrogenase deficiency and combined xanthine dehydrogenase and aldehyde oxidase deficiencies suggests that symptoms of molybdenum cofactor deficiency are mainly due to sulfite oxidase deficiency.

Laboratory Diagnosis

Sulfite can be detected by a dipstick test in urine originally developed to measure sulfite concentrations in wine and other beverages. Fresh urine must be used because sulfite is rapidly and nonenzymatically oxidized to sulfate, resulting in false-negative results. False-positive results can be seen with administration of sulfur-containing drugs such as β-mercaptoethanesulfonate and antibiotics such as ampicillin. S-Sulfocysteine is a more stable and accurate marker of sulfite accumulation. Increased production of S-sulfocysteine is typically more evident in urine than in plasma because of its efficient excretion. S-Sulfocysteine coelutes with other amines very early in ion-exchange/ninhydrin amino acid profiles and is therefore best quantitated using mass spectrometric techniques. Quantitative analysis of other sulfur amino acids may add value to diagnostic evaluation. Decreased plasma cysteine and nearly undetectable homocysteine are characteristic of sulfite excess.

Sulfite oxidase deficiency can be differentiated from molybdenum cofactor deficiency by low plasma and urinary uric acid concentrations in the latter. Demonstration of elevated urinary hypoxanthine and xanthine may be used when uric acid concentrations are equivocal. Activity measurement of sulfite oxidase and xanthine dehydrogenase is not commonly used for further confirmation, but sequence analysis of the *SUOX* gene on chromosome 12 is available.

Treatment and Prognosis

Several therapeutic interventions have been used in an attempt to improve the clinical symptoms of sulfite oxidase deficiencies. Although none have effectively reversed the clinical symptoms, certain therapies have shown some benefit to individual patients. Dietary restriction of sulfur-containing amino acids has achieved considerable improvement of the biochemical profile; however, its effect on neurological function is variable. Molybdenum cofactor deficiency has a better response to dietary restriction than isolated sulfite oxidase deficiency. Treatments using the NMDA antagonist, dextromethorphan, or anticonvulsant medication, vigabatrin, have achieved significant relief of convulsions. A better understanding of the molybdenum cofactor biosynthesis pathway suggests that administration of appropriate precursors might be a possible cure for molybdenum cofactor deficiency. A recent study demonstrated that administration of a synthetic precursor to molybdopterin, cyclic pyranopterin monophosphate, produced metabolic and clinical improvement in a patient who was diagnosed with molybdenum cofactor deficiency *(28)*.

CYSTINURIA

Cystinuria, not to be confused with cystinosis (a defect in lysosomal cystine transport), is unique among inborn metabolic disorders in that it is precipitated by a defect in amino acid transport rather than catabolism. The biochemical abnormalities associated with cystinuria are best appreciated in urine rather than plasma. Cystine is the oxidized homodimer of cysteine and is transported across epithelial membranes with the dibasic amino acids lysine, arginine, and ornithine. Although filtration of these amino acids at the glomeruli is passive, uptake from the renal filtrate is active and performed by numerous multimeric transporter complexes present on the apical and basolateral surface of the renal tubular epithelia. When the filtrate becomes saturated with cystine, stones form leading to tubular obstruction, infection, and chronic renal disease. Most cases of cystinuria originate from mutations in two gene loci.

The disorder has a worldwide incidence of approximately 1 in 10,000 and accounts for 1–2% of all cases of nephrolithiasis and 6-8% in the pediatric population. The goal of treatment is to enhance the solubility of cystine in the renal tubules, thereby decreasing the propensity for stone formation *(29)*.

Clinical Presentation

Presentation of cystinuria is rare in infancy but is evident by the second or third decade of life. Symptoms are those indicating renal stones: colicky lower back and groin pain, recurrent urinary tract infections, and progressive renal failure. Patients usually show little to no signs of malnourishment despite defective absorption of dibasic amino acids from the intestinal lumen and from the glomerular filtrate.

Genetics and Pathogenesis

Greater than 95% of the amino acid load in the glomerular filtrate is reabsorbed in the proximal convoluted tubule by a series of transporters specific for zwitterionic, anionic, and cationic species. At least 50 gene products are involved in the assembly of these transporters *(30)*. Of the four dibasic (cationic) amino acids, cystine is the most sparingly soluble, particularly at pH <7.5. Aqueous solutions of cystine become saturated at concentrations >1,200 μmol/L (300 mg/L). The filtered load of cystine (1 g/day) easily exceeds the limit of solubility given an average daily urine volume of 1–1.5 L if dibasic amino acids are not efficiently reabsorbed.

Two gene loci have been implicated in cystinuria: *SLC3A1* on chromosome 2 and *SLC7A9* on chromosome 19. The heterodimeric transporter formed by these gene products exchanges a luminal cationic transporter for a neutral cytoplasmic one, thus utilizing the energy of the membrane potential to drive transport. Cystine transport is also uniquely driven by a concentration gradient formed as a result of rapid oxidation of cationic cystine to the neutral thiol, cysteine. Approximately two thirds of disease-causing mutations are found in *SLC3A1* with most of the remainder in *SLC7A9*, and the genetic bases for a few cases have not been defined *(31)*. The transporter is expressed on the luminal surface of renal tubular epithelia and the small intestine. Despite the intestinal defect, blood concentrations of the dibasic amino acids remain normal, due in part to direct enteral absorption of smaller peptides. A different combination of gene products (*SLC3A2 + SLC7A7*) is responsible for transport of dibasic amino acids across the basolateral surface into the bloodstream. Mutations in *SLC7A7* are responsible for most disease causing alleles in lysinuric protein intolerance.

Laboratory Diagnosis

Cystinuria is one of the few aminoacidopathies in which urine is the specimen of choice for analysis. Urine from affected individuals may contain colorless, hexagonal cystine crystals. Amino acid profiles of urine reproducibly display increased excretion of cystine, ornithine, lysine, and arginine (Figure 2-11). Increased excretion ranges from two- up to thirtyfold in some cases. Twenty-four-hour urine collections are not necessary for diagnosis. Heterozygotes may display mildly increased excretion typically up to twofold normal.

Treatment and Prognosis

The goal of cystinuria treatment is to decrease the propensity for stone formation, thereby conserving the renal function of affected patients. Approaches to treatment include hydration, alkalinization of urine, and administration of free thiol compounds. Traditional approaches preventing crystallization of cystine include water intake of 3–4 L/day to dilute the gram of cystine filtered and consumption of citrate or bicarbonate to raise urine pH and increase the solubility of cystine. In practice, compliance with extreme hydration is poor and sustaining urine pH above 7.5 is difficult. Modern pharmacologic treatment of cystinuria uses thiol compounds that undergo disulfide exchange with cystine to form

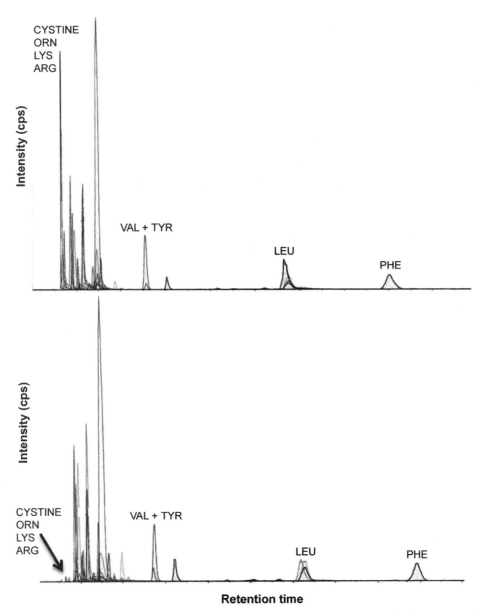

Figure 2-11   LC-MS/MS total ion chromatogram (C8) of urine from patient with cystinuria (upper) and normal patient (lower).

soluble cysteine-containing compounds. These agents include Penicillamine (3-mercapto-D-valine) and Thiola (2-mercaptopropionylglycine) *(32)*. Side effects such as rash, joint pain, fever, and pancytopenia occur in up to half of patients treated and often limit the dose and duration of therapy. Despite these efforts, approximately 50% of patients experience recurrent nephrolithiasis necessitating stone removal via percutaneous or other noninvasive approaches (e.g., lithotripsy).

REFERENCES

1. Beach EF, Munks B, Robinson H. The amino acid composition of animal tissue protein. J Biol Chem 1943;148:431–9.

2. Frame E. The levels of individual free amino acids in the plasma of normal man at various intervals after a high-protein meal. J Clin Invest 1958;37:1710–23.

3. Oladipo OO, Weindel AL, Saunders AN, Dietzen DJ. Impact of premature birth and critical illness on neonatal range of plasma amino acid concentrations determined by LC-MS/MS. Mol Genet Metab 2011;104:476–9.

4. Deyl Z, Hyanek J, Horakova M. Profiling of amino acids in body fluids and tissues by means of liquid chromatography. J Chromatogr 1986;379:177–250.

5. Dietzen DJ, Weindel AL, Carayannopoulos MO, Landt M, Normansell ET, Reimschisel TE, Smith CH. Rapid comprehensive amino acid analysis by liquid chromatography/tandem mass spectrometry: comparison to cation exchange with post-column ninhydrin detection. Rapid Commun Mass Spectrom 2008;22:3481–8.

6. Donlon J, Levy H, Scriver CR. Chapter 77. Hyperphenylalaninemia: phenylalanine hydroxylase deficiency. In: Valle D, Beaudet AL, Vogelstein B, Kinzler KW, Antonarakis SE, Ballabio A, eds. Scriver's Online Metabolic & Molecular Bases of Inherited Disease. McGraw-Hill, published January 2006; updated March 28, 2011. http://www.ommbid.com (Accessed February 2012).

7. Blau N, Thöny B, Cotton RGH, Hyland K. Disorders of tetrahydrobiopterin and related biogenic amines. In: Valle D, Beaudet AL, Vogelstein B, Kinzler KW, Antonarakis SE, Ballabio A, eds. The Online Metabolic & Molecular Bases of Inherited Disease. http://www.ommbid.com (Accessed February 2012).

8. Trefz FK, Burton BK, Longo N, Casanova MM, Gruskin DJ, Dorenbaum A, et al. Efficacy of saptropterin dihydrochloride in increasing phenylalanine tolerance in children with phenylketonuria: a phase III, randomized, double-blind, placebo-controlled study. J Pediatr 2009;154:700–7.

9. Mitchell GA, Grompe M, Lamber M, Tanguay RM. Hypertyrosinemias. In: Valle D, Beaudet AL, Vogelstein B, Kinzler KW, Antonarakis SE, Ballabio A, eds. Scriver's Online Metabolic & Molecular Bases of Inherited Disease. McGraw-Hill, published January 2006; updated March 28, 2011. http://www.ommbid.com (Accessed February 2012).

10. Kayser MA, Introne W, Gahl WA. Alkaptonuria. In: Valle D, Beaudet AL, Vogelstein B, Kinzler KW, Antonarakis SE, Ballabio A, eds. Scriver's Online Metabolic & Molecular Bases of Inherited Disease. McGraw-Hill, published January 2006; updated March 28, 2011. http://www.ommbid.com (Accessed February 2012).

11. Niederwieser A, Matasovic A, Tippett P, Danks DM. A new sulfur amino acid, named Hawkinsin, identified in a baby with transient tyrosinemia and her mother. Clin Chim Acta 1977;76:345–56.

12. Lindstedt S, Home E, Lock EA, Jjalmarson O, Strandvik B. Treatment of hereditary tyrosinaemia type 1 by inhibition of 4-hdyroxyphenylpyruvate dioxygenase. Lancet 1992;340:813–7.

13. Chuang DT, Wynn RM, Shih VE. Maple syrup urine disease (branched-chain ketoaciduria). In: Valle D, Beaudet AL, Vogelstein B, Kinzler KW, Antonarakis SE, Ballabio A, eds. Scriver's Online Metabolic & Molecular Bases of Inherited Disease. McGraw-Hill, published January 2006; updated March 28, 2011. http://www.ommbid.com (Accessed February 2012).

14. Chuang DT. Molecular studies of mammalian branched-chain alpha-keto acid dehydrogenase complexes: domain structures, expression, and inborn errors. Ann NY Acad Sci 1989;573:137–54.

15. Matthews DE, Ben-Galim E, Haymond MW, Bier DM. Alloisoleucine formation in maple syrup urine disease: isotopic evidence for the mechanism. Pediatr Res 1980;14:854–7.

16. Grillo MA, Colombatto S. S-adenosylmethionine and its products. Amino Acids 2008;34:187–93.

17. Mudd SH, Levy HL, Kraus JP. Disorders of transulfuration. In: Valle D, Beaudet AL, Vogelstein B, Kinzler KW, Antonarakis SE, Ballabio A, eds. Scriver's Online Metabolic & Molecular Bases of Inherited Disease. McGraw-Hill, published January 2006; updated March 28, 2011. http://www.ommbid.com (Accessed February 2012).

18. Rosenblatt DS, Cooper BA. Inherited disorders of vitamin B12 utilization. Bioessays 1991;12:331–4.

19. Oladipo OO, Spreitsma L, Dietzen DJ, Shinawi M. Increased homocysteine in a patient diagnosed with Marfan syndrome. Clin Chem 2010;56:1665–8.

20. Hamosh A, Johnston MV. Nonketotic hyperglycinemia. In: Valle D, Beaudet AL, Vogelstein B, Kinzler KW, Antonarakis SE, Ballabio A, eds. Scriver's Online Metabolic & Molecular Bases of Inherited Disease. McGraw-Hill, published January 2006; updated March 28, 2011. http://www.ommbid.com (Accessed February 2012).

21. Dinopoulos A, Matsubara Y, Kure S. Atypical variants of nonketotic hyperglycinemia. Mol Genet Metab 2005;86:61–9.

22. Langosch D, Becker CM, Betz H. The inhibitory glycine receptor: a ligand-gated chloride channel of the central nervous system. Eur J Biochem 1990;194:1–8.

23. Thomson AM. Glycine modulation of the NMDA receptor/channel complex. Trends Neurosci 1989;12:349–53.

24. Johnson JL, Duran M. Molybdenum cofactor deficiency and isolated sulfite oxidase deficiency. In: Valle D, Beaudet AL, Vogelstein B, Kinzler KW, Antonarakis SE, Ballabio A, eds. Scriver's Online Metabolic & Molecular Bases of Inherited Disease. McGraw-Hill, published January 2006; updated March 28, 2011. http://www.ommbid.com (Accessed February 2012).

25. Tan WH, Eichler F, Hoda S, Lee MS, Baris H, Hanley CA, et al. Isolated sulfite oxidase deficiency: a case report with a novel mutation and review of the literature. Pediatrics 2005;116:757–66.

26. Schwarz G, Mendel RR, Ribbe MW. Molybdenum cofactors, enzymes and pathways. Nature 2009;460: 839–47.

27. Leimkuhler S, Charcosset M, Latour P, Dorche C, Kleppe S, Scaglia F, et al. Ten novel mutations in the molybdenum cofactor genes MOCS1 and MOCS2 and in vitro characterization of a MOCS2 mutation that abolishes the binding ability of molybdopterin synthase. Hum Genet 2005;117:565–70.

28. Veldman A, Santamaria-Araujo JA, Sollazzo S, Pitt J, Gianello R, Yaplito-Lee J, et al. Successful treatment of molybdenum cofactor deficiency type A with cPMP. Pediatrics 2010;125;e1249–54.

29. Palacin M, Goodyer P, Nunes V, Gasparini P. Cystinuria. In: Valle D, Beaudet AL, Vogelstein B, Kinzler KW, Antonarakis SE, Ballabio A, eds. Scriver's Online Metabolic & Molecular Bases of Inherited Disease. McGraw-Hill, published January 2006; updated March 28, 2011. http://www.ommbid.com (Accessed February 2012).

30. Broer S, Palacin M. The role of amino acid transporters in inherited and acquired diseases. Biochem J 2011;436:193–211.

31. Mattoo A, Goldfarb DS. Cystinuria. Semin Nephrol 2008;28:181–91.

32. Dolin DJ, Asplin JR, Flagel L, Grasso M, Goldfarb DS. Effect of cystine-binding thiol drugs on urinary cystine capacity in patients with cystinuria. J Endourol 2005;19:429–32.

Chapter 3

Organic Acid Disorders

Stanley F. Lo, Jessica A. Scott-Schwoerer, and William J. Rhead

Organic acidemias or acidurias are a class of disorders characterized by the excretion of organic acids in the urine. This class of inborn error is typically caused by a deficiency in enzymatic activity involved with the catabolism of amino acids. The clinical presentation usually presents itself during the neonatal or infantile period. Typical complaints at presentation include vomiting, lethargy, poor feeding, and seizures. Common laboratory findings at the time of presentation include metabolic acidosis, hypoglycemia, hyperammonemia, lactic acidemia, and ketosis *(1)*.

Diagnosis of these disorders requires urine organic acid testing. Urine organic acid analysis by a gas chromatograph (GC)/mass spectrometer (MS) using a capillary column method represents the standard of analysis or detection and quantitation of acidic amino acid and fatty acid metabolites in urine. Although there are several methods to identify organic acids in urine, the most commonly used extraction method *(2)* requires extraction with an organic solvent, such as ethyl acetate, followed by chemical derivation into trimethylsilyl (TMS) compounds. The GC is used to separate the TMS compounds that flow into the MS and are fragmented. Each compound is identified by their fragmentation pattern. Mass spectra libraries assist in identifying compound fragmentation patterns. Unfortunately, many neutral and positively charged compounds of interest to metabolic physicians and biochemical geneticists are not detected using this classical technique.

A second method for organic acid identification uses the enzyme urease *(3, 4)*. Pretreatment of urine samples with urease permits TMS derivatization of virtually all organic molecules in urine and other body fluids. In this method, the urine is treated with urease to remove urea, the most abundant compound in urine. Then the urease and other proteins are precipitated and the remaining sample is derivatized into TMS compounds. Samples and 11 deuterated organic acid, amino acid, and carbohydrate internal standards are introduced into the GC/MS (Figure 3-1) and identification is accomplished with the assistance of mass spectral libraries. This method can quantitate 55 organic acid metabolites, 39 amino acids, 10 acylglycines, 12 sugars and carbohydrates, 7 neurotransmitters, and 5 purines and pyrimidines during a single 45-min run. Although the method is very laborious, the value in identifying many more biochemical compounds warrants that this method be seriously considered for organic acid testing.

For both methods, identification of fragmentation patterns of different compounds uses a mass spectral library. Diagnosis is not limited to the newborn period. Many variants of these disorders can be identified from infancy into childhood. Samples collected during periods of metabolic decompensation or acute illness have the advantage of likely producing abnormal organic acid profiles, whereas those collected during periods of nonacute illness may or may not produce an abnormal profile. See Table 3-1 for a summary of laboratory testing for acid disorders.

PROPIONIC ACIDEMIA

Propionic acidemia (PA) has a prevalence of approximately 1 in 100,000 live births. It is caused by a deficiency in the enzymatic activity of propionyl-coenzyme A (CoA) carboxylase. This enzyme

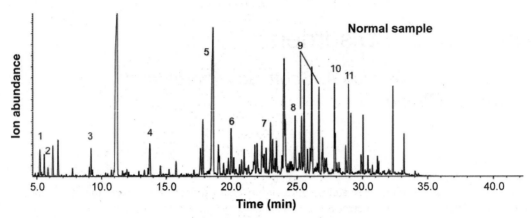

Figure 3-1 GC/MS total ion chromatogram of normal patient. Internal standards, in order of elution: (1) L-lactate-d$_3$, (2) pyruvate-^{13}C$_3$, (3) methyl-d$_3$-malonic acid, (4) DL-serine-d$_3$, (5) creatine-d$_3$, (6) L-phenyl-d$_5$-alanine, (7) orotic-^{15}N$_2$, acid, (8) sebacic-d$_4$ acid, (9) D-glucose-^{13}C$_6$ (two peaks), (10) myo-inositol-d$_6$, and (11) L-trytophan-d$_5$.

converts propionyl-CoA to D-methylmalonyl-CoA (Figure 3-2). Propionyl-CoA is a catabolic product of the amino acids isoleucine, leucine, methionine, and threonine. A minor pathway generating propionyl-CoA is from cholesterol and odd-chain fatty acids.

Clinical Presentation

PA, also called propionyl-CoA carboxylase (PCC) deficiency, is characterized by massive metabolic decompensation (5). Most commonly occurring in the neonatal period, these decompensations are rapid and severe. If left undiagnosed and untreated, they are often fatal to the neonate. The presentation is nonspecific and includes lethargy, poor feeding, vomiting, and hypotonia. Hyperammonemia, lactic and metabolic acidosis, increased plasma glycine and alanine, and ketosis are usually present. Outside of the neonatal period, frequent metabolic decompensations occur as well as seizures, vomiting, and hepatomegaly. Children with the later-onset form may experience poor growth, developmental delay, or varying forms of intellectual disability.

Genetics and Pathogenesis

PA is an autosomal-recessive disease. Mutations involve either of the two genes encoding PCC, *PCCA* or *PCCB*. Mutations in these genes lead to decreased enzymatic activity of PCC, resulting in the accumulation of propionyl-CoA. PCC is a biotin dependent enzyme; thus, defects in the biotin utilization pathway involving biotinidase and holocarboxylase synthase will have a clinical and biochemical overlap with PA.

Laboratory Diagnosis

Newborn screening can identify patients with PA. Elevations in C3 acylcarnitine indicate a positive screen requiring follow-up confirmatory testing. Follow-up testing through urine organic acid testing should present increased concentrations of 3-hydroxypropionic acid, methyl citrate, propionylglycine (Figure 3-3), and tiglylglycine in PA. Plasma glycine concentrations are commonly increased, as well as lactic acid and ammonia. Plasma acylcarnitine testing will show increased C3 acylcarnitine. Confirmatory testing is accomplished by enzyme analysis in fibroblasts or leukocytes. Sequencing of *PCCA* and *PCCB* may also be considered.

Table 3-1 Summary of Laboratory Testing for Organic Acid Disorders

Disorder	Newborn screening bloodspot abnormality	Laboratory findings	Confirmatory test
Propionic acidemia	Elevated C3 acylcarnitine	PAC—elevated C3 acylcarnitine; UOA—methylcitric acid, 3-hydroxypropionic acid, propionylglycine, tiglylglycine	Enzyme analysis of propionyl-CoA carboxylase; sequencing of *PCCA/PCCB*
Methylmalonic acidemia	Elevated C3 acylcarnitine	PAC—elevated C3 acylcarnitine; UOA—methylmalonic acid, methylcitric acid, 3-hydroxypropionic acid	Complementation studies; sequencing of MUT/genes for disorders of cobalamin metabolism
Multiple carboxylase deficiency			
A. Holocarboxylase synthetase deficiency	Elevated C5-OH acylcarnitine.	PAC—mild elevations in C3, C5-OH acylcarnitine; UOA—3-hydroxyisovaleric acid, methylcitric acid, 3-methylcrotonylglycine, propionylglycine	Enzyme analysis of holocarboxylase synthetase; sequencing of *HLCS*
B. Biotinidase	Enzyme analysis		Enzyme analysis of biotinidase; targeted mutation analysis or sequencing of *BTD*
Isovaleric acidemia	Elevated C5 acylcarnitine	PAC—elevated C5 acylcarnitine; UOA—isovalerylglycine, 3-hydroxyisovaleric acid, 4-hydroxyvaleric acid	Targeted mutation analysis or sequencing of *IVA*
Glutaric acidemia type 1	Elevated C5DC acylcarnitine	PAC and UAC—elevated C5-DC acylcarnitine; UOA—3-hydroxyglutaric acid, glutaric acid	Enzyme analysis of glutaryl-CoA dehydrogenase; targeted mutation analysis or sequencing of *GCDH*
3-Methylcrotonyl-CoA carboxylase deficiency	Elevated C5-OH acylcarnitine	PAC and UAC—elevated C5-OH acylcarnitine; UOA—3-methylcrotonylglycine, 3-hydroxyisovaleric acid	Enzyme analysis of 3-methylcrotonyl-CoA carboxylase; sequencing of *MCCC1/MCCC2*

PAC = plasma acylcarnitine (profile), UAC = urine acylcarnitine (specific acylcarnitine tested), UOA = urine organic acids.

39

Treatment and Prognosis

Treatment uses a highly modified protein-restricted diet supplemented with PA precursor-depleted amino acid supplements, L-carnitine, and biotin supplementation *(6)*. The protein-restricted diet limits the abnormal accumulation of propionyl-CoA. Carnitine assists in promoting the excretion of

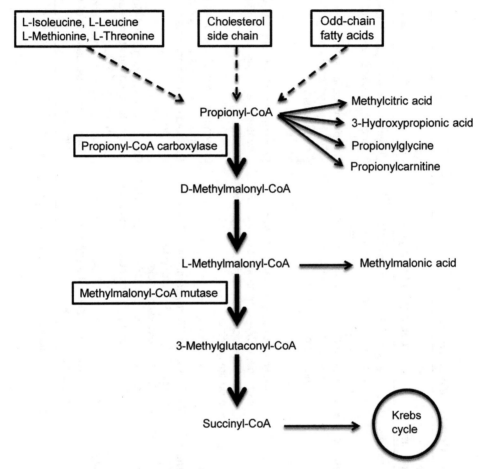

Figure 3-2 Pathway involving propionyl-CoA carboxylase and MCM. Modified with permission from *(7)*.

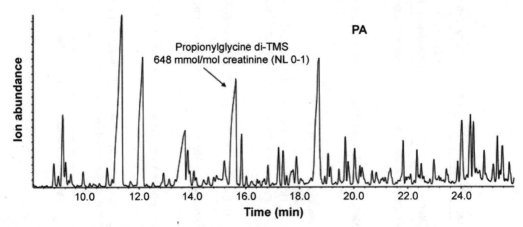

Figure 3-3 GC/MS total ion chromatogram of a PA patient.

propionyl-CoA as propionylcarnitine. Because PCC requires biotin as a cofactor, which is a cofactor for other carboxylases, PA may be identified in patients with multiple carboxylase deficiency. Not all PAs are responsive to biotin, in which case the modified diet is the only treatment. Although outcomes are generally poor, patients identified and treated earlier have a better prognosis than those with later-onset disease. Survival of the early-onset group is not as good as in the late-onset group. In Surtees' study, the median survival age of the early-onset group was 3 years (8). Unfortunately, those identified with late-onset disease typically acquired neurologic damage.

METHYLMALONIC ACIDEMIA

Several disorders are classified under the various methylmalonic acidurias (MMAs), including methylmalonyl-CoA mutase deficiency, 5'-deoxyadenosylcobalamin metabolic defects, and vitamin B12 deficiency (5). Absence of methylmalonyl-CoA mutase (MCM) does not allow methylmalonyl-CoA to be converted to succinyl-CoA (*mut°*). The result of this blockage is an increase in production of methylmalonic and propionic acids, precursors of methylmalonic acid (Figure 3-2). Other MCM mutations lead to fewer reductions in enzymatic activity and constitute another category of mutase deficiency termed *mut⁻*. Defects in the synthesis of 5'-deoxyadenosylcobalamin, a cofactor for the mutase enzyme, are classified into several complementary classes (Figure 3-4). CblA and CblB involve defects in adenosylcobalamin synthesis, resulting in a similar biochemical presentation as observed in mutase deficiency. CblC and CblD are involved in cobalamin reduction, resulting in decreased mutase activity and decreased methionine synthase activity. Methionine synthase converts homocystine to methionine using the methylcobalamin as a cofactor; thus, these defects produce MMA and homocystinemia. CblF is due to defects in transcobalamin degradation that prevent cobalamin from being transported from lysosomes for recycling in the cytoplasm.

Clinical Presentation

Newborns are typically healthy for the first 1–2 weeks of life. *Mut°* and severe *mut⁻* affected individuals typically present with hypotonia, lethargy, and poor feeding. Older infants and children with milder

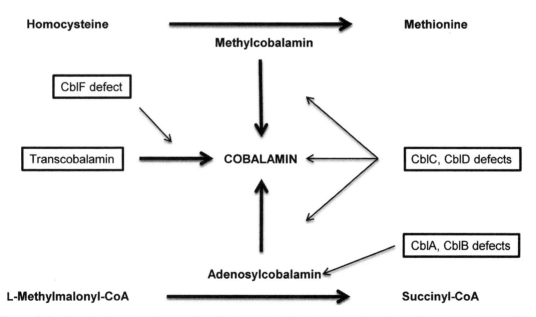

Figure 3-4 Cobalamin metabolism and localization of cobalamin defects. Modified with permission from (7).

mut⁻ mutations will present with poor growth or only during periods of intervening illness. Symptoms will include lethargy, seizures, and hypoglycemia. The CblC form of MMA may present with symptoms related to homocystinuria, including progressive myopathy, thrombosis, and retinal findings.

Genetics and Pathogenesis

The prevalence of MMA is suspected to be between 1 in 50,000 and 1 in 100,000 live births *(9)*. MMA is inherited in an autosomal-recessive manner. Several genes have been identified to cause MMA, including *MUT* (MCM), *MMAA* (methylmalonic aciduria type A protein), *MMAB* (cob(l)yrinic acid *a,c*-diamide adenosyltransferase), *MMACHC* (methylmalonic aciduria and homocystinuria type C protein), and *MCEE* (methylmalonyl-CoA epimerase). Nearly 60% of MMA cases are due to defects in the *MUT* gene. *MUT⁰* disease (78 of the 60%) is the most severe form of MMA because of the complete inactivity of the enzyme. *MUT* disease (22 of the 60%) is less severe because there is some remaining enzymatic activity in these patients. Mutations in *MMAA* (25%), *MMAB* (12%), and *MMADHC* genes also lead to impaired MCM activity and MMA. *MCEE* mutations lead to a mild form of MMA.

Laboratory Diagnosis

Newborn screening can identify patients with MMA. Elevations in C3 acylcarnitine signal a positive screen requiring follow-up confirmatory testing. Follow-up testing for MMA should reveal elevations in methylmalonic acid (Figure 3-5), methyl citrate, and 3-hydroxypropionic acid. Increases in propionylglycine and propionylcarnitine may also be observed. Determination of the different enzymatic subtypes requires additional studies in vitamin B12 responsiveness, ^{14}C propionate incorporation, and cobalamin distribution assays *(9)*. Confirmatory testing is also accomplished through complementation studies. Sequencing of *MUT* and other genes for disorders of cobalamin metabolism may also be done.

Treatment and Prognosis

Treatment for MMA involves a highly modified protein-restricted diet supplemented with PA precursor-depleted amino acid supplements that are adjusted for age and weight. Cobalamin (cyano- or hydoxycobalamin) and L-carnitine supplementation may also be provided. Prolonged periods of fasting should be avoided. Prognosis is related to response to treatment and outcome is dependent on disease subtype, in which *Mut⁰* has the worst prognosis and CblA has the best prognosis. The severity of the other classes range between these two defects. In a study by Nicolaides et al., early-onset cobalamin nonresponders had a median survival of approximately 6 years *(10)*.

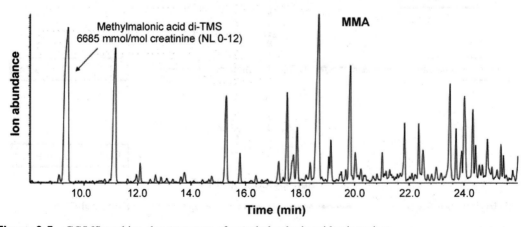

Figure 3-5   GC/MS total ion chromatogram of a methylmalonic acidemia patient.

MULTIPLE CARBOXYLASE DEFICIENCY (HOLOENZYME SYNTHETASE AND BIOTINIDASE)

Multiple carboxylase deficiency includes more than one disorder because of the utilization of biotin as a cofactor for several enzymes *(11)*. Specifically, the enzymes pyruvate carboxylase, propionyl-CoA carboxylase, 3-methylcrotonyl-CoA carboxylase, and acetyl-CoA carboxylase require biotin as an essential, covalently bound cofactor. When the synthesis of biotin cofactor is disrupted, the functional activity of these enzymes is decreased or eliminated, which consequently will have effects on fatty acid synthesis, gluconeogenesis, pyruvate metabolism, and amino acid catabolism. Biotin itself is a water-soluble vitamin derived primarily from the diet. Errors in the metabolism of biotin produce two types of disorders—holocarboxylase synthetase deficiency and biotinidase deficiency

Clinical Presentation

Typical clinical symptoms of holocarboxylase synthetase deficiency include lethargy, hypotonia, seizures, and difficulty feeding and breathing. Other findings include ketoacidosis, hypoglycemia, hyperammonemia, skin rash, and alopecia *(12)*. Onset of symptoms for holocarboxylase synthetase deficiency typically occurs during the neonatal period, although later presentations are common. In biotinidase deficiency, clinical features typically include neurological, dermatological, immunological, and ophthalmological symptoms *(13)*. The onset of symptoms of biotinidase-deficient individuals usually appears during infancy. Although the onset of symptoms for both disorders is usually different, there is considerable temporal and clinical overlap.

Genetics and Pathogenesis

Multiple mutations have been found in the genes for holocarboxylase synthetase and biotinidase. The prevalence of holocarboxylase synthetase deficiency is approximately 1 in 87,000 and for biotinidase it is approximately 1 in 60,000 live births *(13)*. The inheritance pattern of these disorders is autosomal recessive. The mutations in these genes lead to defective enzymes involved in the utilization of biotin. Consequently, enzymes requiring biotin as a cofactor decrease their activity or become inactive.

The biotin cycle is the process by which biotin is utilized and recycled. Enzymes that require biotin as a cofactor, the apocarboxylases, require biotin to be covalently attached through a lysine residue, thereby forming the fully active holocarboxylases (pyruvate carboxylase, PCC, 3-methylcrotonyl-CoA carboxylase, and acetyl-CoA carboxylase). The enzyme responsible for covalently attaching biotin to the apocarboxylases is holocarboxylase synthetase. The biotin cycle involves recycling biotin from the holocarboxylases by proteolytic degradation by which the biotin is cleaved from the lysine side chain by the enzyme biotinidase, resulting in the release of free biotin for use in holocarboxylase synthesis.

Laboratory Diagnosis

Newborn screening for biotinidase deficiency is available *(14, 15)*. Screening of holocarboxylase synthetase deficiency can be identified by elevations of C5-hydroxyacylcarnitine. Follow-up testing using urine organic acid analysis will reveal increases in 3-hydroxyisovaleric acid, methylcitric acid, 3-methylcrotonylglycine, and propionyl glycine. Confirmatory testing is done by determining enzymatic activity, DNA sequence analysis, or targeted mutation analysis of either enzyme.

Treatment and Prognosis

Fortunately, patients with holocarboxylase synthetase deficiency or biotinidase deficiency can both be treated with oral biotin. Most patients are responsive to biotin, resulting in the reversal of symptoms. If treatment is initiated before the onset of neurological symptoms, prognosis is very good. Unfortunately, once vision and hearing symptoms are present, they are usually irreversible.

ISOVALERIC ACIDEMIA

Isovaleric acidemia (IVA) is caused by a deficiency of the enzyme isovaleryl-CoA dehydrogenase (IVD). Loss of IVD function results in the accumulation of isovaleryl-CoA by preventing its oxidation to 3-methylcrotonyl-CoA (Figure 3-6). This catalytic step is part of the catabolic pathway of leucine. IVA is the first organic acidemia diagnosed by GC/MS *(2)* and is readily detected with tandem mass spectrometry (MS/MS) *(16)*.

Clinical Presentation

There are two forms of IVA—an acute neonatal form and a chronic intermittent form. The biochemical defect is the same for both. The difference in clinical presentation is not determined by the causative mutation, but it is a consequence of catabolic stress and other factors *(17)*. Neonates with the acute form begin to exhibit signs and symptoms within the first few days of life. Poor feeding, vomiting, and lethargy are apparent, and the foul "odor of sweaty feet" is commonly found. Laboratory findings demonstrate increased ketones, metabolic acidosis, increased lactate, and hyperammonemia. Other findings include thrombocytopenia, neutropenia, pancytopenia, and hypocalcemia *(18–21)*. Neonates that survive the acute episode will then fall into the chronic intermittent form of disease and their development may be normal *(20–22)*.

In the chronic intermittent form of IVA, presentation occurs within the first year of life. Similar to the acute form, vomiting, lethargy, acidosis with ketonuria, and the odor of sweaty feet are

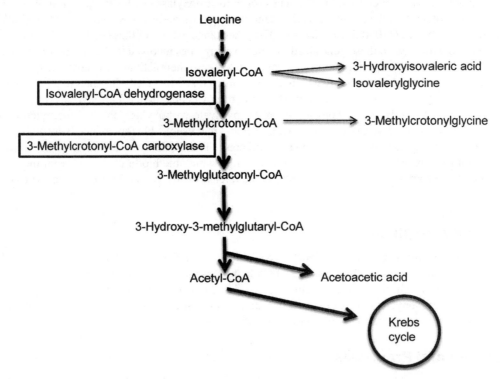

Figure 3-6   Leucine metabolism involving isovaleryl-CoA dehydrogenase and 3-methylcrotonyl-CoA carboxylase. Modified with permission from *(7)*.

commonly found at presentation. It is common for patients with IVA to have some form of developmental delay and mental retardation along with an aversion to protein-rich foods *(23)*. With the improvements in early diagnosis, normal development of individuals with IVA is more common than in the past.

Genetics and Pathogenesis

IVA has a prevalence of 1 in 250,000 and is an autosomal-recessive disorder characterized by mutations in the IVD gene. The protein product is a homotetramer. IVD is initially synthesized in the cytoplasm as a 45,000-g/mol precursor. With posttranslational modification and transfer into the mitochondria, a 43,000-g/mol mature protein is created. The combination of four mature polypeptides forms IVD. The molecular heterogeneity of IVD has been classified into six classes. Class I mutations generate a mixture of the precursor and mature peptides, suggesting the presence of point mutations and normal processing. Class II, III, and IV mutations generate smaller proteins of the precursor and mature forms, suggesting the presence of point mutations and deletions. Classes V and VI do not form any detectable protein product because of either an inability to translate mRNA and the formation of unstable mRNA or defective transcription.

Laboratory Diagnosis

Newborn screening using MS/MS is used to detect elevations in C5 acylcarnitine. Although the characteristic odor of sweaty feet due to increased concentrations of isovaleric acid is commonly identified during acute episodes, it is not completely specific for IVA because a similar odor is identifiable in glutaric acidemia type II (GAII; multiple acyl-CoA dehydrogenase deficiency). In IVA, gas chromatography/mass spectroscopy for urine organic acid testing will specifically identify isovalerylglycine (Figure 3-7). During acute episodes, concentrations of urinary isovalerylglycine are 100–500 times normal. In remission, concentrations range from normal to 10 times normal. Plasma acylcarnitine analysis is a complementary test for IVA diagnosis. Identification of C5 acylcarnitine suggests the presence of isovalerylcarnitine, although an isobaric isomer, 2-methylbutyrylcarnitine, may also be present. However, the isomer is typically accompanied with an increased C4- and C16-acylcarnitines if GA2 (multiple acyl-CoA dehydrogenase deficiency) is present. DNA analysis for specific IVD mutations as well as sequencing is available for confirmatory testing. Confirmatory testing by enzymatic analysis on fibroblasts can also be done.

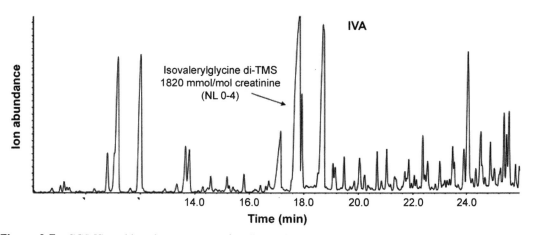

Figure 3-7   GC/MS total ion chromatogram of an IVA patient.

Treatment and Prognosis

If no neurological damage has occurred before the initiation of treatment with a leucine-restricted diet and glycine and/or carnitine, then prognosis for normal development is good.

GLUTARIC ACIDEMIA TYPE I

Glutaric acidemia type I (GAI), also called glutaryl-CoA dehydrogenase deficiency, is a disorder of the catabolic pathways of lysine, hydroxylysine, and tryptophan (Figure 3-8). Increased concentrations of these amino acids and their breakdown products can cause damage to the basal ganglia, leading to dystonia and dyskinesia *(24)*.

Clinical Presentation

Development can be normal throughout the first year of life, but macrocephaly is commonly present. Noticeable chronic symptoms may include difficulty feeding and irritability. After 5 years of age, onset of symptoms is rare. Initial presentation, typically between 4 and 18 months of age, is usually an acute, irreversible, encephalopathic, stroke-like episode acquired concurrently with another illness, infection, fasting, or minor trauma. Loss of head control, hypotonia, and seizures can evolve rapidly. Other irreversible neurological symptoms follow including dystonia, opisthotonus, and rigidity. These

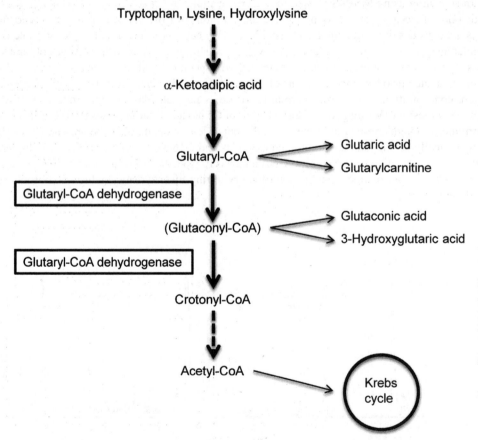

Figure 3-8   Catabolism of tryptophan, lysine, and hydroxylysine involving glutaryl-CoA dehydrogenase. Modified with permission from *(7)*.

symptoms previously suggested cerebral palsy, but with the development of newborn screening for GAI, this catastrophic presentation is less common. If metabolic crises recur, dyskinesia and dystonia may worsen and become very severe. Fortunately, regardless of neurological symptoms, intellect is generally preserved. Individuals with GAI exhibit a wide range of neurological complications.

Genetics and Pathogenesis

The GAI gene is inherited in an autosomal-recessive manner and occurs in approximately 1 in 30,000 to 1 in 100,000 births. In some homogeneous populations, the incidence of disease can be as frequent as 1 in 225 births (25). Heterozygous carriers are essentially normal. Mutations in the glutaryl-CoA dehydrogenase gene (GCDH) prevent the catabolism of lysine, hydroxylysine, and tryptophan. Decreased enzymatic activity leads to the accumulation of glutaric acid, 3-hydroxyglutaric acid, glutaconic acid, and glutarylcarnitine. GCDH is approximately 7 kb long and has 11 exons (26). The protein product is approximately 4,500 g/mol. Over 100 mutations have been identified, and enzymatic activity typically ranges from 0 to 10% in GAI tissues from GAI patients. No correlation between specific mutations and clinical severity has been demonstrated.

Laboratory Diagnosis

Diagnosis can be determined by detecting increased glutaric acid and 3-hydroxyglutaric acid in urine organic acid analysis (Figure 3-9). 3-Hydroxyglutaric acid is usually but not always detectable, but if identified, it is pathognomic for GAI. Complementary testing using MS/MS for plasma acylcarnitines reveals increased C5-DC acylcarnitine. This is method is also used to detect glutarylcarnitine in dried blood spots for newborn screening. Confirmatory testing can be done by enzymatic analysis using ^{14}C-labeled glutaryl-CoA and measuring the release of ^{14}-carbon dioxide (CO_2) (27). Specific mutation detection and genetic sequencing of GCDH is also available for confirmatory testing.

Treatment and Prognosis

Treatment uses carnitine supplementation as well as immediate and vigorous treatment of illnesses with antipyretics, fluids, insulin, and glucose. When treated properly, >80% of GAI patients developed normally (28). It is unclear if dietary restriction of protein, lysine, and tryptophan provides any benefit, although many centers restrict dietary intake of these amino acids.

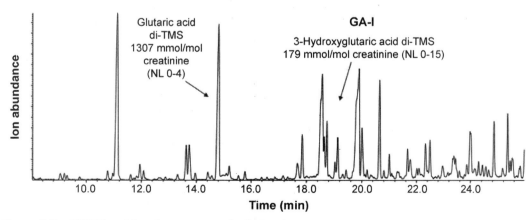

Figure 3-9 GC/MS total ion chromatogram of a GAI patient.

3-METHYLCROTONYL-COA CARBOXYLASE DEFICIENCY

As with other biotin-dependent carboxylases, the isolated deficiency of 3-methylcrotonyl-CoA carboxylase (3-MCC) must be distinguished from the biotin-responsive disorders holocarboxylase synthetase or biotinidase deficiencies as well as other isolated carboxylase deficiencies. In isolated 3-MCC deficiency, also called 3-methylcrotonylglycinuria, the catabolism of leucine is impaired and this enzyme is unable to convert 3-methylcrotonyl-CoA to 3-methylglutaconyl-CoA (Figure 3-6).

Clinical Presentation

There is a large range of clinical presentations for 3-MCC, ranging from clinically benign to severe disease and death. The most severely affected patients can present with metabolic acidosis, hypoglycemia, and hyperammonemia *(17)*. Other laboratory findings include elevated hepatic transaminases, moderate ketonuria, and plasma carnitine deficiency *(29)*. Initial signs may include poor feeding, vomiting, and lethargy. Untreated 3-MCC patients may present with failure to thrive, Reye-like symptoms, hypotonia, seizures, coma, developmental delay, and possibly death.

Genetics and Pathogenesis

Prevalence is approximately 1 in 50,000 live births. Inheritance of this disorder is autosomal recessive. 3-MCC is composed of two subunits encoded by two genes. The gene *MCCC1* codes for methylcrotonyl-CoA carboxylase subunit a, and *MCCC2* codes for methylcrotonyl-CoA carboxylase subunit β.

Laboratory Diagnosis

Newborn screening with MS/MS can identify 3-MCC by detecting isobaric isomers of C5 hydroxyacylcarnitine. Because five metabolic diseases can generate high concentrations of an isobaric acylcarnitine with the same mass as 3-methylcrotonylcarnitine on MS/MS screening, follow-up testing is required to determine which disorder is responsible for the positive screen. Diagnosis is made by urine organic acid testing demonstrating increased concentrations of 3-hydroxyisovaleric acid and 3-methylcrotonylglycine (Figure 3-10). If methylcitrate, 3-hydroxypropionic acid, and lactate are present, multiple carboxylase deficiency must be considered. Diagnosis of isolated 3-MCC may also be confirmed by plasma acylcarnitine analysis and the identification of significant elevations

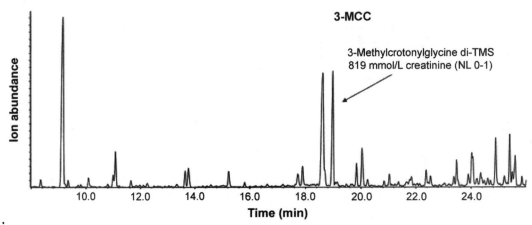

Figure 3-10   GC/MS total ion chromatogram of a 3-MCC-deficient patient.

Table 3-2 Summary of Other Organic Acid Disorders—Major Clinical Findings, Enzyme and Biological Function, and Gene

Disorder	Major clinical findings	Enzyme and biological function	Gene
β-Ketothiolase deficiency (T2) (30)	Episodic severe ketoacidosis usually with stress, possible hyperlacticacidemia	Mitochondrial acetoacetyl-CoA thiolase—involved in ketogenesis and ketolysis, involved in catabolism of isoleucine	ACAT1
3-Methylglutaconic aciduria—type I (32)	Variable—developmental delay, failure to thrive—neurological, no hyperammonemia, no acidosis	3-Methylglutaconic dehydratase—involved in leucine degradation	AUH
3-Methylglutaconic aciduria—type II (Barth syndrome) (32,33)	Dilated cardiomyopathy, skeletal myopathy, neutropenia, growth deficiency	Protein predicted to be acyltransferases involved in remodeling of cardiolipin	TAZ (Tafazzin)
3-Methylglutaconic aciduria—type III (Costeff syndrome) (32,34)	Optic atrophy, choreoathetoid movements	Optic atrophy 3 protein—unknown function	OPA3
3-Methylglutaconic aciduria—type IV (32)	Variable neurologic features, cardiomyopathy	Unknown	Unknown
3-Methylglutaconic aciduria—type V (32)	Dilated cardiomyopathy, ataxia	Unknown	DNAJC19
2-Methylbutyryl-CoA dehydrogenase deficiency, acyl-CoA dehydrogenase short/branched chain (35)	Variable presentation from asymptomatic to life threatening, poor feeding, lethargy, vomiting, irritable, difficulty breathing, seizures, and coma. Increase frequency in Hmong population	2-Methylbutyryl-CoA dehydrogenase—involved in degradation of isoleucine	ACADSB (or SBCAD)
Fumarase deficiency, fumaric aciduria (36)	Severe neurological abnormalities—brain malformations, developmental delay, hypotonia, microcephaly, failure to thrive, minor seizures, unusual facial features, hepatosplenomegaly, polycythemia, leukopenia; no acute crises	Fumarate hydratase/fumarase—catalyzes the conversion of fumarate to malate within the citric acid cycle	FH
Malonic aciduria (37–39)	Variable presentation—developmental delay, hypotonia, seizures, diarrhea, vomiting, hypoglycemia, acidosis, cardiomyopathy	Malonyl-CoA decarboxylase—first step in fatty acid biosynthesis	MLYCD
L-2-Hydroxyglutaric aciduria (32)	Abnormalities in cerebellum, seizures, intellectual disability, macrocephaly	L-2-Hydroxyglutarate dehydrogenase; toxic effect of L-2-hydroxyglutarate on central nervous system	L2HGDH
D-2-Hydroxyglutaric aciduria (32)	Variable presentation (mild and severe), developmental delay, seizures, hypotonia, abnormalities in the cerebrum, cardiomyopathy	D-2-Hhydroxyglutarate dehydrogenase	D2HGDH
Canavan disease (ASPA deficiency or aspartoacylase deficiency) (32,40)	Developmental delay, macrocephaly, lack of head control, hypotonia, blindness	Aspartoacylase—catalyzes the conversion of N-acetylaspartic acid to aspartic acid and acetate	ASPA

49

Table 3-3 Summary of Other Organic Acid Disorders—Laboratory Findings and Treatment

Disorder	Laboratory findings	Treatment
β-Ketothiolase deficiency (T2) (30)	UOA: 2-methyl-3-hydroxybutyrate, 2-methylacetylacetate, tiglylglycine. PAC: elevated C5-OH (3-hydroxyisovalerylcarnitine) enzyme: confirm with enzyme testing on fibroblast. Molecular DNA testing available	Acute—glucose infusion and treat acidosis but beware of hypernatremia with aggressive alkanization. Chronic—mild protein restriction, avoid fasting and early treatment with illness, carnitine if low
3-Methylglutaconic aciduria (31)—type I (32)	UOA: 3-methylglutaconic acid, 3-methylglutaric acid; type 1 also has elevation in 3-hydroxyisovaleric acid. Molecular DNA testing available	Type 1—consider leucine restriction, carnitine supplementation
3-Methylglutaconic aciduria—type II (Barth syndrome) (32,33)	UOA: 3-methylglutaconic acid, 3-methylglutaric acid. Molecular DNA testing available	No specific treatment (fatty acid therapy under investigation)
3-Methylglutaconic aciduria—type III (Costeff syndrome) (32,34)	UOA: 3-methylglutaconic acid, 3-methylglutaric acid. Molecular DNA testing available	No specific treatment
3-Methylglutaconic aciduria—type IV (32)	UOA: 3-methylglutaconic acid, 3-methylglutaric acid. Molecular DNA testing available	No specific treatment
3-Methylglutaconic aciduria—type V (32)	UOA: 3-methylglutaconic acid, 3-methylglutaric acid. Molecular DNA testing available	No specific treatment
2-Methylbutyryl-CoA dehydrogenase deficiency, acyl-CoA dehydrogenase short/branched chain (35)	UOA: 2-methylbutyrylglycine. PAC: elevated C5 (2-methylbutyrylcarnitine)	Variable—no treatment to avoid prolonged periods of time without eating, low-protein diet, restricted isoleucine intake, carnitine
Fumarase deficiency, fumaric aciduria (36)	UOA: fumaric acid. Enzyme: activity assay from fibroblasts, lymphoblasts, or leucocytes. Molecular genetic testing available	No specific treatment
Malonic aciduria (37–39)	UOA: malonic acid. PAC: C3DC (malonylcarnitine). Molecular DNA testing available	No consensus for dietary treatment. Long-chain triglyceride restricted/medium-chain triglyceride supplemented diet has been suggested
ʟ-2-Hydroxyglutaric aciduria (32)	UOA: 2-hydroxyglutaric acid (chirality not determined)	No specific treatment
ᴅ-2-Hydroxyglutaric aciduria (32)	UOA: 2-hydroxyglutaric acid (chirality not determined)	No specific treatment
Canavan disease (ASPA deficiency or aspartoacylase deficiency) (32,40)	UOA: N-acetylaspartic acid. Molecular DNA testing for ASPA available	No specific treatment

PAC = plasma acylcarnitine (profile), UOA = urine organic acids.

50

of 3-hydroxyisovalerylcarnitine *(41)*. Confirmatory testing is done by enzyme activity analysis of 3-MCC in leukocytes. To distinguish 3-MCC from multiple carboxylase deficiency, normal activity of at least one carboxylase should be demonstrated. Genetic sequencing of *MCCC1* and *MCCC2* may also be used for confirmatory testing.

Treatment and Prognosis

The spectrum of clinical disease is broad. Some individuals remain asymptomatic throughout their lifetime. Others begin to have symptoms as early as 3 months of age and commonly before 3 years of age. Treatment may require the restriction of leucine and carnitine supplementation because carnitine deficiency occurs secondary to urinary loss of 3-methylcrotonyl-carnitine. Glycine may also be administered to remove 3-MCC as 3-methylcrotonylglycine *(42)*. Development is typically normal with treatment. Without treatment recurring metabolic crises may occur, especially during illness, and developmental delay, seizures, coma, or death may result.

OTHER ORGANIC ACID DISORDERS

Many other organic disorders have been identified and are not discussed in this chapter. Tables 3-2 and 3-3 show several of these less prevalent disorders.

REFERENCES

1. Seashore MR. Updated December 22, 2009. The organic acidemias: an overview. In: GeneReviews at Gene-Tests: Medical Genetics Information Resource (database online). Copyright, University of Washington, Seattle, 1997-2011. http://www.genetests.org (Accessed February 2012).
2. Sweetman L. Organic acid analysis. In: Hommes F, ed. Techniques in Diagnostic Human Biochemical Genetics: A Laboratory Manual. New York: John Wiley & Sons, 1991:646pp.
3. Shoemaker J, Elliot W. Automated screening of urine samples for carbohydrates, organic and amino acids after treatment with urease. J Chromatography 1991;562:125–38.
4. Lo SF, Young V, Rhead WJ. Identification of urine organic acids for the detection of inborn errors of metabolism using urease and gas chromatograph-mass spectrometry (GC-MS). In: Garg U, Hammett-Stabler CA, eds. Clinical Applications of Mass Spectrometry: Methods and Protocols. New York: Humana Press, 2010:433–43.
5. Fenton WA, Gravel RA, Rosenblatt DS. Chapter 191. Disorders of propionate and methylmalonate metabolism. In: Valle D, Beaudet AL, Vogelstein B, Kinzler KW, Antonarakis SE, Ballabio A, eds. Scriver's Online Metabolic & Molecular Bases of Inherited Disease. McGraw-Hill, published January 2006; updated March 28, 2011. http://www.ommbid.com (Accessed February 2012).
6. Standing Committee on the Scientific Evaluation of Dietary Reference Intakes, Institute of Medicine Dietary Reference Intakes for Thiamin, Riboflavin, Niacin, Vitamin B6, Folate, Vitamin B12, Pantothenic Acid, Biotin, and Choline. Washington, DC: National Academy Press, 1999:245–54.
7. Jones PM, Rakheja D. Quick Guide to Organic Acid Interpretation. Washington, DC: AACC Press, 2011:147pp.
8. Surtees RA, Matthews EE, Leonard JV. Neurologic outcome of propionic acidemia. Pediatr Neurol 1992;8:333–7.
9. Manoli I, Venditti CP. Updated September 28, 2010. Methylmalonic acidemia. In: GeneReviews at Gene-Tests: Medical Genetics Information Resource (database online). Copyright, University of Washington, Seattle, 1997-2011. http://www.genetests.org (Accessed February 2012).
10. Nicolaides P, Leonard J, Surtees R. Neurological outcome of methylmalonic acidemia. Arch Dis Child 1998;78:508–12.
11. Wolf B. Chapter 156. Disorders of biotin metabolism. In: Valle D, Beaudet AL, Vogelstein B, Kinzler KW, Antonarakis SE, Ballabio A, eds. Scriver's Online Metabolic & Molecular Bases of Inherited Disease. New York: McGraw-Hill, published January 2006; updated March 28, 2011. http://www.ommbid.com (Accessed February 2012).

12. Roth KS, Rang W, Foremann JW, Rothman R, Segal S. Holocarboxylase synthetase deficiency: a biotin-responsive organic acidemia. J Pediatr 1980;96:845–9.
13. Wolf B. Updated March 15, 2011. Biotinidase deficiency. In: GeneReviews at GeneTests: Medical Genetics Information Resource (database online). Copyright, University of Washington, Seattle, 1997-2011. http://www.genetests.org (Accessed February 2012).
14. Heard GS, Secor McVoy JR, Wolf B. A screening method for biotinidase deficiency in newborns. Clin Chem 1984;30:125–7.
15. Pettit DA, Amador PS, Wolf B. The quantitation of biotinidase activity in dried blood spots using microtiter transfer plates identification of biotinidase-deficient and heterozygous individuals. Anal Biochem 1989;179:371–4.
16. Millington DS, Kodo N, Norwood DL, Roe CR. Tandem mass spectrometry: a new method for acylcarnitine profiling with potential for neonatal screening for inborn errors of metabolism. J Inherit Metab Dis 1990;13:321–4.
17. Sweetman L, Williams JC. Chapter 93. Branched chain organic acidurias. In: Valle D, Beaudet AL, Vogelstein B, Kinzler KW, Antonarakis SE, Ballabio A, eds. Scriver's Online Metabolic & Molecular Bases of Inherited Disease. New York: McGraw-Hill, published January 2006; updated March 28, 2011. http://www.ommbid.com (Accessed February 2012).
18. Fischer AQ, Challa VR, Burton BK, McLean WT. Cerebellar hemorrhage complicating isovaleric academia: a case report. Neurology 1981;31:746–8.
19. Mendiola J, Robotham JL, Liehr JG, Williams JC. Neonatal lethargy due to isovaleric acidemia and hyperammonemia. Texas Med 1984;80:52–4.
20. Wilson WG, Audenaert SM, Squillaro EJ. Hyperammonemia in a preterm infant with isovaleric acidemia. J Inherit Metab Dis 1984;7:71.
21. Kelleher JF, Yudkoff M, Hutchison R, August CS, Cohn RM. The pancytopenia of isovaleric acidemia. Pediatrics 1980;65:1023–7.
22. Cohn RM, Yudkoff M, Rothman R, Segal S. Isovaleric academia: use of glycine therapy in neonates. N Engl J Med 1978;299:996–9.
23. Gerdes AM, Gregersen N, Lúdvigsson P, Güttler F. A Scandinavian case of isovaleric acidemia. J Inherit Metab Dis 1988;11:218–20.
24. Goodman SI, Frerman FE. Chapter 95. Organic acidemias due to defects in lysine oxidation: 2-ketoadipic acidemia and glutaric acidemia. In: Valle D, Beaudet AL, Vogelstein B, Kinzler KW, Antonarakis SE, Ballabio A, eds. Scriver's Online Metabolic & Molecular Bases of Inherited Disease. New York: McGraw-Hill, published January 2006; updated March 28, 2011. http://www.ommbid.com (Accessed February 2012).
25. Greenberg CR, Reimer D, Singal R, Triggs-Raine B, Chudley AE, Dilling LA, et al. A G-to-T transversion at the +5 position of intron 1 in the glutaryl-CoA dehydrogenase gene is associated with the Island Lake variant of glutaric acidemia type 1. Hum Mol Genet 1995;4:493–5.
26. Biery BJ, Stein DE, Morton DH, Goodman SI. Gene structure and mutations of glutaryl-coenzyme A dehydrogenase: impaired association of enzyme subunits due to an A421V substitution causes glutaric acidemia (type I) in the Amish. Am J Human Genet 1996;59:1006–11.
27. Besrat A, Polan CE, Henderson LM. Mammalian metabolism of glutaric acid. J Biol Chem 1969;244:1461–7.
28. Hoffmann GF, Athanassopoulos S, Burlina AB, Duran M, de Klerk JB, Lehnert W, et al. Clinical course, early diagnosis, treatment, and prevention of disease in glutaryl-CoA dehydrogenase deficiency. Neuropediatrics 1996;27:115–23.
29. Tsai MY, Johnson DD, Sweetman L, Berry SA. Two siblings with biotin-resistant 3-methylcrotonyl-coenzyme A carboxylase deficiency. J Pediatr 1989;115:110–3.
30. Fukao T. Beta-ketothiolase deficiency. Orphanet encyclopedia, September 2001:1–11. http://www.orpha.net/data/patho/GB/uk-T2.pdf (Accessed January 2012).
31. Gunay-Aygun M. 3-Methylglutaconic aciduria: a common biochemical marker in various syndromes with diverse clinical features. Mol Genet Metab 2005;84:1–3.
32. OMIM®, Online Mendelian Inheritance in Man®. Baltimore, MD: McKusick-Nathans Institute of Genetic Medicine, Johns Hopkins University, Updated February 13, 2012. http://omim.org/ (Accessed February 2012).
33. Barth PG, Valianpour F, Bowen VM, Jam J, Duran M, Vaz FM, Wanders RJ. X-linked cardioskeletal myopathy and neutropenia (Barth Syndrome): an update, Am J Med Genet A 2004;126A:349–54.
34. Gunay-Aygun M, Gahl W, Anikster Y. Updated March 31, 2009. 3-Methylglutaconic aciduria type 3. In: GeneReviews at GeneTests: Medical Genetics Information Resource (database online). Copyright, University of Washington, Seattle, 1997-2011. http://www.genetests.org (Accessed February 2012).

35. Matern D, He M, Berry SA, Rinaldo P, Whitley CB, Madsen PP, et al. Prospective diagnosis of 2-methylbutyryl-CoA dehydrogenase deficiency in the Hmong population by newborn screening using tandem mass spectrometry. Pediatrics 2003;112:74–8.

36. Shih V. Updated June 2, 2009. Fumarate hydratase deficiency. In: GeneReviews at GeneTests: Medical Genetics Information Resource (database online). Copyright, University of Washington, Seattle, 1997-2011. http://www.genetests.org (Accessed February 2012).

37. Salomons GS, Jakobs C, Pope LL, Errami A, Potter M, Nowaczyk M, et al. Clinical, enzymatic and molecular characterization of nine new patients with malonyl-coenzyme A decarboxylase deficiency. J Inherit Metab Dis 2007;30:23–8.

38. Zammit VA. The malonyl-CoA-long-chain acyl-CoA axis in the maintenance of mammalian cell function. Biochem J 1999;343(Pt 3):505–15.

39. Footitt EJ, Stafford J, Dixon M, Burch M, Jakobs C, Salomons GS, Cleary MA. Use of a long-chain triglyceride-restricted/medium-chain triglyceride-supplemented diet in a case of malonyl-CoA decarboxylase deficiency with cardiomyopathy. J Inherit Metab Dis 2010 Jun 15. [Epub ahead of print] doi 10.1007/s10545-010-9137-z.

40. Matalon R, Michals-Matalon K. Updated August 11, 2011. Canavan disease. In: GeneReviews at GeneTests: Medical Genetics Information Resource (database online). Copyright, University of Washington, Seattle, 1997-2011. http://www.genetests.org (Accessed February 2012).

41. van Hove JL, Rutledge SL, Nada MA, Kahler SG, Millington DS. 3-Hydroxyisovalerylcarnitine in 3-methylcrotonyl-CoA carboxylase deficiency. J Inherit Metab Dis 1995;18:592–601.

42. Rolland MO, Divry P, Zabot MT, Guibaud P, Gomez S, Lachaux A, et al. Isolated 3-methylcrotonyl-CoA carboxylase deficiency in a 16-month-old child. J Inherit Metab Dis 1991;14:838–9.

Chapter 4

The Urea Cycle Disorders and Hyperammonemias

Laurie D. Smith and Uttam Garg

The urea cycle disorders comprise several conditions that present with hyperammonemia, all related to enzymatic dysfunction or deficiency of transport molecules involved in the ability of the cell to detoxify ammonia generated by protein metabolism. Six of these disorders directly affect function of the urea cycle (carbamoyl phosphate synthetase deficiency, ornithine transcarbamoylase deficiency, argininosuccinate synthetase deficiency, argininosuccinate lyase deficiency, arginase deficiency, and *N*-acetylglutamate synthetase deficiency) whereas three affect transport of urea cycle intermediates (lysinuric protein intolerance [LPI], hyperammonemia-hyperornithinemia-homocitrullinuria [HHH] syndrome, and citrin deficiency). The urea cycle occurs in two different intracellular compartments—the cytosol and the mitochondrion—and is fully functional only in the liver. The overall function of the urea cycle is as the final common pathway for excretion of waste nitrogen by converting ammonia, which is toxic to the cell, to urea, which is relatively nontoxic and excreted in the urine *(1)*. The urea cycle is shown in Figure 4-1. Although other inherited conditions such as certain fatty acid oxidation defects and organic acidurias can lead to hyperammonemia, unless caused by a defect in the urea cycle, this is caused by secondary inhibition of the cycle.

CLINICAL PRESENTATION

Although historically considered a condition that presents with overwhelming illness in the neonatal period, there is actually considerable variation in the presentation of the disorders with onset of symptoms ranging from the neonatal period to late in life *(2, 3)*. However, these disorders are more likely to present at times associated with metabolic stress, including illness that results in protein catabolism, the neonatal period, late infancy, puberty, and postpartum. The patterns of clinical presentation are quite similar and characteristic given that most are related to the presence of hyperammonemia, although arginase deficiency, lysinuric protein intolerance, HHH syndrome, and citrin deficiency have other presenting signs and symptoms in addition to hyperammonemia.

The intrinsic, inherited disorders of the urea cycle include carbamoyl phosphate synthetase (CPS) deficiency, ornithine transcarbamoylase (OTC) deficiency, argininosuccinate synthetase deficiency (citrullinemia), argininosuccinate lyase deficiency (argininosuccinic aciduria), arginase deficiency, and *N*-acetylglutamate synthetase (NAGS) deficiency. These can present neonatally, in infancy, or in older patients.

The neonatal presentation is typically one of an initially healthy neonate with a normal birth weight who becomes ill after a very short time interval, sometimes <24 h. Because neonates have a relatively limited repertoire of responses to catabolic stress (poor feeding, vomiting, tachypnea, or lethargy/irritability), they often are initially diagnosed with sepsis. There is often a transient mild metabolic alkalosis. Neonates rapidly deteriorate with the appearance of neurologic and autonomic symptoms, including hypotonia with loss of reflexes, hypo- or hyperthermia, apnea, and somnolence. Without rapid intervention, seizures, coma, peripheral circulatory failure, cerebral edema, liver failure, and multisystem organ failure can ensue. Cerebral and pulmonary hemorrhage can also ensue, complicating the recognition of an underlying metabolic cause. Even with intensive interventions, the outcome may be poor.

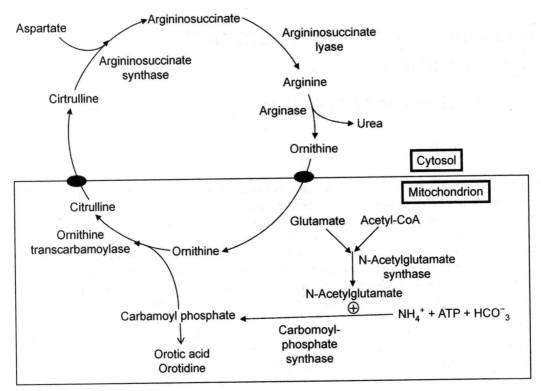

Figure 4-1   Urea cycle.

Presentation in infancy is usually more variable and less acute, with anorexia, cyclic vomiting, lethargy, and failure to thrive associated with poor developmental progress. There is often nonspecific liver enlargement. Behavioral problems or irritability may also be present. A urea cycle disorder can sometimes be confused with severe gastroesophageal reflux or cow's milk protein intolerance. The diagnosis is often not considered until there is an acute encephalitic event.

Children and adults usually present with a more chronic picture, although an acute encephalopathic event may be the initially recognized symptom. A careful history may reveal protein aversion and self-selection of a vegetarian, low-protein diet. Again, symptoms usually develop after metabolic stress such as infection, anesthesia, or protein catabolism as can be seen postpartum (4), although a specific trigger may not always be identified. More chronic symptoms associated with these disorders include protein aversion (self-selected vegetarian diet), headaches and migraines, abnormal movements (tremor, asterixis), dysarthria, lethargy, dizziness, and lethargy. Symptoms may also include a history of hyperactive, aggressive, or self-injurious behavior as well as psychiatric symptoms. Stroke-like episodes and seizures have also been described. Abdominal pain and vomiting along with failure to thrive may also be associated symptoms. Elevated liver function tests may be noted in routine laboratory testing.

Arginase deficiency, lysinuric protein intolerance, HHH syndrome, and citrin deficiency differ somewhat in their presentation, although all lead to dysfunction of the urea cycle and subsequent hyperammonemia (1).

Arginase deficiency typically presents with episodic hyperammonemia that is not of rapid onset. Affected individuals may be identified because of slowing of linear growth during childhood. Plateauing of cognitive abilities with subsequent loss of developmental milestones is seen, resulting in severe intellectual disability. Severe spasticity ensues and may be accompanied by tremor, ataxia, and choreoathetosis with eventual loss of ambulation and bowel and bladder control.

Lysinuric protein intolerance usually presents after weaning of an affected infant from breast milk to infant formulas. Initial clinical findings may include recurrent episodes of vomiting and diarrhea, stupor, and coma after a protein-rich meal; poor feeding; aversion to protein-rich foods; failure to thrive; hepatosplenomegaly; and hypotonia. With time, other complications may become apparent, such as poor growth, osteoporosis, progressive interstitial lung parenchymal changes, pulmonary alveolar proteinosis, progressive glomerular or proximal renal tubular disease, and bone marrow involvement (anemia, leucopenia, thrombocytopenia, erythroblastophagocytosis). Liver and pancreatic involvement can also be seen. Plasma ammonia concentrations tend to be normal in the fasting state, rising after a protein-rich meal. Urinary excretion of orotic acid may also be seen, along with increased urinary excretion of the cationic amino acids lysine, arginine, and ornithine. It is interesting to note that plasma concentrations of thyroxine-binding globulin, lactate dehydrogenase, and ferritin are elevated in this disorder. Nonspecific hematologic findings include normo- or hypochromic anemia, leucopenia, and thrombocytopenia.

HHH syndrome also presents similarly to the intrinsic urea cycle disorders with hyperammonemia *(5, 6)*. Hyperammonemia is intermittent and associated with vomiting, lethargy, and coma. Somewhat different from the intrinsic disorders, growth and intellectual development are universally affected, with spasticity and seizures being common. Adults with partial activity may self-select low-protein diets.

Citrin deficiency, also known as citrullinemia type II, actually has two phenotypic presentations *(7)*. The first is characterized by adult-onset recurrent episodes of hyperammonemia, usually sometime during the second to fifth decades. Neuropsychiatric symptoms are common (delirium, aggression, irritability, disorientation, memory loss, seizures, flapping tremor). The second is seen in children <12 months of age and presents as transient intrahepatic cholestasis, diffuse fatty liver, and hepatic fibrosis. Other findings may include low birth weight, growth retardation, hemolytic anemia, hepatomegaly, hypoproteinemia, decreased coagulation factors, and hypoglycemia. This usually resolves by 1 year of age, with development, around the age of 2 years, of aversion to sugar-rich and carbohydrate rich foods. These individuals may then develop the more typical neuropsychiatric symptoms at a later age.

GENETICS AND PATHOGENESIS

All of the urea cycle disorders and related transport disorders are inherited in an autosomal-recessive fashion except for OTC deficiency, which is inherited in an X-linked fashion. Manifesting female carriers of OTC are not uncommon.

Carbamoylphosphate synthetase I (CPSI) deficiency is the most severe of the urea cycle disorders and is caused by mutations in the *CPS1* gene located at chromosome 2q35. CPSI is the first enzyme of the urea cycle and results in the condensation of bicarbonate (HCO_3^-) with ammonium (NH_4^+) to form carbamyl phosphate. It requires *N*-acetylglutamate as a cofactor for the reaction to occur. The enzyme is active in the mitochondria of the liver. Inability to form carbamoyl phosphate results in inactivity of the urea cycle because it is required to condense with ornithine to form citrulline. Those with complete absence of enzymatic function rapidly develop severe hyperammonemia in the newborn period.

OTC deficiency results from mutations in the *OTC* gene located at Xp21.1. The enzyme is also known as OTC. Absence of this enzyme results in urea cycle dysfunction because carbamoyl phosphate cannot condense with ornithine to form citrulline. This reaction also occurs within the mitochondria. Affected males present quite similarly to individuals with CPSI deficiency. As an X-linked disorder, approximately 15% of carrier females develop hyperammonemia in their lifetime, requiring medical interventions.

Citrullinemia type I results from deficiency of the cytoplasmic enzyme argininosuccinate synthase (ASS). This enzyme, encoded by the *ASS1* gene on 9q34, is necessary for the condensation of aspartic acid with citrulline to form argininosuccinic acid. Deficiency of this enzyme also disrupts function of the urea cycle, although waste nitrogen may be incorporated into other urea cycle intermediates.

Argininosuccinicaciduria results from a deficiency of argininosuccinate lyase (ASL) activity. The *ASL* gene is located at 7cen-q11.2. The enzyme deficiency occurs after all points in the urea cycle at which waste nitrogen has been incorporated into urea cycle intermediates; thus, rapid-onset hyperammonemia is usually seen in the newborn period.

Arginase deficiency is caused by mutations in the *ARG1* gene, which is located on 6q23. Rapid-onset hyperammonemia is not the rule for this disorder. High concentrations of arginine in the central nervous system have been implicated in encephalopathic processes that likely contribute to the pathogenesis of the disorder.

NAGS deficiency is caused by defects in the *NAGS* gene, which localizes to chromosome 17q21.3. Symptoms are very similar to CPS1 deficiency because CPS1 requires *N*-acetyl glutamate for its activity.

LPI is caused by mutations in the *SLC7A7* gene. The product of this gene, which is located at 14q11.2, is a cationic (dibasic) amino acid transporter (Y+L amino acid transporter 1). Deficiency of this transporter results in a functional deficiency of the urea cycle secondary to depletion of arginine and ornithine. Deficiency of lysine probably contributes to the poor growth, skeletal manifestations, and immune dysfunction associated with this disorder.

HHH syndrome, which is more commonly seen in individuals of French-Canadian background, results from a deficiency of ornithine translocase activity. The gene *ORNT1* (also known as *SLC25A15*) is localized to 13q14 and has been identified as an inner mitochondrial membrane ornithine transporter. Defects in this transporter lead to the severely compromised transport of ornithine, one of the urea cycle intermediates, into the mitochondrial compartment, resulting in elevated cytoplasmic and decreased mitochondrial ornithine concentrations. Ornithine is thus unavailable for condensation with carbamoyl phosphate to generate citrulline.

Citrullinemia type II (CTLN2) results from a deficiency of the aspartate glutamate carrier, citrin. This protein is encoded by the *SLC25A13* gene, localized to chromosome 7q21.3. Although described in other populations, mutations have been most commonly identified in those of Japanese descent. Citrin is a member of the malate aspartate shuttle and is important for the synthesis of urea from ammonia. It is postulated that citrin deficiency results in limitation of transport of mitochondrial aspartate into the cytosol and thus interferes with the generation of argininosuccinate by argininosuccinate synthase in the cytosolic compartment. This results in elevated citrulline, the precursor to argininosuccinic aciduria *(6)*.

LABORATORY DIAGNOSIS

Algorithms for the diagnosis of urea cycle disorders have been described *(1, 8, 9)*. It must be emphasized that routine tests are generally not helpful in establishing a diagnosis in conditions that present with hyperammonemia. Electrolytes, glucose, renal function tests, hepatic function tests, blood pH, and basic hematologic and coagulation tests may be helpful in the management of the acutely ill patient.

The most important factor in establishing the diagnosis of hyperammonemia is to consider the diagnosis. The most important diagnostic test is the measurement of plasma ammonia concentrations. Acutely ill patients with urea cycle disorders will usually have ammonia concentrations >150 μmol/L, and often these concentrations are significantly higher. Ammonia concentrations may normalize when patients are well or well managed on a low-protein, high-carbohydrate diet. Blood samples for ammonia testing should be collected from a stasis-free vein (no tourniquet) and placed immediately on ice. Plasma should be separated and analyzed within 30 min or stored frozen. Grossly icteric, hemolyzed, or lipemic samples should be rejected.

Plasma and urine amino acid profiles are important diagnostic tests for the diagnosis and confirmation of urea cycle defects. Fasting samples are required for proper interpretation of plasma amino acid profiles. Fasting is generally defined as 3 h in infants to 6 months of age; 3–6 h in infants 6–12 months of age; and 6–12 h in patients older than 12 months of age. Fasting is not necessary for urine amino acid profiles. Blood for plasma amino acid profiles is collected in a heparin or ethylenediaminetetraacetic acid (EDTA)-containing tube. Plasma should be separated from cells within 1–2 h and stored frozen. All urea cycle disorders present with elevations of alanine and glutamine. Plasma and/or urine amino acid profiles are usually diagnostic for citrullinemia, argininosuccinic aciduria, and arginase deficiency as well as lysinuric protein intolerance and HHH (Table 4-1). Representative amino acid profiles for several urea cycle defects are shown in Figures 4-2 to 4-5.

Urine organic acid profiles are helpful in differentiating urea cycle disorders from several of the organic acidemias such as propionic, methylmalonic, and isovaleric acidemias that may also present with hyperammonemia. Most, although not all, urea cycle defects have identifiable elevations of urine orotic acid. However, orotic acid is low or normal in CPS1 and NAGS deficiencies. Orotic acid can generally be identified on a urine organic acid profile. Sometimes it may be necessary to perform a separate assay to identify and quantify urinary orotic acid. In the past, quantification of orotic acid after a protein load or allopurinol administration was used to identify females who were heterozygous for X-linked OTC after a deficient patient was identified in the family. For the most part, these studies have been superseded by molecular analyses. Quantification of orotic acid can also be helpful in the evaluation of hereditary orotic aciduria. For orotic acid concentrations and urine organic acid profiles, 5–10 mL of urine should be collected, without preservatives, and stored frozen. A representative organic acid profile from a patient with OTC is shown in Figure 4-6.

Acylcarnitine profiles can be useful to differentiate hyperammonemia secondary to an organic acidemia from that caused by a urea cycle disorder. This testing should be considered during the initial workup of a patient presenting with hyperammonemia. For further discussion, please see Chapter 3 on organic acidemias/acidurias.

Other findings that may help to direct one toward a diagnosis include elevated lactic acid concentrations and lactic to pyruvic acid ratios and paradoxical postprandial elevation of glutamine in HHH; increased lactate dehydrogenase, ferritin, and thyroxine binding globulin in LPI; and increased theronine:serine ratios and increased pancreatic secretory trypsin inhibitor in citrin deficiency. Elevated liver transaminases are often seen but are a nonspecific finding as is hepatomegaly. Neonatal intrahepatic cholestasis, caused by citrin deficiency, may also present with the biochemical findings of elevated galactose, methionine, phenylalanine, threonine, tyrosine, total/direct bilirubin, total bile acids, and plasma α-fetoprotein. Most of these disorders are now confirmed by identification of pathologic mutations in the associated genes.

TREATMENT

A full discussion of the management of hyperammonemia is beyond the scope of this handbook (for review, see references 10 and 11). Management of acute hyperammonemia includes discontinuation of oral protein intake or amino acid infusions and provision of high-energy intake as 10–25% glucose orally, if tolerated, or intravenously at 8–10 mg/kg body weight/min with the addition of insulin if necessary. Intravenous L-arginine-HCl should be provided at 2 mmol/kg body weight as a loading dose over 90 min and then as a continuous infusion over 24 h. Practically speaking, this is equivalent to 2 mL/kg of a 10% solution that should be piggybacked into the intravenous glucose infusion. Nitrogen scavengers should be considered. Ammonul®, a commonly used nitrogen scavenger, is a combination of sodium benzoate and sodium phenylacetate. A loading dose of 250 mg/kg body weight of each in 25–35 mL/kg 10% dextrose solution should be given as a loading dose over 90 min followed by a continuous infusion over 24 h. Consideration should also be given to the use of carbamylglutamate at 200 mg/kg divided in three oral doses. The use of this compound may obviate the need for eventual hemodialysis in cases of NAGS and partial CPSI deficiency (12). If the initial ammonia is >500 μmol/L or if the ammonia does not fall within 2 h after starting the treatment, then hemodialysis should be considered.

Table 4-1 Laboratory Changes in Various Hyperammonemia Disorders

Disorder	NH$_4$	Arginine (P)	Ornithine (P)	Citrulline (P/U)	Alanine (P)	Glutamine (P)	Arginiosuccinic (U)	Orotic acid (U)	Homocitrulline (U)	Dibasic amino acids (U)	BUN
CPS1	↑-↑↑	↓-N		↓-N	↑	↑		↓-N			↓
OTC	N-↑↑	→		↓-N	↑	↑		↑-↑↑			↓
Citrullinemia I	↑↑	↓↓		↑↑↑	↑	↑		↑-↑↑			↓
Citrin deficiency (CTLN2)	↑	N-↑		↑		↑	↑				
Argininosuccinic aciduria	↑-↑↑	↓		↑	↑	↑	↑↑↑	N-↑↑			↓
Arginase deficiency	N-↑↑	↑↑↑		↑	↑	↑	↑	↑-↑↑		↑	↓
NAGS deficiency	↑-↑↑	↓		↓-N	↑	↑		↓-N		↑	↓
LPI	↑-↑↑	↓	↓	↑	↑	↑		↑-↑↑		↑↑	
HHH	↑-↑↑	Normal	↑	Normal	↑	↑		↑	↑↑		

LPI: decreased plasma lysine, arginine, and ornithine levels; increased plasma glutamine, alanine, serine, proline, citrulline, and glycine; increased urine orotic acid; serum lactate dehydrogenase activity increased; and increased serum ferritin and thyroxin-binding globulin.

Citrin deficiency: increased threonine:serine ratio, increased pancreatic secretory trypsin inhibitor, secondary deficiency of ASS, neonatal intrahepatic cholestasis, increased galactose, methionine, phenylalanine, threonine, tyrosine, total/direct bilirubin, total bile acids, and plasma α-fetoprotein.

HHH: increased lactic acid, increased lactate:pyruvate ratio, postprandial hyperammonemia, and glutamine may paradoxically elevated with protein restriction.

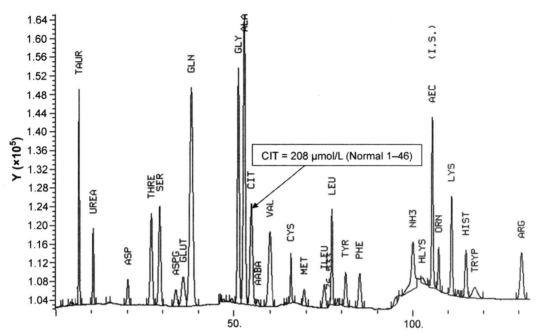

Figure 4-2 Plasma amino acid profile from a patient with citrullinemia. Glutamine and citrulline are elevated. The sample preparation involved addition of internal standard S-(2-aminoethyl)-L-cysteine to the sample and precipitation of proteins using sulfosalicylic acid. The analysis of supernatant involved a Biochrom 30 amino acid analyzer, an ion-exchange column, lithium-citrate-buffered mobile phases, and postcolumn ninhydrin derivatization.

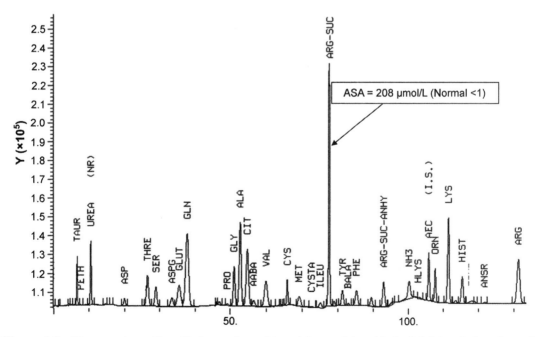

Figure 4-3 Plasma amino acid profile in a patient with argininosuccinic aciduria. Brief description of sample preparation and analysis is given in Figure 4-2.

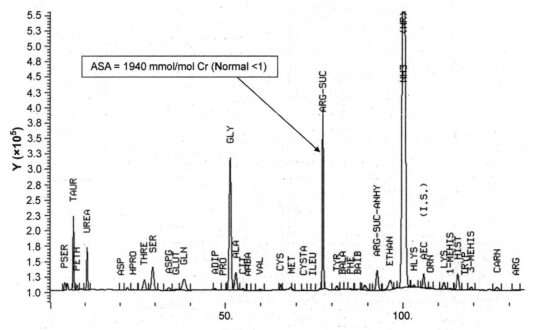

Figure 4-4   Urine amino acid profile in a patient with argininosuccinic aciduria. In addition to an argininosuccinic acid peak, an argininosuccinic anhydride peak is also seen. A brief description of sample preparation and analysis is given in Figure 4-2.

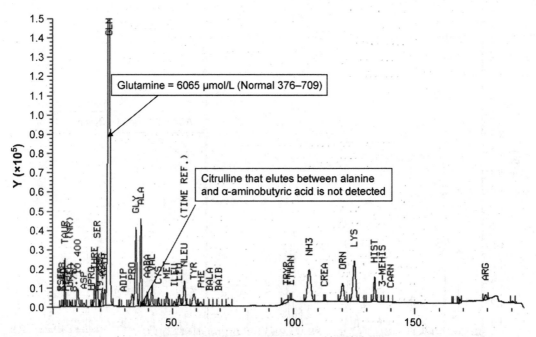

Figure 4-5   Plasma amino acid profile in a patient with OTC deficiency. Glutamine is highly elevated and citrulline is undetectable. The sample preparation involved addition of the internal standard norleucine to the sample and precipitation of proteins using sulfosalicylic acid. The analysis of supernatant involved a Dionex amino acid analyzer, an ion-exchange column, lithium-citrate-buffered mobile phases, and postcolumn ninhydrin derivatization.

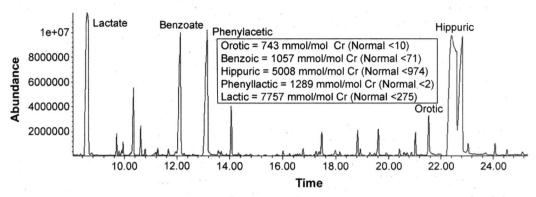

Figure 4-6 Urine organic acids profile from a patient with OTC deficiency. Very high hippuric and benzoic acids are due to benzoate therapy. The sample preparation involved addition of tropic and α-ketocaproic acids as internal standards, use of hydroxylamine to form the oxime derivatives of the ketoacids, acidification of samples, extraction of organic acids with ethylacetate, and formation of trimethylsilyl (TMS) derivatives of organic acids using *N,O*-bis(trimethylsilyl)trifluoroacetamide (BTSFA) with trimethylchlorosilane (TMCS) and pyridine. The analysis was performed using gas chromatography/mass spectrometry.

Long-term management revolves around provision of a low-protein diet with supplementation of essential amino acids as a medical beverage along with minerals, vitamins, and trace elements. Pharmacologic management includes the use of ammonia scavengers such as sodium benzoate and/or sodium phenylbutyrate *(1, 13)*. Currently, only the latter compound is approved by the U.S. Food and Drug Administration (FDA) for the treatment of hyperammonemia. Arginine should also be given, except in the case of arginase deficiency and LPI. Because the latter disorder results in cellular inability to absorb or reabsorb (as in the kidney tubules) cationic anions, arginine supplementation is ineffective. This can be circumvented by provision of citrulline (0.1–0.5 g/kg before or during three to five meals) along with protein restriction. Management of citrin deficiency revolves around a lipid and protein-rich, low-carbohydrate diet. Liver transplantation is considered an option for treatment of severe CPS or OTC deficiency, for citrin deficiency, for patients with argininosuccinic aciduria who develop liver cirrhosis, and for patients who have recurrent symptomatic hyperammonemic episodes even with optimal medical interventions and management. Recent studies have demonstrated that the 5-year posttransplant survival rate for patients with urea cycle disorders is approximately 80% *(14)*. Arginine deficiency is not corrected with transplantation, despite correction of hyperammonemia. Thus, arginine supplementation remains necessary. Gene therapy, although widely discussed as a possible future treatment, is not yet a reality.

PROGNOSIS

The overall prognosis for the urea cycle disorders depends on the age of the patient, the condition at the time of diagnosis, and the amount of residual enzyme activity. Those who present in the newborn period with symptomatic hyperammonemia have a poorer prognosis; those who survive have some degree of handicap. Even for those who are treated prospectively, there may be significant complications with the risk of metabolic decompensation and recurrent hyperammonemic episodes. The prognosis for LPI is more guarded, especially because of marked osteoporosis, pancytopenia, and disturbed immune function. Varicella infection can be fatal. Interstitial pulmonary disease with alveolar proteinosis and renal insufficiency are rare, but recognized, complications *(15)*. The prognosis for HHH also varies among individuals, depending on the age of presentation. Growth delay, along with learning disabilities, especially speech, developmental delays, ataxia, and intermittent confusion are part of the disorder and may have a more favorable outcome with early detection and treatment *(6)*. The prognosis for citrin deficiency is much more guarded. Yasuda et al. *(16)* found that in adult-onset patients, almost all had serious and recurring symptoms with disorientation, drowsiness progressing to coma, and death ensuing within a few years of symptom onset secondary to cerebral edema. In the neonatal form of the disorder, intrahepatic cholestasis usually resolves between 5 and 7 months of age *(17)*; however, gradual progression to CTLN2 is observed over the next 10–20 years.

ACKNOWLEDGMENT

The authors are thankful to David Scott for his assistance with the preparation of the figures in this chapter.

REFERENCES

1. Leonard JV. Disorders of the urea cycle and related enzymes. In: Fernandez J, Saudubray JM, van den Berghe G, Walter JH, eds. Inborn Metabolic Diseases: Diagnosis and Treatment, 4th ed. Heidelberg, Germany: Springer Medizin Verlag, 2006:265–72.
2. Braissant O. Current concepts in the pathogenesis of urea cycle disorders. Mol Genet Metab 2010;100 Suppl 1:S3–12.
3. Nassogne MC, Heron B, Touati G, Rabier D, Saudubray JM. Urea cycle defects: management and outcome. J Inherit Metab Dis 2005;28:407–14.
4. Arn PH, Hauser ER, Thomas GH, Herman G, Hess D, Brusilow SW. Hyperammonemia in women with a mutation at the ornithine carbamoyltransferase locus. A cause of postpartum coma. N Engl J Med 1990;322: 1652–5.
5. Shih VE, Baumgartner MR. Disorders of ornithine metabolism. In: Fernandez J, Saudubray JM, van den Berghe G, Walter JH, eds. Inborn Metabolic Diseases: Diagnosis and Treatment, 4th ed. Heidelberg, Germany: Springer Medizin Verlag, 2006:288.
6. Debray FG, Lambert M, Lemieux B, Soucy JF, Drouin R, Fenyves D, et al. Phenotypic variability among patients with hyperornithinaemia-hyperammonaemia-homocitrullinuria syndrome homozygous for the delF188 mutation in SLC25A15. J Med Genet 2008;45:759–64.
7. Saheki T, Kobayashi K, Iijima M, Nishi I, Yasuda T, Yamaguchi N, et al. Pathogenesis and pathophysiology of citrin (a mitochondrial aspartate glutamate carrier) deficiency. Metab Brain Dis 2002;17:335–46.
8. Steiner RD, Cederbaum SD. Laboratory evaluation of urea cycle disorders. J Pediatr 2001;138:S21–9.
9. Bowker R, Green A, Bonham JR. Guidelines for the investigation and management of a reduced level of consciousness in children: implications for clinical biochemistry laboratories. Ann Clin Biochem 2007;44:506–11.
10. Urea Cycle Disorders Conference group. Consensus statement from a conference for the management of patients with urea cycle disorders. J Pediatr 2001;138:S1–5.
11. Haberle J. Clinical practice: the management of hyperammonemia. Eur J Pediatr 2011;170:21–34.
12. Daniotti M, la Marca G, Fiorini P, Filippi L. New developments in the treatment of hyperammonemia: emerging use of carglumic acid. Int J Gen Med 2011;4:21–8.
13. Batshaw ML, MacArthur RB, Tuchman M. Alternative pathway therapy for urea cycle disorders: twenty years later. J Pediatr 2001;138:S46–54; discussion S54–5.
14. Lee B, Goss J. Long-term correction of urea cycle disorders. J Pediatr 2001;138:S62–71.
15. Sebastio G, Sperandeo MP, Andria G. Lysinuric protein intolerance: reviewing concepts on a multisystem disease. Am J Med Genet C Semin Med Genet 2011;157:54–62.
16. Yasuda T, Yamaguchi N, Kobayashi K, Nishi I, Horinouchi H, Jalil MA, et al. Identification of two novel mutations in the SLC25A13 gene and detection of seven mutations in 102 patients with adult-onset type II citrullinemia. Hum Genet 2000;107:537–45.
17. Tamamori A, Okano Y, Ozaki H, Fujimoto A, Kajiwara M, Fukuda K, et al. Neonatal intrahepatic cholestasis caused by citrin deficiency: severe hepatic dysfunction in an infant requiring liver transplantation. Eur J Pediatr 2002;161:609–13.

Chapter 5

Disorders of the Carnitine Cycle and Mitochondrial Fatty Acid Oxidation

Patricia M. Jones and Michael J. Bennett

Mitochondrial fatty acid oxidation (FAO) is one of the metabolic pathways that provides caloric support during periods of increased energy demand such as prolonged fasting or muscular exertion when glycogen reserves are depleted. The pathway can be divided into four components: (1) carnitine transport and the carnitine cycle; (2) oxidation of long-chain fatty acids at the inner mitochondrial membrane; (3) oxidation of medium- and short-chain fatty acids in the mitochondrial matrix; and (4) ketogenesis or utilization of the end product, acetyl-CoA, in the tricarboxylic acid (TCA) cycle (Figure 5-1). The pathway shows a degree of tissue specificity because ketogenesis can only take place in the liver. High-energy-requiring tissues such as cardiac and skeletal muscle directly oxidize the acetyl-CoA whereas liver generates and circulates ketone bodies as an energy source for tissues such as brain that cannot generate energy through this pathway *(1)*.

Genetic defects of the pathway lead to a failure to generate this essential energy, and the signs and symptoms reflect intolerance to high energy demands. In liver, the fatty acids that are channeled for eventual ketone body formation accumulate and produce steatosis, which may lead to liver failure with the biochemical hallmark of hypoglycemia and inappropriately low ketone body formation (hypoketotic hypoglycemia), elevated plasma liver enzymes, and hyperammonemia. In skeletal muscle, there may be initial muscle weakness, which may lead to frank rhabdomyolysis and elevated creatine kinase (CK) concentrations when stressed. The release of myoglobin during rhabdomyolysis may precipitate acute renal failure. Disorders in the pathway may also represent a significant cause of adult-onset rhabdomyolysis in individuals not showing hepatic or cardiac symptoms. Cardiac signs associated with disorders include progressive dilated cardiomyopathy. For some disorders, there is also an associated renal tubular acidosis that may not always be recognized with the severe systemic complications *(2)*.

1. *Carnitine transport and the carnitine cycle:* Carnitine is an essential component for transporting long-chain fatty acids into the mitochondria. Carnitine is mostly derived from the diet, but a de novo biosynthetic pathway also exists for which genetic defects have not been described. The concentration of carnitine inside of cells is 50 times greater than the concentration in plasma, a gradient that is maintained by the plasma membrane carnitine transporter. Muscle and renal tubules have a high-affinity carnitine transport system maintained by the OCTN2 carnitine transporter. Long-chain fatty acids, predominantly of chain lengths C16–C18, are transported into the cell via fatty acid transporter systems and activated to the corresponding acyl-CoAs by acyl-CoA synthetases at the outer mitochondrial membrane. Acyl-CoA species cannot cross the inner mitochondrial membrane. Carnitine palmitoyltransferase 1 (CPT1) converts the acyl-CoAs to acylcarnitines, which can be delivered to the mitochondrial matrix by the action of carnitine:acylcarnitine translocase (CACT). Once inside of the mitochondria, carnitine palmitoyltransferase 2 converts the acylcarnitines back into acyl-CoAs for the purpose of oxidation. CACT is bidirectional and free carnitine is delivered back to the cytosol for further reactions.

2. *Long-chain FAO at the inner mitochondrial membrane:* Long-chain acyl-CoA species enter the fatty acid β-oxidation cycle first through the action of the membrane-associated very-long-chain acyl-CoA dehydrogenase (VLCAD), which introduces a double bond in the 2,3 position to form

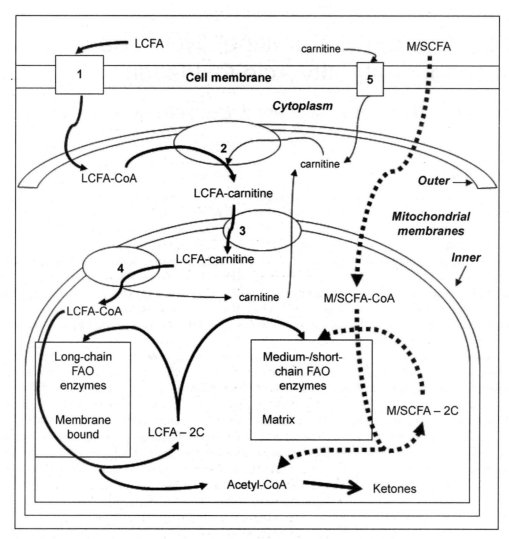

Figure 5-1 Diagram of mitochondrial fatty acid β-oxidation (FAO). Long-chain fatty acids (LFCA) are shown with the four steps necessary to transport them into the mitochondria: 1 = long-chain fatty acid transporter, 2 = carnitine palmitoyl transferase I (CPT-I), 3 = carnitine:acylcarnitine translocase (CACT), 4 = carnitine palmitoyl transferase II (CPT II). 5 = carnitine transporter is also depicted. The medium- and short-chain fatty acids (M/SCFA) can cross directly into the mitochondria. The long-chain and medium/short-chain FAO enzymes include acyl-CoA dehydrogenase, 2,3-enoyl-CoA hydratase, 3-hydroxyacyl-CoA dehydrogenase, and 3-keto-thiolase. The long-chain forms of these enzymes are bound to the inner mitochondrial membrane and the medium-/short-chain forms are found in the matrix. The β-oxidation by these enzymes results in a product that is two carbons shorter (LCFA – 2C and M/SCFA – 2C), which recycles back through the pathway, plus acetyl-CoA.

an enoyl-CoA. The electrons generated from this reduction are transferred to the respiratory chain at the level of coenzyme Q via the actions of electron transfer flavoprotein (ETF) and electron transfer flavoprotein dehydrogenase (ETFDH). The enoyl-CoA is hydrated by a long-chain enoyl-CoA hydratase (LHYD) to form a 3-hydroxyacyl-CoA species, which in turn is reduced to form a 3-ketoacyl-CoA by the action of long-chain 3-hydroxyacyl-CoA dehydrogenase (LCHAD), and finally this is thiolytically cleaved by a long-chain 3-ketoacyl-CoA thiolase (LKAT) to form acetyl-CoA and a two-carbon shortened acyl-CoA, which re-enters the cycle. The latter three enzymes are part of a multienzyme complex known as the mitochondrial trifunctional protein (mTFP).

3. *Medium and short-chain FAO in the mitochondrial matrix:* At around carbon chain length C10 there is transfer of substrate from the membrane to the matrix and complete oxidation of the now medium-chain species by a family of related enzymes with different chain-length specificities. These include medium-chain acyl-CoA dehydrogenase (MCAD), an as yet unclassified hydratase, medium- and short-chain 3-hydroxyacyl-CoA dehydrogenase (M/SCHAD), short-chain acyl-CoA dehydrogenase (SCAD), and short-chain 3-keto-acyl-CoA thiolase (SKAT, also known as β-ketothiolase).

4. *Ketogenesis:* Hepatic ketone body formation from the acetyl-CoA derived by FAO requires the presence of two additional enzymes: 3-hydroxy-3-methylglutaryl-CoA synthase (HMG-CoA synthase), which forms 3-hydroxy-3-methylglutaryl-CoA from acetoacetyl-CoA and acetyl-CoA, and 3-hydroxy-3-methylglutaryl-CoA lyase (HMG-CoA lyase), which converts HMG-CoA to acetoacetate and acetyl-CoA. Acetoacetate is converted to the other two ketone bodies, predominately to 3-hydroxybutyric acid via β-hydroxybutyrate dehydrogenase, with some spontaneous formation of acetone.

Genetic defects have been identified for most of the enzymes and transport proteins described above, which will now be defined individually *(3, 4)*. Many of the defects can now be identified presymptomatically by the use of newborn screening *(5)* and frequently the outcomes are much better than those when patients were only identified as a result of symptomatic presentation. As a result, clinicians are not always exposed to the worst-case scenario of profound metabolic decompensation. For the purpose of this chapter, we will define that worst-case situation as well as milder presentations to ensure that the reader is aware of the potential severity of disorders in the pathway. Table 5-1 summarizes the disorders that will be discussed in this chapter and the tests commonly used in their diagnosis.

CARNITINE TRANSPORTER (CARNITINE UPTAKE) DEFECT

The carnitine transporter defect differs from other disorders of FAO in that it defines a defect that results in secondary abnormalities in FAO. The primary defect results in massive renal loss of carnitine due to reabsorption failure, reduced tissue carnitine content, and insufficient carnitine to support FAO *(6)*.

Clinical Presentation: Symptomatic Presentation

Most patients who presented clinically, before early diagnosis, did so in the first year of life with progressive muscle weakness, hypotonia, and cardiomyopathy. Children would die of heart failure in the first few years of life. Rarely, patients also presented with a more acute history of liver failure associated with hypoketotic hypoglycemia leading to coma and death *(7)*. With early diagnosis, this is one of the easiest and most rewarding metabolic conditions to treat. Early recognition and identification of the carnitine loss can be remedied by carnitine supplementation. This is the only disorder for which carnitine therapy is rationally justified and early introduction of carnitine supplementation prevents the skeletal and cardiac signs and symptoms and helps support ketogenesis. Even patients who are diagnosed symptomatically in unscreened populations have complete reversal of the pathological hallmarks. Of developing interest are the increasing numbers of previously asymptomatic mothers with a carnitine transport defect who give birth to infants with positive newborn screens as a result of reduced availability of transplacental carnitine *(8)*. The infants do well without carnitine supplementation because they do not have renal loss. The long-term outcome for the mothers is not yet established.

Genetics and Pathogenesis

The carnitine transporter defect is inherited as an autosomal-recessive trait. The *SLC22A5* gene is located on chromosome 5q31.1-q32. Carriers have lower than normal blood concentrations of total carnitine but appear to be without symptoms *(9)*. Pathogenesis results from the reduced intracellular carnitine content and secondary failure of FAO.

Table 5-1 Disorders of Fatty Acid β-Oxidation

Disorder	Newborn screening blood spot abnormality	Other useful testing/findings	Confirmatory test
Carnitine transporter defect	Very low free carnitine	↓ Plasma total and free carnitine	Sequence *SLC22A5* gene Fibroblast carnitine uptake studies
Carnitine palmitoyltransferase 1 (CPT1)	Elevated free carnitine and elevated ratio of free carnitine to long-chain acylcarnitine	↑ Plasma total carnitine with ↓ acyl fraction	Enzyme analysis (fibroblast, leukocyte) Sequence *CPT1A* gene
Carnitine:acylcarnitine translocase (CACT)	Elevated C16-, C18-, and C18:1-carnitines (overlaps with CPT2), low free carnitine	↑ Plasma C16, C18, C18:1 acylcarnitines ↑ NH₃	Sequence *SLC25A20* gene Functional fibroblast transport assay
Carnitine palmitoyltransferase 2 (CPT2)	Elevated C16-, C18-, and C18:1-carnitines for early-onset form (overlaps with CACT and VLCAD)	↑ Plasma C16, C18, C18:1 acylcarnitines ↑ CK, myoglobinuria	Enzyme analysis (fibroblasts) Sequence *CPT2* gene
Very-long-chain acyl-CoA dehydrogenase (VLCAD)	Elevated C14- and C14:1-carnitines (overlaps with CPT2)	↑ Plasma C14:1, C14:2 acylcarnitines (may be normal when well)	Enzyme analysis (fibroblasts) Sequence *ACADVL* gene
Mitochondrial trifunctional protein (MTP, TFP) and long-chain 3-hydroxyacyl-CoA dehydrogenase (LCHAD)	Elevated C16-OH-, C18-OH-, and C18:1-OH-carnitines	Serum 3-OH fatty acid analysis—↑ C14-C18 3-hydroxy fatty acids (3-OHFA) Urine organic acid (UOA)—C10–C14 3-OH dicarboxylic aciduria	Enzyme analysis of three long-chain enzymes (fibroblasts) *HADA* common G1528C mutation Sequence *HADA* and *HADB* genes if G1528 negative
Medium-chain acyl-CoA dehydrogenase (MCAD)	Elevated C8-, C10-, and C10:1-carnitines	UOA—hexanoylglycine, suberyl glycine, ± C6–C10 dicarboxylic aciduria	Molecular testing for *ACADM* K304E common mutation Sequence *ACADM* gene if K304E negative

Medium/short-chain 3-hydroxyacyl-CoA dehydrogenase (M/SCHAD)	Elevated C4-OH carnitine	3-OH fatty acid analysis—↑ C6-C10 3-OHFA; UOA—3-hydroxyglutaric acid	Enzyme analysis (fibroblasts); Sequence *SCHAD* gene
Short-chain acyl-CoA dehydrogenase (SCAD)	Elevated C4-carnitine	UOA—ethylmalonic acid, methylsuccinic acid, butyrylglycine	Sequence *ACADS* gene
3-Hydroxy-3-methylglutaryl-CoA (HMG-CoA) synthase		↓ Glucose, ↓ ketones on fasting	Sequence *HMGCS2* gene
3-Hydroxy-3-methylglutaryl-CoA (HMG-CoA) lyase	Elevated C5-OH-carnitine	↓ Glucose, ↓ ketones on fasting, ↑ lactate, ↑ NH_3; UOA—3-OH-3-methylglutaric, 3-OH-isovaleric, 3-methylglutaconic, 3-methylglutaric	Enzyme analysis (fibroblasts, leukocytes); Sequence *HMGCL* gene
Multiple acyl-CoA dehydrogenases (MADD, glutaric acidemia type 2)	Multiple acylcarnitine species elevated, including C5DC, C4, C8, and C14:1	UOA—glutaric acid, ethylmalonic acid, dicarboxylic acids, multiple acylglycines including isovaleryl-, isobutyryl-, butyryl-, 2-methylbutyryl, hexanoyl-, and suberyl-glycine. ↑ C4–C8 acylcarnitines, ↑ C5DC acylcarnitine	Enzyme analysis of ETF and ETFDH activity (fibroblasts); Sequence *ETFA*, *ETFB*, and *ETFDH* genes

Laboratory Diagnosis

For newborn screening purposes, most programs monitor the total amount of free carnitine (C0). A positive screen or symptomatic patient should be further evaluated in the laboratory by the measurement of total and free carnitine in plasma. The total carnitine concentration is frequently less than 5 µmol/L (normal 25–50). Patients who have already been therapeutically given a high dose of carnitine may show excessive urinary excretion of carnitine, typically in the several thousand micromolar range, but urinary excretion may appear normal or even low when plasma concentrations are very low. Confirmation of the diagnosis is typically made by sequencing the causative gene (*SLC22A5*). Occasionally a DNA change of unknown significance will be identified. This is best evaluated by measurement of carnitine uptake in cultured skin fibroblasts *(10)*.

Treatment and Prognosis

As mentioned above, this disorder is exquisitely responsive to high-dose carnitine therapy. Patients diagnosed in the newborn period may go through life being free of symptoms. Patients who are diagnosed clinically may have complete reversal of the effects. However, for symptomatic patients who have hypoglycemic episodes, there may be residual neurological damage. The outcomes for the mothers who have been diagnosed as a result of their infant's positive screen remain unanswered because these individuals have spent a lifetime with very low carnitine concentrations but appear to have been asymptomatic into adulthood. Longer-term evaluations are required to know if these patients will develop signs and symptoms in later life.

CARNITINE PALMITOYLTRANSFERASE 1 (CPT1) DEFICIENCY

CPT1 enzyme activity regulates the entry of fatty acids into the mitochondria. In liver, the enzyme is inhibited postprandially when concentrations of malonyl-CoA are high. CPT1 activity is activated during periods of fasting when malonyl-CoA concentrations are low. The enzyme takes long-chain acyl-CoA species, mostly of chain lengths C16–C18, and converts them to acylcarnitines for eventual transport into the mitochondria. There are three distinct genetic forms of CPT1. CPT1A is expressed in liver and kidney, CPT1B is found in cardiac and skeletal muscle, and CPT1C is found in brain. Only CPT1A deficiency has been described to date. This enzyme is also the one that is expressed in cultured skin fibroblasts, making this a suitable material for diagnostic purposes.

Clinical Presentation

CPT1A deficiency presents only as a defect of fasting intolerance *(11)*. Precipitation of a catabolic event can be induced by starvation or increased caloric loss due to gastrointestinal illness. The clinical phenotype is that of hepatic failure associated with hypoglycemia and failure of ketogenesis very much like Reye syndrome and similar to the presentation that is classically associated with MCAD deficiency. There may be modest hyperammonemia and transaminitis. Patients may also demonstrate renal tubular acidosis during periods of decompensation. Unlike other defects of long-chain FAO, the disorder does not have cardiac or skeletal muscle signs and symptoms.

Genetics and Pathogenesis

CPT1A deficiency is inherited as an autosomal-recessive disorder. Most patients in the literature appear to have unique mutations in the *CPT1A* gene and very low residual enzyme activity *(11)*. A variant of CPT1A, the P479L variant, is very common in individuals of Inuit ancestry in Alaska, Canada, and Greenland. The variant has high residual (20% of normal) enzyme activity, which is not inhibited by malonyl-CoA and therefore represents a CPT1 variant that is permanently activated *(12)*. The clinical significance of the P479L variant is presently unknown *(13)*. It may represent an adaptive advantage to ancient Inuit lifestyles or could be the result of a founder effect in individuals from isolated communities.

Laboratory Diagnosis

CPT1A deficiency represents the only disorder of FAO that has elevated concentrations of free carnitine. The total carnitine concentration may also be elevated. Diagnosis by newborn screening relies on monitoring a ratio of free carnitine to a long-chain acylcarnitine (usually C16:0) in dried blood spots. The sensitivity of this assay has not yet been established. When a patient with CPT1A deficiency is well, the measurement of urine organic acids, plasma nonesterified fatty acids, and ketone bodies (3-hydroxybutyrate) may be uninformative. When there is metabolic decompensation, the urine may demonstrate nonspecific hypoketotic dicarboxylic aciduria and inappropriately low plasma 3-hydroxybutyrate concentration. There are no specific biomarkers for CPT1A deficiency. Diagnosis can be confirmed by enzyme assay or by molecular testing of the *CPT1A* gene, which is located on chromosome 11q13.1-q13.5. Because of the high degree of private mutations in non-Inuit individuals, whole gene sequencing is required. For the Inuit P479L variant, a simple polymerase chain reaction (PCR)-based screen is available *(14)*.

Treatment and Prognosis

Metabolic decompensation in an unrecognized case of CPT1A deficiency can produce profound and potentially fatal hypoglycemia and liver damage. Survivors of the severe hypoglycemia can suffer irreversible neurological damage. However, with early recognition of the defect in subsequent siblings or by newborn screening, and with a clinical strategy to prevent the onset of increased flux through the FAO pathway by providing carbohydrate energy support (glucose), all of the adverse effects can be ameliorated and there are no severe effects. Clinical outcome for patients with known CPT1A deficiency and disease management by preventing the onset of fasting FAO are likely to be very good. There are no long-term neurological complications described in well-treated individuals *(11)*.

CARNITINE:ACYLCARNITINE TRANSLOCASE (CACT) DEFICIENCY

CACT deficiency is one of the rarer defects of inherited long-chain FAO. It was initially described as a very severe form of fasting intolerance with unremitting hyperammonemia and early death. More recent observations have shown it to be a disorder with a wider spectrum of presentation. The disorder results in failure to transport acylcarnitines into the inner mitochondrial matrix and subsequent lack of any substrate for FAO. This disorder can also be detected presymptomatically by newborn screening of blood spot acylcarnitine profiles.

Clinical Presentation

Unlike CPT1A, CACT is expressed in all tissues, in particular those with high energy demands. In the most severe form of CACT deficiency, patients present with multisystem involvement of liver, skeletal muscle, cardiac muscle, and kidney. The liver disease includes fasting-induced hepatic encephalopathy with associated steatosis and the biochemical hallmarks of hypoglycemia, hypoketonemia, and persistent hyperammonemia *(15)*. Many of the earliest cases were fatal. Subsequently, milder forms of CACT deficiency were described with milder systemic disease including modest liver disease and mild muscle weakness *(16)*. There is no long-term experience with surviving patients with this milder form of the disease so long-term outcomes remain unknown.

Genetics and Pathogenesis

CACT is an autosomal-recessive disorder that results from mutations in the *CACT* gene on chromosome 3p21. The disease process results from failure to deliver long-chain acylcarnitines into the mitochondrial matrix for eventual conversion to acyl-CoAs for high-energy tissues. Failure of energy production in high-energy tissues results in multisystem failure. For example, the heart requires fatty acids as energy substrates even when not fasting, and many patients die with cardiac failure.

Laboratory Diagnosis

For newborn screening purposes, blood spot acylcarnitines in CACT deficiency demonstrate accumulation of the primary physiological fatty acylcarnitine species being mostly of chain lengths C16:0, C18:2, and C18:1(5). Unfortunately, this pattern is also seen with carnitine palmitoyltransferase 2 (CPT2) deficiency (see below) and a laboratory differentiation between the two disorders is required for confirmation of a positive acylcarnitine result *(5)*. Confirmation of a positive screen requires follow-up with a plasma acylcarnitine profile and then further differentiation of either defect using a functional transport assay in cultured fibroblasts (for CACT deficiency), an enzyme assay for CPT2 deficiency, or molecular testing of both genes. DNA variants of unknown significance will require a functional assay to help determine significance *(17)*.

Treatment and Prognosis

Treatment is primarily designed to prevent the onset of significant flux through the pathway during periods of metabolic stress, which may include fasting, febrile illness, or loss of calories through the gastrointestinal tract. Calories should be provided in the form of carbohydrate, either dextrose for rapid protection or slow-release carbohydrate in the form of cornstarch for sustained provision of calories. The prognosis for the more severe forms of the defect remains poor because the hyperammonemia is difficult to control and few, if any, long-term survivors have been described. Although the milder forms of the disorder appear to have better outcomes, the numbers of patients are relatively small, and no long-term observational studies have yet been performed.

CARNITINE PALMITOYLTRANSFERASE 2 (CPT2) DEFICIENCY

CPT2 converts the acylcarnitines that are delivered into the mitochondrial matrix by CACT into acyl-CoAs, which are the substrates for the cyclical b-oxidation pathway. CPT2 is a membrane-associated protein that forms a super complex with other membrane-associated FAO proteins and components of oxidative phosphorylation *(18)*. Like CACT, CPT2 is systemic and is present in all cell types that perform FAO.

Clinical Presentation

CPT2 deficiency has variable presentation. The three distinct disease phenotypes include newborn presentation with acute multisystem failure associated with developmental abnormalities, a later-onset fasting-induced multisystem disease of infancy, and a late-childhood through adult-onset myopathic form of the disease. In the newborn with the dysmorphia variant of CPT2 deficiency, the outcome is almost always that of neonatal demise with fulminant liver and cardiac failure. The infants are myopathic and have renal and cerebral anomalies at autopsy including cystic changes to both organs *(19)*. The infantile disorder presents with fasting-induced multiorgan failure, including hepatic encephalopathy, hypertrophic cardiac disease, and skeletal myopathy. With early diagnosis and appropriate management this form of CPT2 deficiency can be successfully managed. However, progressive cardio-myopathy and skeletal muscle weakness may still occur in some patients despite early diagnosis and intervention. The late-onset form of CPT2 deficiency is purely myopathic. Individuals generally do not have a history of liver or cardiac disease. Some patients may have a history of relative exercise intolerance. Onset of symptoms is usually induced by vigorous exercise. This is frequently a cause of muscle disease leading to rhabdomyolysis in young adults suddenly undergoing high-intensity exercise as a result of athletic training or as a result of military training. The rhabdomyolysis may itself lead to acute renal failure due to rapid myoglobin release from muscle. Withdrawal from intense exercise appears to ameliorate the muscle symptoms.

Genetics and Pathogenesis

CPT2 deficiency results from mutations in the *CPT2* gene on chromosome 1p32. There is a distinct genotype:phenotype correlation with the three distinct types of clinical presentation. Most individuals with the neonatal form of the disease have null mutations and do not produce a functional protein. The observation of developmental defects in these patients implies that CPT2 may be required for normal development in utero. The late-onset disease tends to have missense mutations that lead to production of a protein with reduced but not absent activity such as the commonly identified S113L mutation. It is believed that there is sufficient residual activity in homozygotes for S113L to spare hepatic and cardiac involvement and skeletal muscle is only affected at times of vigorous exercise and increased demand on muscular energy sources. CPT2 deficiency may be the most common metabolic cause of myopathy in man and could be significantly underdiagnosed because not all individuals will encounter the precipitating metabolic stress and they may go undetected but suffer with milder exercise intolerance. The later infantile form of the disease usually occurs in individuals who are compound heterozygotes for the severe and milder types of mutation. However, there is evidence to suggest that even in family members carrying the same mutations, presentations may vary and metabolic modifiers may exist. There are also cases of symptomatic heterozygotes carrying a severe allele such as the Q413fs frame-shift mutation.

Laboratory Diagnosis

As described above for CACT, diagnosis in the newborn period is indicated by abnormal elevation of C16, C18:1, and C18:2 acylcarnitines in a blood spot test and similar elevations in a plasma acylcarnitine profile (Figure 5-2). For the severest form of CPT2 deficiency, this pattern may be masked by multiple other elevated long-chain acylcarnitine species. For asymptomatic patients with the intermediate form of the disease, these abnormalities should persist, and if symptomatic, multiple long-chain species should be elevated similar to the most severe form. Newborn screening for the late-onset form may not be sufficiently sensitive to detect all cases and some may be missed. The relative elevations of acylcarnitines in the late-onset form are lower than the other two forms. A positive screen for this form may be followed up by a normal confirmatory test, particularly if the infant is well nourished. Multiple tests may be required, but a positive screen that is not immediately confirmed should still retain suspicion for a true diagnosis. The observation of elevated C16, C18:1, and C18:2 acylcarnitines in a confirmatory test requires further investigation to determine if this is CPT2 or CACT deficiency. This testing may include enzymatic and/or molecular testing.

Treatment and Prognosis

The prognosis for the severest form of CPT2 deficiency is uniformly bad with early infant death. The late-onset myopathic CPT2 deficiency requires little treatment other than not to submit the patient to extreme muscular exertion. Liver and muscle do not seem to be involved, although regular testing of

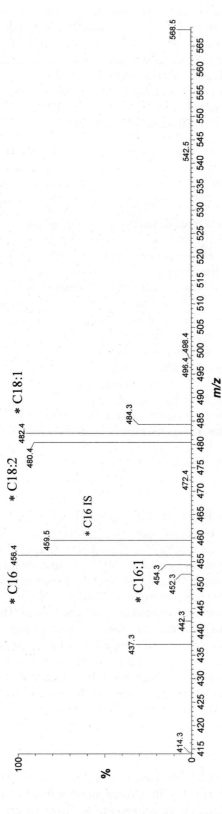

Figure 5-2 Acylcarnitine scan from a patient with CPT2 deficiency showing elevated concentrations of C16-, C18:1-, and C18:2-carnitines. CACT deficiency shows a very similar pattern. Acylcarnitine scans are generated from tandem mass spectrometer runs of samples extracted as follows: 20 μL of serum or plasma is added to 300 μL of internal standards in acetonitrile. After vortexing, centrifuging, and evaporating to dryness under nitrogen at 37 °C, 100 μL of butanolic HCl is added and allowed to react for 15 min at 65 °C. The samples are evaporated to dryness again under nitrogen at 37 °C, dissolved in 100 μL of 80% acetonitrile:water, and are then ready for injection on the tandem mass spectrometer.

hepatic and cardiac function is generally recommended. Prognosis is excellent for these individuals unless there has been an episode of acute renal failure. The prognosis for patients with the intermediate form of the disease is less clear. For some patients, with good management, acute episodes of metabolic decompensation may be avoided. For other patients, there are frequent admissions of multisystem failure. Even apparently well-controlled patients may develop progressive cardiac disease and skeletal myopathy and still be prone to hepatic encephalopathy (20).

VERY-LONG-CHAIN ACYL-COA DEHYDROGENASE (VLCAD) DEFICIENCY

The acyl-CoA dehydrogenases are the enzymes that catalyze the first step in the four-step mitochondrial fatty acid β-oxidation spiral. These enzymes oxidize saturated, straight-chain fatty acids. There are three main chain-length-specific isoforms (VLCAD, MCAD, and SCAD), although these enzymes have somewhat overlapping chain-length specificity. VLCAD uses acyl-CoA species with carbon chain lengths of 14–22 carbons. Similar to all enzymes of FAO that are specific for long-chain fatty acids, VLCAD is bound to the inner mitochondrial membrane. Long-chain fatty acids that have been shuttled into the mitochondrion by the carnitine shuttle and activated back to acyl-CoA are the substrates for VLCAD, which catalyzes the removal of two hydrogens and the formation of a double bond between carbons 2 and 3 of the acyl chain.

Clinical Presentation

The clinical features of VLCAD deficiency are similar to those of CPT2 deficiency, no doubt because with both conditions, tissues cannot use physiological long-chain fatty acids as a source of energy. There are three basic phenotypes of VLCAD deficiency: a severe neonatal, a milder childhood, and an adult-onset form. In the severe neonatal form, cardiomyopathy and hepatomegaly are the primary findings and the mortality rate is high. Infants who survive the early severe crises will have recurrent episodes and significant fasting intolerance. The main clinical feature of the mild childhood form is hypoketotic hypoglycemia, with the second most common clinical feature being hepatomegaly. Some of these milder cases may also show cardiomyopathy and/or rhabdomyolysis or myoglobinuria. This form of VLCAD usually presents with milder metabolic decompensations that occur relatively infrequently, and it has infrequent mortality. As the child gets older, the metabolic decompensations tend to decrease and the disorder becomes essentially muscle-related, similar to the adult-onset form. The adult-onset form generally presents as muscle pain, rhabdomyolysis, and myoglobinura usually triggered by exercise or fasting. The rhabdomyolysis and myoglobinura can lead to acute kidney damage.

Genetics and Pathogenesis

VLCAD deficiency results from mutations in the *ACADVL* gene on chromosome 17p11.13-p11.2. More than 150 mutations have been found that are scattered across all 20 exons of the gene. No prevalent mutations have yet been discovered; however, the most common mutation found, c.884T>C, has been observed most frequently in infants through newborn screening and in approximately 10% of the mild-onset or adult-onset cases. Similar to CPT2 deficiency, there is a distinct genotype:phenotype correlation with the three distinct types of clinical presentation. The severe, neonatal cases tend to have mutations that are null and do not produce a functional protein (21). VLCAD is expressed in all tissues examined, with the highest concentrations found in cardiac and skeletal muscle (22). These tissues have an absolute requirement for fatty acids and for intact FAO to function appropriately, even when not fasting. The milder and adult-onset cases have mutations in which enzyme with residual activity is produced. Under nonstressful conditions, the residual enzyme activity is often sufficient to prevent catabolic crisis. However, under the stress of fasting, intercurrent infections, or increased muscle exercise, the defective enzyme cannot maintain sufficient FAO flux to meet the increased demand.

Laboratory Diagnosis

Laboratory findings in VLCAD deficiency often overlap those seen in CPT2 deficiency, and distinguishing between the two diagnoses is often difficult and may not be possible with acylcarnitine analysis alone. In general, VLCAD deficiency will show abnormal elevations of C14:0, C14:1, and C14:2-carnitines, with C14:1-carnitine often being found in the highest concentration (Figure 5-3). As in CPT2 deficiency, individuals with mild forms of the disorder may be identified using newborn screening and then may show a normal acylcarnitine profile on follow-up testing. Patients with the milder forms of VLCAD deficiency may have normal acylcarnitines during times of low or no metabolic stress. The enzyme defect can be demonstrated by measuring palmitoyl-CoA dehydrogenase activity in skin fibroblasts or lymphocytes, with definitive diagnosis being made by mutational analysis of the VLCAD gene and demonstration of mutations.

Treatment and Prognosis

The treatment for VLCAD deficiency revolves around the prevention of fasting-induced lipolysis and the reduction of the amount of long-chain fatty acids in the diet. Medium-chain fatty acids are often supplemented in the form of medium-chain triglycerides (MCTs) to bypass the metabolic block. In the severe form of the disorder, any slight hypoglycemia will precipitate the multisystem metabolic decompensation that can rapidly lead to death in the neonatal period. In general, treating the hypoglycemia with intravenous (IV) glucose will correct these decompensation episodes if treatment is rapid enough, which may be difficult in neonates unless the underlying disease is known. However, with correct intensive therapy and diet modification, cardiac dysfunction and hypertrophy are reversible in these individuals. In the milder forms, the above treatments work well, and in the adult-onset form prevention of the type of extreme exercise that causes decompensation provides the best treatment.

MITOCHONDRIAL TRIFUNCTIONAL PROTEIN (MTFP) DEFICIENCY AND LONG-CHAIN 3-HYDROXYACYL-COA DEHYDROGENASE (LCHAD) DEFICIENCY

For long-chain fatty acid species, after the VLCAD first step of the FAO spiral, the last three steps involve a LHYD that adds water across the double bond to produce a hydroxyl group on carbon 3, a LCHAD that removes hydrogens and converts the hydroxyl group to a keto group, and a LKAT that cleaves a two-carbon acetyl CoA off the fatty acid and leaves the fatty acid two carbons shorter and ready for the next cycle. These three enzymes work as a heterooctomeric protein multienzyme complex referred to as mTFP. mTFP is also bound to the inner mitochondrial membrane, close to VLCAD, and together they provide an efficient means of oxidizing long-chain fatty acids. There are deficiency states that involve only LCHAD, as well as those that involve the mTFP complex and show reduced or lacking activity of all three enzymes in the complex.

Clinical Presentation

Presentation of LCHAD deficiency can be extremely variable, ranging from chronic, nonspecific failure to thrive and feeding difficulties to liver dysfunction and a Reye syndrome-like presentation of

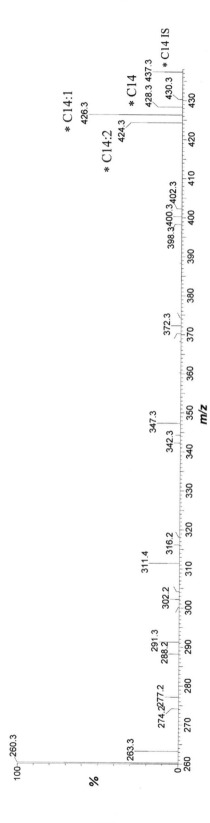

Figure 5-3 Acylcarnitine scan from a patient with VLCAD deficiency demonstrating a classic pattern of elevated C14-, C14:1-, and C14:2-carnitines, with C14:1-carnitine showing the highest concentration.

hepatic encephalopathy to cardiopulmonary arrest and sudden death. Some of the more common signs and symptoms include hypoketotic hypoglycemia with liver dysfunction, hepatomegaly, and hypotonia. Severe presentations can include tachycardic arrhythmias, cardiomyopathy, multiorgan failure, seizures, and coma. Presentations that include feeding difficulties and failure to thrive, jaundice secondary to cholestasis, and asymptomatic neonatal hypoglycemia are probably less common. During childhood, progressively degenerative opthalmologic abnormalities and neuropathies often develop, which is a unique finding among the FAO defects (23). Another important point to note in LCHAD deficiency is its association with maternal liver disease, specifically acute fatty liver of pregnancy (AFLP) and hemolysis (hypertension), elevated liver enzymes, and low platelets (HELLP) syndromes (24, 25). Although HELLP syndrome is a more common complication of pregnancy than AFLP, LCHAD deficiency is much less commonly associated with HELLP syndrome than with AFLP.

Complete TFP deficiency is not as common as isolated LCHAD deficiency. Similar to other long-chain FAO defects, there appears to be three clinical phenotypes with mTFP deficiency, including a severe neonatal form with cardiomyopathy, a milder form with hypoketotic hypoglycemia, and a later-onset myopathic form. Most mTFP-deficient individuals present with the later-onset form and may be diagnosed during the second decade of life. mTFP deficiency usually presents as recurrent skeletal muscle pain and weakness that is often brought on by exercise. Occasionally mTFP deficiency may present with a neonatal onset and a presentation very similar to isolated LCHAD deficiency. The most severe forms of mTFP deficiency are highly associated with neonatal death, and this type of presentation may include a lethal cardiac failure and sudden death with predominate cardiac involvement. mTFP deficiency also has been shown to associate with maternal liver disease, but to a lesser extent than isolated LCHAD deficiency.

Genetics and Pathogenesis

LCHAD deficiency results from mutations in the *HADH-A* gene and mTFP deficiencies result from mutations in the *HADH-A* and/or *HADH-B* genes on chromosome 2p23. The heterooctomeric protein is composed of four α subunits that contain the LCHAD activity and four β subunits that contain the LHYD and LKAT activities. Isolated LCHAD deficiency has a common mutation, G1528C, which is found homozygously in 65% of LCHAD-deficient individuals and compound heterozygously in the remainder. mTFP does not have a common mutation; however, mutations in α or β subunits can lead to mTFP deficiency with enzyme activity reduced in all three enzymes. There appears to be some genotype:phenotype correlation with mTFP deficiency, with missense mutations associated with the milder myopathic form (26). Similar to VLCAD deficiency, inability to use long-chain fatty acids for fuel and the buildup of those long-chain fatty acids as toxic metabolites are believed to be responsible for clinical symptoms. Retinopathy and neuropathies are believed to be linked to the atypical 3-hydroxy long-chain metabolite toxicity.

Laboratory Diagnosis

LCHAD deficiency can be identified on the expanded newborn screen using tandem mass spectroscopy (MS/MS) for acylcarnitine analysis. Abnormal findings on acylcarnitine analysis include elevated concentrations of the long-chain hydroxyacyl-carnitines, especially C16-OH, C18-OH-, and C18:1-OH-carnitines (Figure 5-4). However, it is important to note that LCHAD-deficient individuals often have normal acylcarnitine profiles when they are metabolically stable. This analysis is most useful when the individual is ill. Measuring serum 3-OH-fatty acids may be useful in these cases (27) because the concentrations of C14-C18 3-OH-fatty acids in blood are always elevated in LCHAD deficiency (Figure 5-5). For isolated LCHAD deficiency, samples can be analyzed for the common G1528C mutation to confirm this diagnosis. Analysis of enzyme activity in skin fibroblasts can be used to determine residual activity and to determine the activity of LKAT and LHYD to diagnose TFP deficiency. Molecular

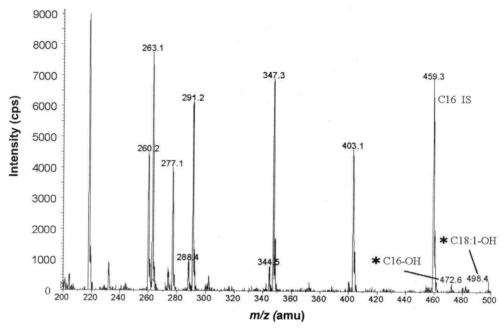

Figure 5-4 Acylcarnitine scan from a patient with LCHAD deficiency showing mildly elevated concentrations of C16-OH- and C18:1-OH-carnitines. This scan demonstrates that in the case of LCHAD the elevations may not be very high unless the patient is decompensated. The scan is from a different instrument but using the same extraction protocol as previously described.

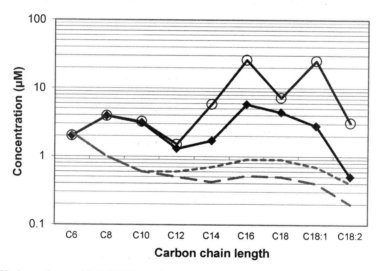

Figure 5-5 3-Hydroxy-fatty acid (3OHFA) analysis results from a patient with LCHAD deficiency showing massively elevated concentrations of C14-OH through C18-OH fatty acids, with C16-OH and C18:1-OH being particularly elevated. The dashed lines are the upper limit of normal for free (long dashes) and total (short dashes) 3-OHFA. Patient results show free (solid diamonds) and total (open circles) 3-OHFAs. This analysis is done via stable isotope dilution electron impact ionization gas chromatography-mass spectrometry (GC/MS) after sample extraction as follows: 10 µL of each of seven 3-OHFA internal standards is added to 0.5 mL of serum or plasma. The sample is acidified with HCl, centrifuged, and the supernatant is then extracted twice with 3 mL of ethyl acetate each time. The ethyl acetate extractions are combined, dried down at 37 °C under nitrogen, and then derivatized with 65 µL of bis(trimethylsilyl)trifluoroacetamide:trimethylchlorosilane, 99:1(BSTFA) for 30 min to 2 h at 75 °C. Derivatized samples are injected onto the GC/MS.

analysis for subunit mutations leading to TFP is available. It is also important to note that women with AFLP should have their newborn immediately and urgently tested for LCHAD deficiency by acylcarnitine analysis and, if necessary, mutational confirmation.

Treatment and Prognosis

Similar to other disorders of long-chain FAO, treatment for LCHAD deficiency includes the prevention of fasting, reduction of the amount of long-chain fatty acids in the diet, and supplementation of the diet with medium-chain fatty acids to provide the necessary energy from fatty acids for those tissues with a high requirement. There has been some suggestion that MCT treatment may not only provide fats with necessary chain lengths, but may also reduce the buildup of the toxic long-chain metabolites *(28)*. In young patients with LCHAD deficiency, sudden death from an acute episode is not uncommon. Treatment of acute crisis with IV glucose is the standard rescue for LCHAD-deficient patients who have metabolically decompensated. Survivors tend to have recurrent decompensations, and as they grow older, other sequelae develop, including retinopathy and peripheral neuropathy. Later there may be episodes of skeletal myopathy and muscle pain. Mortality for severe presentations is high in LCHAD deficiency and morbidity remains high in individuals despite treatments *(29)*.

MEDIUM-CHAIN ACYL-COA DEHYDROGENASE (MCAD) DEFICIENCY

MCAD deficiency is the most commonly diagnosed disorder of FAO. The disorder has a frequency of approximately 1 in 15,000 live births in the United States *(5)*. This defect represents the first defect of the mitochondrial matrix pathway of FAO when acyl-CoA intermediates are transferred from the predominantly membrane-associated long-chain enzyme complex *(18)* to a presumed matrix enzyme complex for the complete oxidation of intermediates of chain length C10 to the final acetyl-CoA end products.

Clinical Presentation

Before the introduction of newborn screening programs for MCAD deficiency, presentation was primarily hepatic and very similar to that described above for CPT1A deficiency. Patients would present with the biochemical hallmarks of fasting-induced hypoketotic hypoglycemia leading to coma, hepatic encephalopathy with modest hyperammonemia, fulminant liver failure, and in some instances sudden and unexpected death in infancy *(30)*. Presentation was typically around the time of weaning and was often associated with mild viral infections and consequent reduced caloric intake. Some of the deaths were so sudden that they were classified initially as sudden infant death syndrome (SIDS). Autopsy evaluation would reveal massive hepatic steatosis and lipid storage in cardiac and skeletal muscle, although cardiac and myopathic presentation was only rarely associated with the defect. MCAD deficiency provided the impetus for including disorders of FAO into newborn screening programs and provides a standard for successful screening. Patients diagnosed with MCAD deficiency very rarely present with acute metabolic decompensation after early diagnosis, and many clinicians today have not encountered the severity of MCAD deficiency. These patients do not have chronic cardiac or skeletal muscle signs and symptoms and appear perfectly normal.

Genetics and Pathogenesis

MCAD deficiency is caused by mutations in the *MCAD* or *ACADM* gene on chromosome 1p32. A common mutation resulting in a K304E amino acid substitution is common in northern Europeans and accounts for most disease alleles. Homozygosity for this mutation results in an unstable peptide without enzymatic activity. Pathogenesis results from failure to completely oxidize medium-chain acyl-CoA species. In liver this results in impaired ketogenesis and insufficient numbers of circulating ketone bodies to support tissues including brain that cannot oxidize fatty acids. Because heart and skeletal muscle do not appear to be part of the clinical phenotype, it is assumed that partial degradation of long-chain fatty acids is sufficient to maintain energy requirements in these tissues. The hepatic encephalopathy is associated with accumulation of macro- and microvesicular lipid storage, which may cause secondary tissue damage.

Laboratory Diagnosis

Newborn screening programs mostly utilize octanoylcarnitine (C8) as the biomarker for MCAD deficiency. Confirmation of a positive screen can be made by performing a more comprehensive acylcarnitine profile on plasma. A characteristic profile of elevated C6, C8, and C10:1 acylcarnitines is pathognomonic for MCAD deficiency in almost all cases even when the patient is clinically well (Figure 5-6). Additional confirmatory metabolite testing to ensure a diagnosis can include measurement of urine acylglycines. Increased hexanoylglycine and suberylglycine excretion is found in patients

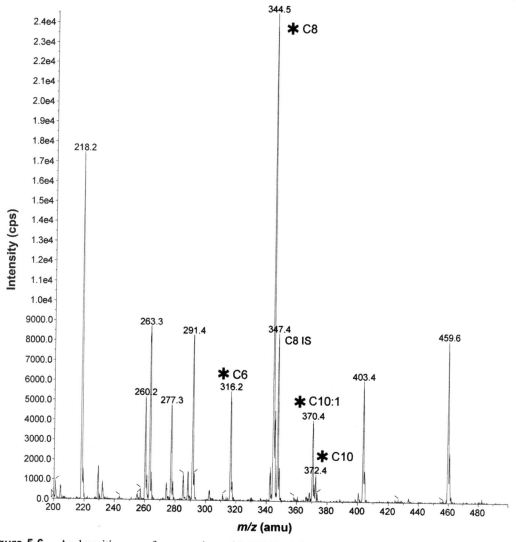

Figure 5-6 Acylcarnitine scan from a patient with MCAD deficiency demonstrating the massive increase in concentration of C8-carnitine as well as elevated concentrations of C10:1-, C10-, and C6-carnitines.

with MCAD deficiency, but these biomarkers are less specific because they are also found in multiple acyl-coA dehydrogenation defects (see below). Quantitative assays for these urinary acylglycines are available, but with appropriate analysis of ion-extracted species hexanoylglycine and suberylglycine can also be seen with urine organic acid analysis (Figure 5-7). Absolute confirmation of a diagnosis is usually performed by molecular testing with initial testing for the common mutation (K304E) and if negative or heterozygous followed by complete gene sequencing.

Critically ill children with MCAD deficiency are rarely seen in a previously screened population because treatment is typically excellent and preventative. However, in unscreened populations and even in older individuals born before screening, there is a risk of severe metabolic decompensation. In this scenario, patients can present in liver failure or coma with profound hypoglycemia with modest hyperammonemia and modest elevation of liver enzymes. Contrary to some belief, urine testing for ketones may be positive. This is because long-chain fatty acids can be partially chain-shortened in MCAD deficiency, and some ketones can be generated. However, analysis of urinary organic acids will reveal an inappropriately hypoketotic medium-chain dicarboxylic acidura with elevated adipic, suberic, and sebacic acids and the unsaturated suberic and sebacic acids. Hexanoylglycine and suberylglycine will also be detected *(31)*.

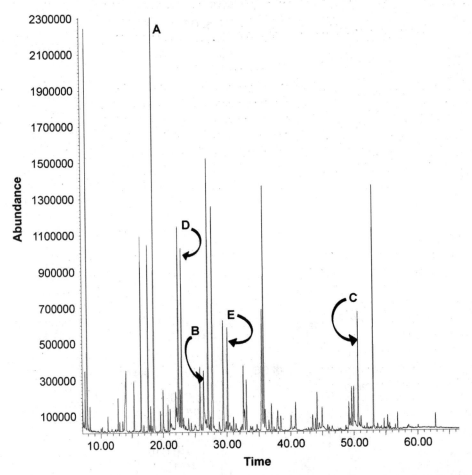

Figure 5-7 Organic acid profile from a patient with MCAD deficiency. A = internal standard, B = hexanoylglycine, C = suberylglycine, D = adipic acid, E = suberic acid. This assay uses GC/MS after sample extraction as follows: volume of urine to be extracted is determined by measuring the urine creatinine and then using a urine volume that will produce a creatinine of roughly 0.1 mg. Twenty-five microliters of 2-phenylbutyric acid is added to each sample as an internal standard. The sample is acidified with 125 μL of HCl and extracted as described for 3-OHFAs after acidification. Derivatization uses 100 μL BSTFA rather than 65 μL.

Treatment and Prognosis

Despite the dire outcome in unscreened populations, treatment of asymptomatic screened individuals is very satisfying *(32)*. Most patients do very well, and there is little or no morbidity associated with long-term follow up. Newborns rarely have developed signs and symptoms before a result being returned from the screening laboratory. This is usually in association with failure to institute early breast-feeding. Treatment is designed to prevent the onset of fasting-induced lipolysis. Frequent feeding regimens are introduced and an emergency regimen of high carbohydrate loading to cover periods of febrile illness or gastrointestinal loss of calories. In unscreened populations there is a high mortality and morbidity associated with unrecognized MCAD deficiency.

MEDIUM/SHORT CHAIN 3-HYDROXYACYL-COA DEHYDROGENASE (M/SCHAD) DEFICIENCY

M/SCHAD deficiency may be the rarest disorder of FAO with approximately 14 known cases. This enzyme is also known simply as SCHAD. Similar to LCHAD, it catalyzes the third step of FAO, the conversion of the 3-hydroxy intermediate to the 3-keto intermediate. M/SCHAD has broad chain-length specificity, using fatty acids with 4–14 carbons. Similar to other medium- and short-chain length-specific enzymes, it is a mitochondrial matrix enzyme that does not appear to be membrane bound. The enzyme is abundantly expressed in many tissues in mammals. Deficiency in this enzyme function is also one of the rare causes of congenital hyperinsulinism *(33)*.

Clinical Presentation

The presentation of M/SCHAD deficiency is highly variable, and the extent of the clinical presentation is unclear because of the few reported cases. Presentation within the first year of life may be rapidly fatal, and M/SCHAD deficiency has been shown as the cause of some cases of SIDS *(34)*. Biochemical and clinical findings include hypotonia, hypoglycemia, and hepatic steatosis. M/SCHAD deficiency has also presented as fulminant liver failure. Similar to other FAO defects, recurrent hypketotic hypoglycemic episodes occur, often accompanied by seizures. In general, cardiomyopathies and skeletal muscle myopathies are not associated with M/SCHAD deficiency. Unique among FAO disorders, M/SCHAD deficiency is associated with hyperinsulinemic hypoglycemia and is one of the rare causes of congenital hyperinsulinism.

Genetics and Pathogenesis

Mutations in the *SCHAD* gene (also called the *HADH* or *HAD* gene) are found in M/SCHAD deficiency, although M/SCHAD enzyme deficiencies have been established in individuals with no demonstrable mutations in the gene. In patients with reported mutations, the mutations have been homozygous. In cases of congenital hyperinsulinism caused by M/SCHAD deficiency, mutations in the *SCHAD* gene that lead to a lack of protein production have been found to produce a gain of function and upregulation of glutamate dehydrogenase (GDH) activity. Hyperinsulinsim in these cases appears to be a direct result of loss of SCHAD inhibition of GDH activity *(35)*.

Laboratory Diagnosis

To date, prospective diagnosis of M/SCHAD deficiency has not been demonstrated by newborn screening, but the condition is regarded as a secondary target. The biochemical abnormality most commonly seen is an elevated concentration of 3-hydroxybutyryl carnitine (C4-OH) on acylcarnitine analysis by MS/MS. Urine organic acids may show elevated amounts of 3-hydroxyglutarate. Enzyme assays often show reduced activity; however, significant residual activity is usually present. Serum 3-hydroxy-fatty acid analysis may show elevated medium- and short-chain 3-hydroxy fatty acids, but this finding is not specific for M/SCHAD deficiency. Molecular genetic analysis of the *SCHAD* gene sequence is necessary for definitive diagnosis.

Treatment and Prognosis

Frequent feedings and overnight infusion of carbohydrates are the usual treatments for M/SCHAD deficiency; however, this is sometimes insufficient to prevent the recurrent hypoglycemic episodes. Hypoglycemia may be difficult to control. Treatment with diazoxide used to treat the hyperinsulinemic hypoglycemia of infancy has been reported as effective in cases in which there is clear hyperinsulinism *(36)*. M/SCHAD deficiency appears to have a good prognosis for normal development if diagnosed early and if the intractable hypoglycemic events are controlled as much as possible.

SHORT-CHAIN ACYL-COA DEHYDROGENASE (SCAD) DEFICIENCY

SCAD deficiency is clinically heterogeneous and is not a well-understood disorder. The enzyme catalyzes the first step of FAO with a substrate specificity for C4 and C6 saturated straight-chain fatty acids. Affected individuals with biochemical markers of the disease and decreased enzyme activity may not show obvious mutations in the gene. Instead, they often demonstrate polymorphic sequence variations, suggesting that other factors are necessary for manifestation of the disorder or suggesting that changes in the gene may predispose to the development of the disorder.

Clinical Presentation

Clinical presentation of SCAD deficiency is extremely heterogeneous, ranging from neonatal metabolic acidosis progressing to death, to teenagers whose only symptoms are recurrent episodes of vomiting, to asymptomatic individuals identified with newborn screening with an elevated butyryl carnitine concentration. Initial clinical presentation may occur before the age of 3 years old or even in infancy within the first few days of life. However, SCAD-deficient individuals often present in childhood with mainly neurological and muscular symptoms and developmental delay *(37)*. There are increasing numbers of reports based on patients who are identified through newborn screening who never develop signs and symptoms of disease. It is thought by many that SCAD deficiency is benign and that the initial cases were identified because of the high frequency of the polymorphic gene variations in the general population and that any clinical phenotype may be unrelated to SCAD deficiency. Some newborn screening programs have dropped SCAD screening because of these concerns.

Genetics and Pathogenesis

SCAD deficiency is caused by mutations in the *ACADS* gene on chromosome 12p22-qter. Less than 12 mutations that cause classic SCAD deficiency have been reported in the literature; however, two common polymorphic variants are found frequently that seem to confer some level of susceptibility for the disease when accompanied by other, as-yet-unknown factors. The two variants c.625G>A and c.511C>T are found in almost 14% of the general population and found in a predominance of patients with ethylmalonic aciduria. Despite this prevalence, only those individuals who have other, currently unknown genetic factors or suffer certain environmental stresses will have clinical disease. There is some evidence that the defective enzyme in this disorder misfolds under certain stresses, causing the deficient activity *(38)*. Because this enzyme is at the end of the FAO spiral, most of the energy has already been produced from the oxidized fatty acid when it reaches this four- to six-carbon stage, therefore symptoms of energy deficiency found in other FAO disorders are not commonly found in SCAD deficiency. The enzyme deficiency causes a buildup of butyryl-CoA, which can be carboxylated to ethylmalonic acid. Pathogenic effects may be related to the toxic accumulation of butyric and ethyl-malonic acid intermediates rather than a lack of appropriate energy production as is seen with other FAO disorders.

Laboratory Diagnosis

SCAD deficiency is indicated by elevated concentrations of butyryl carnitine on acylcarnitine analysis by MS/MS (Figure 5-8). Because butyryl and isobutyryl carnitines cannot be differentiated by this analysis, isobutyryl-CoA dehydrogenase deficiency will need to be considered when C4-carnitine is elevated. Urine organic acid analysis can be used to help to sort out these two disorders. Findings of increased excretion of ethylmalonic acid, especially in the presence of methylsuccinic acid and

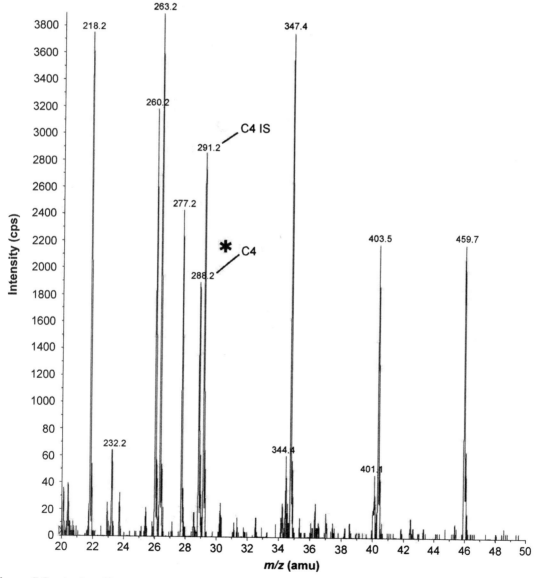

Figure 5-8   Acylcarnitine scan from a patient with SCAD deficiency demonstrating an increased concentration of C4-carnitine.

butyrylglycine, are suggestive of SCAD deficiency. The presence of isobutyrylglycine would be indicative of isobutyryl-CoA dehydrogenase deficiency. Analysis of enzyme activity for SCAD is hampered by overlapping substrate specificity between SCAD and the other acyl-CoA dehydrogenases, particularly MCAD. Definitive diagnosis requires full sequencing of the *ACADS* gene and the finding of inactivating mutations. Finding the polymorphic variants will not be fully useful until a better understanding is achieved of the other factors involved in the susceptibility conferred by these variants.

Treatment and Prognosis

Treatment strategies for SCAD deficiency are not clearly defined, but similar to other FAO disorders, avoiding prolonged fasting and quickly treating metabolic decompensations may be valuable. Prognosis is variable depending on presentation, with many cases being asymptomatic despite many of the cases not having a specific treatment. Longer-term prospective evaluation of cases may determine the significance of this disorder and optimal treatment if required.

HMG-COA SYNTHASE AND HMG-COA LYASE DEFICIENCIES

HMG-CoA synthase and HMG-CoA lyase are enzymes involved in ketone synthesis. HMG-CoA synthase converts acetoacetyl-CoA to HMG-CoA, and then HMG-CoA lyase converts HMG-CoA to acetoacetate. Defects in either enzyme lead to the inability to form the ketones acetoacetate, acetone, and β-hydroxybutyrate. These enzymes are thus involved in handling the acetyl-CoA products of FAO. Defects in these ketogenic enzymes show a clinical picture similar to other FAO deficiencies significant for hypoketotic hypoglycemia. Although HMG-CoA synthase is active only in the liver, HMG-CoA lyase enzyme assays can be performed using leukocytes and skin fibroblasts. HMG-CoA lyase is also a step in the leucine degradative pathway.

Clinical Presentation

Deficiencies in the ketogenic enzymes often show up in the first few days of life and tend to be episodic thereafter. Any amount of fasting may precipitate an attack, and in the neonatal period those decompensations may be life-threatening. Infants who survive the early critical decompensations may show episodes that become less frequent as the child gets older. Occasionally milder forms of these disorders may present in later childhood or even in adulthood, but essentially always in response to metabolic stress states such as infections, dehydration, or fasting. HMG-CoA synthase deficiency often presents with severe hypoketotic hypoglycemia leading to hypoglycemic encephalopathy after relatively short fasting periods, which can progress rapidly to coma. Mild hepatomegaly is often present. HMG-CoA lyase deficiency usually presents nonspecifically with hypotonia, vomiting, lethargy, severe metabolic acidosis, and profound hypoglycemia *(39)*. Hyperammonemia may be present. Hepatomegaly is usually present with elevated transaminases, and the disorder may be misdiagnosed as Reye syndrome.

Genetics and Pathogenesis

HMG-CoA synthase deficiency is caused by mutations in the *HMGCS2* gene on chromosome 1p13-p12. HMG-CoA lyase deficiency is an autosomal-recessive disorder caused by homozygous or compound heterozygous mutations in the *HMGCL* gene on chromosome 1pter-p33. In both cases the end product of the FAO spiral, acetyl-CoA, cannot be converted into ketone bodies, which are normally used by the body for a supplemental fuel for the brain during fasting as well as a means of storing acetyl-CoA until enzyme systems can handle the excess produced by FAO. Without the availability of ketones during hypoglycemic events, the brain may have an inadequate fuel source and will sustain damage. Individuals with these defects may proceed rapidly to coma after a relatively short fasting period. Hepatomegaly may be present with accumulation of lipids in the hepatocytes.

Laboratory Diagnosis

HMG-CoA lyase deficiency can be identified on the newborn screen and appears as an elevated C5-OH-carnitine concentration. Unfortunately multiple other inborn errors of metabolism also show up on the newborn screen with an elevated C5-OH carnitine, including 3-methylcrotonyl carboxylase deficiency, β-ketothiolase deficiency, multiple CoA carboxylase deficiency, and 2-methyl-3-hydroxybutyryl-CoA dehydrogenase deficiency. Follow-up testing will be necessary. HMG-CoA lyase deficiency may show elevated lactate and ammonia in the blood, and the urine organic acid profile will show elevated 3-hydroxy-3-methylglutaric, 3-hydroxy-isovaleric, 3-methylglutaconic, and 3-methylglutaric acids. An acylcarnitine profile will often show elevated 3-methylglutarylcarnitine (C6DC) as well as C5-OH-carnitine concentrations. Diagnosis of HMG-CoA lyase deficiency can be confirmed by enzyme analysis in fibroblasts or lymphocytes and detection of a mutation on *HMGCL* gene analysis. At least 28 mutations in this gene have been documented, with some mutations being highly population-specific *(40)*.

HMG-CoA synthase deficiency has fewer diagnostic biomarkers than lyase deficiency. The only common laboratory tests with abnormal results in HMG-CoA synthase deficiency may be a low serum glucose and nonspecific dicarboxylic aciduria in urine organic acid analysis. HMG-CoA synthase deficiency shows a normal or nonspecific acylcarnitine profile *(41)*. Diagnosis is confirmed for HMG-CoA synthase deficiency by sequence analysis of the *HMGCS2* gene. Deficiencies in the ketogenic enzymes may need to be assessed during fasting, when no ketones will be produced. A controlled fast may be necessary and if so it should be performed in a specialized metabolic unit. Disorders of FAO can be fatal when fasting results in failure of processes and pathways and/or production of toxic metabolites.

Treatment and Prognosis

Treatment of acute cases is supportive, with IV glucose being the predominant treatment. With HMG-CoA lyase deficiency, long-term management may include dietary modifications with moderate protein restriction, specifically restriction of leucine, which is normally metabolized to the substrate for HMG-CoA lyase. Critical to management is providing plenty of calories in the form of supplemental carbohydrates, especially during intercurrent illnesses. Individuals with defects in ketogenic enzymes may have normal growth and development as long as any early severe decompensations have not caused brain damage. The frequency of episodes tends to decrease with age.

MULTIPLE ACYL-COA DEHYDROGENATION DEFECTS (MADD)

MADD (also known as glutaric aciduria type 2) represents a group of secondary defects of FAO and of some organic acid metabolic pathways. All mitochondrial acyl-CoA dehydrogenases transfer their reducing equivalent through electron transfer sequentially to ETF and then to ETFDH (also known as ETF-QO) and finally into the respiratory chain at the level of coenzyme Q. Defects of either ETF or ETF-QO lead to impaired electron transfer from multiple pathways, including all three acyl-CoA dehydrogenases of FAO (VLCAD, MCAD, and SCAD). Of the non-FAO pathway acyl-CoA dehydrogenases involved in this group of disorders, isovaleryl-CoA dehydrogenase of the leucine metabolic pathway and glutaryl-CoA dehydrogense of lysine and tryptophan metabolism are the most significant. The specific individual disorders are covered in the organic acidemia section.

Most importantly and sometimes not completely understood, the acyl-CoA dehydrogenases themselves are normally expressed and active in MADD if measured in an in vitro system that provides electron carriers.

Clinical Presentation

Three distinct presentations have been described for MADD *(42)*. It was initially described as a severe and often fatal neonatal disease with multisystem failure and polycystic changes to brain and kidney similar to that seen in the most severe form of CPT2 deficiency (type 1). The condition is also remarkable for many patients having an odor that was similar to that observed in isovaleric acidemia, unfortunately termed the odor of sweaty feet. Other infantile forms of MADD were described without the organ dysgenesis but with many of the severe metabolic consequences, including liver failure, cardiac hypertrophy, skeletal myopathy, and renal tubular acidosis and still associated with the unusual odor (type 2). A third, milder presentation (type 3) is of a later-onset disorder precipitated by catabolic stress with hepatic encephalopathy similar to that seen in primary FAO defects, with slowly progressive cardiomyopathy and milder skeletal muscle weakness *(3)*.

Genetics and Pathogenesis

Three distinct genes are responsible for MADD. The genes for the a and b subunits of ETF (*ETFA* and *ETFB*) are located on chromosomes 15q23-25 and 19q13.3, respectively, and that for ETF-QO is on chromosome 4q32-ter. Mutations in any of these genes can produce all three clinical phenotypes that typically are determined by the severity of a mutation. Truncating or null mutations in any of the genes can produce the severest phenotype whereas missense mutations tend to predominate in milder disease. The pathogenesis of MADD results from failure of the multiple acyl-CoA dehydrogenase enzymes. The many similarities between MADD and FAO defects result primarily from functional deficiencies of VLCAD and MCAD (the clinical role of SCAD is not clear). The unusual odor arises from a functional defect of isovaleryl-CoA dehydrogenase (isovaleric acidemia), and the involvement of glutaryl-CoA dehydrogenase may be responsible for any neurological deficit similar to glutaric acidemia type 1, but that has not been established convincingly (see Chapter 3 on organic acid disorders).

Laboratory Diagnosis

MADD is one of the conditions that can potentially be diagnosed in the newborn period by blood spot acylcarnitine assays. The presence of multiple acylcarnitine species including isovaleryl-, glutaryl-, C8 (MCAD), and C14:1 (VLCAD) are strong indicators of a defect. However, in clinical practice, the onset of the more severe type 1 and 2 forms of MADD is in the immediate perinatal period with multisystem organ failure and may easily predate any screening efforts. Analysis of plasma acylcarnitines will give a characteristic profile and urine organic acid analysis will have a distinctive pattern of organic acids, including elevated glutaric acid; medium-chain dicarboxylic acids characteristic of FAO defects; and multiple acylglycine species including isovalerylglycine, butyryl and isobutyryl glycine, 2-methylbutyryl glycine, hexanoylglycine, and suberylglycine. Many of these compounds may be seen on a total ion chromatogram, but this may also require selected ion monitoring for detection. Quantitative urine acylglycine analysis may be required for less clear organic acid profiles. The milder forms of MADD may pose more of a diagnostic challenge because newborn screening may not always detect a defect and measurement of metabolite profiles may be normal when the patient is not stressed. Ultimate confirmation of a diagnosis of any type of MADD may need a combination of enzyme analysis and gene sequencing. Most mutations associated with these rare conditions are private and no common mutations are known.

Treatment and Prognosis

Patients with type 1 MADD do not survive the perinatal period. Type 2 patients also do very poorly as a result of the multiple abnormal metabolic pathways. The outcome for patients with type 3 MADD is somewhat better. Because the defect involves fatty acid and amino acid degradative pathways, appropriate nutritional management and prevention of fasting during febrile illness is very difficult to achieve. ETF and ETF-QO are flavoproteins, and high-dose riboflavin therapy has been attempted with little published success. Most patients are placed on riboflavin because it is otherwise a cheap and harmless approach.

REFERENCES

1. Snider MD, McGarry JD, Hanson RW. Lipid metabolism: synthesis, storage and utilization of fatty acids and triacylglycerols. In: Devlin TM, ed. Textbook of Biochemistry with Clinical Correlations, 6th ed. Hoboken, NJ: Wiley-Liss, 2006:662–94.
2. Rinaldo P, Matern D, Bennett MJ. Fatty acid oxidation disorders. Annu Rev Physiol 2002;64:477–502.
3. Strauss AW, Andresen BS, Bennett MJ. Mitochondrial fatty acid oxidation defects. In: Sarafoglou K, Hoffmann GF, Roth KS, eds. Pediatric Endocrinology and Inborn Errors of Metabolism. New York: McGraw Hill, 2009:51–70.
4. Sansaricq C, Pardo-Reoyo S. Ketone synthesis and utilization defects. In: Sarafoglou K, Hoffmann GF, Roth KS, eds. Pediatric Endocrinology and Inborn Errors of Metabolism. New York: McGraw Hill, 2009:119–25.
5. Schulze A, Matern D, Hoffmann GF. Newborn screening. In: Sarafoglou K, Hoffmann GF, Roth KS, eds. Pediatric Endocrinology and Inborn Errors of Metabolism. New York: McGraw Hill, 2009:17–36.
6. Stanley CA, Bennett MJ, Longo N. Plasma membrane carnitine transporter defect. In: Valle D, Beaudet AL, Vogelstein B, Kinzler KW, Antonarakis SE, Ballabio A, eds. Scriver's Online Metabolic & Molecular Bases of Inherited Disease. McGraw Hill, November 2011. http://www.ommbid.com (Accessed April 30, 2012).
7. Longo N, Amat Di San Filippo C, Pasquali M. Disorders of carnitine transport and the carnitine cycle. Amer J Med Genet C Semin Med Genet 2006;142:77–85.
8. Schimmenti LA, Crombez EA, Schwahn BC, Heese BA, Wood TC, Schroer RJ, et al. Expanded newborn screening identifies maternal primary carnitine deficiency. Mol Genet Metab 2007;90:441–5.
9. Stanley CA, DeLeeuw S, Coates PM, Vianey-Liaud C, Divry P, Bonnefont JP, et al. Chronic cardiomyopathy and weakness or acute coma in children with a defect in carnitine uptake. Ann Neurol 1991;30:709–16.
10. Tein I, De Vivo DC, Bierman F, Pulver P, De Meirleir LJ, Cvitanovic-Sojat L, et al. Impaired skin fibroblast carnitine uptake in primary carnitine deficiency manifested by childhood carnitine-responsive cardiomyopathy. Pediatr Res 1990;28:247–55.
11. Bennett MJ, Narayan SB, Santani A. Updated September 7, 2010. Carnitine palmitoyltransferase 1A deficiency. In: GeneReviews at GeneTests: Medical Genetics Information Resource (database online). Copyright, University of Washington, Seattle, 1997-2011. http://www.genetests.org (Accessed February 2012).
12. Brown NF, Mullur RS, Subramanian I, Esser V, Bennett MJ, Saudubray J-M, et al. Molecular characterization of liver-type carnitine palmitoyltransferase I (L-CPT I) deficiency in six patients: insights into function of the native enzyme. J Lipid Res 2001;42:1134–42.
13. Greenberg CR, Dilling LA, Thompson GR, Seargeant LE, Haworth JC, Phillips S, et al. The paradox of the carnitine palmitoyltransferase type Ia P479L variant in Canadian Aboriginal populations. Mol Genet Metab 2009;96:201–7.
14. Park JY, Narayan SB, Bennett MJ. Molecular assay for detection of the common carnitine palmitoyltransferase 1A 1436(C>T) mutation. Clin Chem Lab Med 2006;44:1090–1.
15. Rubio-Gozalbo ME, Bakker JA, Waterham HR, Wanders RJ. Carnitine-acylcarnitine translocase deficiency, clinical, biochemical and genetic aspects. Mol Aspects Med 2004;25:521–32.
16. Iacobazzi V, Pasquali M, Singh R, Matern D, Rinaldo P, Amat di San Filippo C, et al. Response to therapy in carnitine/acylcarnitine translocase (CACT) deficiency due to a novel missense mutation. Am J Med Genet 2004;126:150–5.
17. Dietzen, DJ, Rinaldo P, Whitley RJ, Rhead WJ, Hannon WH, Garg U. National Academy of Clinical Biochemistry Laboratory Medicine Practice Guidelines: Follow-up testing for metabolic diseases identified by expanded newborn screening using tandem mass spectrometry; executive summary. Clin Chem 2009;55:1615–26.

18. Wang Y, Mohsen AW, Mihalik SJ, Goetzman ES, Vockley J. Evidence for physical association of mitochondrial fatty acid oxidation and oxidative phosphorylation complexes. J Biol Chem 2010;285:29834–41.
19. Bonnefont JP, Djouadi F, Prip-Buus C, Gobin S, Munnich A, Bastin J. Carnitine palmitoyltransferases 1 and 2: biochemical, molecular and medical aspects. Mol Aspects Med 2004;25:495–520.
20. Weiser T. Updated October 6, 2011. Carnitine palmitoyltransferase II deficiency. In: GeneReviews at Gene-Tests: Medical Genetics Information Resource (database online). Copyright, University of Washington, Seattle, 1997-2011. http://www.genetests.org (Accessed February 2012).
21. Andresen BS, Olpin S, Poorthuis BJHM, Scholte HR, Vianey-Saban C, Wanders R, et al. Clear correlation of genotype with disease phenotype in very-long-chain acyl-CoA dehydrogenase deficiency. Am J Hum Genet 1999;64:479–94.
22. Zhou C, Blumberg B. Overlapping gene structure of human VLCAD and DLG4. Gene 2003;305:161–6.
23. Harding CO, Gillingham MB, van Calcar SC, Wolff JA, Verhoeve JN, Mills MD. Docosahexaenoic acid and retinal function in children with long-chain 3-hydroxyacyl-CoA dehydrogenase deficiency. J Inher Metab Dis 1999;22:276–80.
24. Treem WR, Rinaldo P, Hale DE, Stanley CA, Millington DS, Hyams JS, et al. Acute fatty liver of pregnancy and long-chain hydroxyacyl-coenzyme A dehydrogenase deficiency. Hepatology 1994;19:339–45.
25. Ibdah JA, Bennett MJ, Rinaldo P, Zhao Y, Gibson B, Sims HF, Strauss AW. A fetal fatty-acid oxidation disorder as a cause of liver disease in pregnant women. New Eng J Med 1999;340:1723–31.
26. Spiekerkoetter U, Sun B, Khuchua Z, Bennett MJ, Strauss AW. Molecular and phenotypic heterogeneity in mitochondrial trifunctional protein deficiency due to beta-subunit mutations. Hum Mutat 2003;21:598–607.
27. Jones PM, Quinn R, Fennessey PV, Tjoa S, Goodman SI, Fiore S, et al. Improved stable isotope dilution-gas chromatography-mass spectrometry method for serum or plasma free 3-hydroxy-fatty acids and its utility for the study of disorders of mitochondrial fatty acid b-oxidation. Clin Chem 2000;46:149–55.
28. Jones PM, Butt Y, Bennett MJ. Accumulation of 3-hydroxy-fatty acids in the culture medium of long-chain L-3-hydroxyacyl CoA dehydrogenase and mitochondrial trifunctional protein deficient skin fibroblasts: implications for medium chain triglyceride dietary treatment of LCHAD deficiency. Pediatr Res 2003;53:783–7.
29. den Boer MEJ, Wanders RJA, Morris AAM, Ijlst L, Heymans HSA, Wijburg FA. Long-chain 3-hydroxyacyl-CoA dehydrogenase deficiency: clinical presentation and follow-up of 50 patients. Pediatrics 2002;109:99–104.
30. Matern D, Rinaldo P. Updated January 19, 2012. Medium-chain acyl-CoA dehydrogenase deficiency. In: GeneReviews at GeneTests: Medical Genetics Information Resource (database online). Copyright, University of Washington, Seattle, 1997-2011. http://www.genetests.org (Accessed February 2012).
31. Bennett MJ. The laboratory diagnosis of inborn errors of mitochondrial fatty acid oxidation. Ann Clin Biochem 1990;27:519–31.
32. Wilcken B, Haas M, Joy P, Wiley V, Chaplin M, Black C, et al. Outcome of neonatal screening for medium-chain acyl-CoA dehydrogenase deficiency in Australia: a cohort study. Lancet 2007;369:37–42.
33. Kelly A, Stanley CA. Hyperinsulinism. In: Sarafoglou K, Hoffmann GF, Roth KS, eds. Pediatric Endocrinology and Inborn Errors of Metabolism. New York: McGraw Hill, 2009:38–50.
34. Bennett MJ, Spotswood SD, Ross KF, Comfort S, Koonce R, Boriack RL, et al. Fatal hepatic short-chain L-3-hydroxyacyl-coenzyme A dehydrogenase deficiency: clinical, biochemical, and pathological studies on three subjects with this recently identified disorder of mitochondrial beta-oxidation. Pediat Dev Path 1999;2:337–45.
35. Li C, Chen P, Palladino A, Narayan S, Russell LK, Chen J, et al. Mechanism of hyperinsulinism in short-chain 3-hydroxyacyl-CoA dehydrogenase deficiency involves activation of glutamate dehydrogenase. J Biol Chem 2010;285:31806–18.
36. Molven A, Matre GE, Duran M, Wanders RJ, Rishaug U, Njølstad PR, et al. Familial hyperinsulinemic hypoglycemia caused by a defect in the SCHAD enzyme of mitochondrial fatty acid oxidation. Diabetes 2004;53:221–7.
37. Van Maldegem BT, Duran M, Wanders RJ, Niezen-Konig KE, Hogeveen M, Ijlst L, et al. Clinical, biochemical and genetic heterogeneity in short-chain acyl-coenzyme A dehydrogenase deficiency. JAMA 2006;296:943–52.
38. Pedersen CB, Kolvraa S, Kolvraa A, Stenbroen V, Kjeldsen M, Ensenauer R, et al. The ACADS gene variation spectrum in 114 patients with short-chain acyl-CoA dehydrogenase (SCAD) deficiency is dominated by missense variations leading to protein misfolding at the cellular level. Hum Genet 2008;124:43–56.
39. Gibson KM, Breuer J, Nyhan WL. 3-Hydroxy-3-methylglutaryl-coenzyme A lyase deficiency: review of 18 reported patients. Europ J Pediat 1988;148:180–6.

40. Pie J, Lopez-Vinas E, Puisac B, Menao S, Pie A, Casale C, et al. Molecular genetics of HMG-CoA lyase deficiency. Mol Gen Metab 2007;92:198–209.
41. Aledo R, Mir C, Dalton RN, Turner C, Pie J, Hegardt FG, et al. Refining the diagnosis of mitochondrial HMG-CoA synthase deficiency. J Inherit Met Dis 2006;29:207–11.
42. Loehr JP, Goodman, SI, Frerman FE. Glutaric acidemis type II: heterogeneity of clinical and biochemical phenotypes. Pediatr Res 1990;27:311–5.

Chapter **6**

Disorders of Carbohydrate Metabolism

Angela Ferguson, Laurie D. Smith, and Uttam Garg

Carbohydrates play important structural and metabolic roles. They are structural components of glycoproteins and nucleic acids and act as a major source of energy. In energy metabolism, glucose is the most important carbohydrate, with tightly maintained blood concentrations. During fasting, glucose is primarily produced from glycogen. Postprandially, excess glucose is stored in muscles and the liver as an energy reserve in the form of glycogen. Various other carbohydrates such as galactose and fructose are converted to glucose. Mutations in the enzymes involved in carbohydrate metabolism cause various disorders, ranging from completely benign to fatal. This chapter focuses on disorders of carbohydrate metabolism, including galactosemia, glycogen storage diseases, and disorders of fructose metabolism.

GALACTOSEMIA

The major carbohydrate found in breast milk and infant formula is lactose, a disaccharide of glucose and galactose. The Leloir pathway, which consists of galactokinase (GALK), galactose-1-phosphate-uridyltransferase (GALT), and galactose-1,4-epimerase (GALE), is responsible for the metabolism of galactose (Figure 6-1). Mutations in any of the three enzymes involved results in galactosemia with a range of clinical symptoms. Deficiency of GALT is life-threatening and is termed "classical galactosemia" *(1)*. Deficiencies of GALK and GALE are relatively rare. The former tends to have milder clinical features whereas the latter may present with either milder clinical features or as a severe form similar to classical galactosemia.

Clinical Presentation

Clinical symptoms occur within the first few days of life because of galactose, galactose-1-phosphate, and galactitol intoxication *(1)*. These include failure to thrive, feeding difficulties, vomiting, liver dysfunction leading to jaundice and coagulation defects, renal tubular dysfunction, cerebral edema, vitreous hemorrhage, formation of cataracts due to galactitol formation, and *Escherichia coli* sepsis *(1)*. Long-term complications include mental retardation and premature ovarian failure *(1)*. Multiple neurological symptoms including ataxia, tremor, speech apraxia, and cognitive impairment are also seen *(1)*.

Patients with GALE deficiency can be asymptomatic, have poor feeding and minimal accumulation of galactose metabolites with poor growth and hypotonia, or they can have a course very similar to GALT deficiency *(2–4)*. Patients with GALK deficiency accumulate high concentrations of galactose in their blood stream and tissues when on a regular diet, but once they are on a galactose-restricted diet, they have no long-term complications *(4)*. Cataracts are also seen in patients with GALK deficiency, but they self-resolve with dietary restriction if implemented early *(3–5)*.

Genetics and Pathogenesis

GALT deficiency is an autosomal-recessive condition with an incidence of 1 in 23,000 to 1 in 47,000 *(1, 3)*. The *GALT* gene is localized to chromosome 9p13 *(3)*. There are more than 230 different

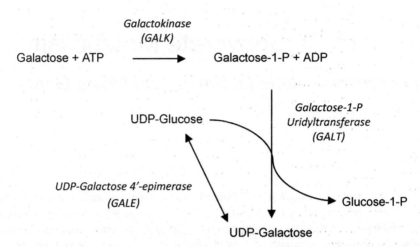

Figure 6-1   The Leloir pathway of galactose metabolism. Enzymes defective in galactosemia are italicized.

identified mutations in GALT that have less than 5% GALT enzyme activity, with the most common mutation in Caucasians being Q188R *(1)*. The Duarte variant, N314D, has up to 25% residual activity. Individuals with this mutation are phenotypically normal, even when compound heterozygosity with a more severe mutation is present *(1)*.

GALK deficiency is an autosomal-recessive condition and very rare, with an estimated incidence of 1 in 100,000 *(4)*. *GALK* is found on chromosome 17q24 *(3)*.

GALE deficiency is inherited in an autosomal-recessive fashion and is also very rare, with an unknown incidence *(4)*. *GALE* is found on chromosome 1p36 *(3)*.

Laboratory Diagnosis

Galactosemia is screened for in most newborn screening programs, commonly by screening for GALT activity in dried blood spots *(1, 3)*. In addition to GALT, some newborn screening laboratories measure total galactose. However, because of the high false-positive rate, most newborn screening laboratories have dropped this assay. It is important to keep in mind that if newborn screening is done by GALT assay alone, galactosemia due to GALK and GALE deficiency will be missed. Screening for GALT activity does not require prior ingestion of lactose, but it can be confounded if the neonate has received a blood transfusion because the enzyme activity is intracellular *(3)*. Confirmation of putative positive newborn screening results includes determination of GALT enzyme activity and galactose-1-phosphate in erythrocytes *(1, 3)*. In classical galactosemia GALT activity is generally less than 5% of controls. GALT activity can be measured by the assays involving the following reactions:

$$\text{UDPG} + \text{Galactose-1-phosphate} \rightarrow \text{UDP galactose} + \text{glucose-1-phosphate}$$

Disappearance of uridine diphosphoglucose (UDPG) is measured by the following reaction catalyzed by UDPG dehydrogenase.

$$\text{UDPG} + \text{H}_2\text{O} + 2\text{NAD+} \rightarrow \text{UDP glucuronic acid} + 2\text{H}^+ + 2\text{NADH}$$

The testing may also include measurements of galactitol and galactonate in urine. Molecular analysis involving targeted mutational analysis or gene sequencing may be performed to confirm the diagnosis and to screen for certain variants such as Duarte. Laboratory findings in GALT deficiency include conjugated and unconjugated hyperbilirubinemia, elevated transaminases, hypoglycemia, clotting abnormalities, metabolic acidosis, galactosuria, glucosuria, phosphaturia, hypophosphatemia, and hemolytic anemia *(6)*. A urine screening test for reducing substances may be positive in patients with any form of galactosemia. Testing urine for reducing substances is not sensitive or specific enough to generate a diagnosis, but it can raise clinical suspicion that will lead to further evaluation *(7)*.

Treatment and Prognosis

Treatment for galactosemia is lifelong dietary restriction of lactose and galactose. Neonates are switched to a lactose-free infant formula as soon as a diagnosis is suspected and maintained on a lactose-free formula if the diagnosis is confirmed *(1)*. Because many other foods contain hidden lactose and galactose, a metabolic dietician plays a significant role in the lifelong management of these patients. Approximately 75% of female patients develop ovarian dysfunction due to hypogonadotropic hypogonadism, but no fertility problems have been reported in male patients *(1)*. Gonadotropin concentrations (luteinizing hormone and follicle stimulating hormone) should be determined on a yearly basis after the age of 10 and pubertal development should be monitored *(1)*. Affected individuals are at a higher risk of developing osteoporosis later in life because of dietary restriction of milk and milk products, and inclusion of calcium and vitamin D supplements is recommended, along with regular monitoring of bone density. Speech therapy is essential for treatment of apraxia of speech, but some patients are completely refractory to therapy *(1)*.

GLYCOGEN STORAGE DISEASES

Glycogen storage diseases (GSDs) are a group of disorders of glycogen metabolism with mutations in enzymes that regulate the synthesis or degradation of glycogen, resulting in abnormal glycogen structures or concentrations *(1, 8)*. Figure 6-2 illustrates the main pathway of glycogen metabolism, along with the GSD that results from a specific enzyme deficiency. The organs most commonly involved include the liver and muscles; thus, the most common presenting symptoms are hypoglycemia and muscle cramps and weakness *(1, 8)*. To date, multiple different disorders have been identified, and in the different disorders, glycogenolysis, gluconeogenesis, or production of ketone bodies and lactate may be impaired *(3)*. The different GSDs are listed in Table 6-1.

Clinical Presentation

Disorders of glycogen storage mostly manifest in muscle and liver symptoms. In the disorders that mainly affect the liver, hepatomegaly and hypoglycemia are the major symptoms *(1)*. When GSDs that involve muscle are suspected, elevated lactate in blood or urine might be found, along with an elevated lactate/pyruvate ratio *(9)*.

   GSD 0 is caused by a deficiency of glycogen synthase activity. The lack of glycogen synthase leads to a decrease in liver glycogen, and carbohydrates are converted to lactate. Symptoms include postprandial hyperglycemia and hyperlacticacidemia alternating with fasting hypoglycemia and hyperketonemia *(8)*. Most children are asymptomatic unless they are fasting because of illness. Lethargy, pallor, nausea, vomiting, and seizures after a nighttime fast are all seen because of the hypoglycemia *(10)*.

   Glucose 6-phosphate is a key metabolic intermediate in the homeostatic regulation of blood glucose concentrations. Two inborn errors of glycogen metabolism directly affect glucose 6-phosphate concentrations: GSD Ia (glucose-6-phosphatase deficiency) and GSD Ib (glucose-6-phosphate translocase deficiency). GSD I is the most severe of the GSDs because of the complete blockage of glucose production from the liver. Infants present with severe fasting hypoglycemia, lactic acidemia, and hepatomegaly *(10–12)*. Patients who remain untreated can have failure to thrive, protuberant abdomen, and delayed motor development. Other characteristics of the disorder include nephromegaly, obesity, tachypnea, short stature, gout, osteoporosis, renal failure, pulmonary hypertension, and platelet dysfunction. Even with treatment, hepatomegaly and truncal obesity do not resolve. Cognitive development is not affected unless the patient suffers multiple hypoglycemic seizures. Most patients with

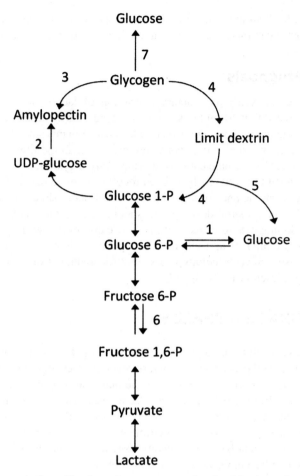

Figure 6-2   Glycogen metabolism. Numbers denote enzymes involved in the pathway and Roman numerals indicate the GSD that occurs when that enzyme is deficient: 1 = glucose-6-phosphatase (Ia), 2 = glycogen synthase (0), 3 = glycogen branching enzyme (IV), 4 = glycogen phosphorylase (V, VI), 5 = glycogen debranching enzyme (III), 6 = phosphofructokinase (VII), and 7 = α-glucosidase (II).

GSD I have GSD Ia (von Gierke disease), accounting for 80% of those diagnosed *(8)*. Patients with GSD Ib also have hematologic abnormalities, inflammatory bowel disease, and neutropenia, leading to recurrent bacterial infections. By adulthood, hepatic adenomas develop, but they are usually benign *(1)*.

GSD II (Pompe disease), a deficiency of α-glucosidase activity, can present at varying times through life. The infantile form has presenting symptoms by 6 months of age, which include severe axial hypotonia, hypertrophic cardiomyopathy, respiratory insufficiency, frequent respiratory infections, delayed motor milestones, hepatomegaly, and macroglossia *(12)*. The childhood forms are progressive and include proximal muscle weakness involving the respiratory muscles but not cardiac muscles. The juvenile/adult forms progress slowly and include proximal muscle weakness in the lower extremities *(12)*.

GSD III (Cori disease) patients have muscle and liver involvement, but symptoms can be quite variable. This disorder results from a deficiency of debranching enzyme (amylo-1,6-glucosidase) activity. Hepatomegaly, fasting hypoglycemia with ketosis, and hyperlipidemia are the most common features *(8, 10)*. These patients also have hepatomegaly, hyperlipidemia, and early growth retardation *(9)*. Liver fibrosis occurs early in the disease process but does not lead to active liver disease. GSD III can be subdivided into two groups: IIIa, the combined hepatic-myogenic form, affects the liver and muscle and

Table 6-1 Glycogen Storage Diseases

Type	Gene	Defect	Laboratory abnormalities	Tissue for enzyme analysis	Molecular testing
Ia	G6PC	Glucose-6-phosphatase	↓ Glucose, ↑ lactic acid, ↑ lipids, ↑ uric acid, ↓ ketone bodies	Liver	Available
Ib	SLC37A4	Glucose-6-phosphate translocase	↓ Glucose, ↑ lactic acid, ↑ lipids, ↑ uric acid, ↑ ketone bodies	Liver	Available
II	GAA	α-Glucosidase	↑ CK, ↑ aldolase, ↑ serum transaminases, ↑ lactate dehydrogenase, ↑ urine oligosaccharides	Lymphocytes, liver, muscle, fibroblasts, amniocytes, chorionic villi	Available
III	AGL	Glycogen debrancher enzyme	↓ Glucose, ↑ serum transaminases, ↑ CK, ↑ lactic acid (postprandial), ↑ urine oligosaccharides	Liver, muscle, fibroblasts	Available
IV	GBE1	Glycogen branching enzyme	↑ Serum transaminases, ↑ bilirubin ↑ prothrombin time	Liver, muscle, fibroblasts, white blood cells	Available
V	PYGM	Myophosphorylase	↑ CK, ↑ uric acid, abnormal nonischemic forearm test (no rise in lactic acid after exercise)	Muscle	Available
VI	PYGL	Hepatic phosphorylase	↓ Glucose, ↑ serum transaminases, ↑ fasting ketone bodies, ↑ triglycerides, ↑ cholesterol	Liver	Available
VII	PFKM	Muscle phosphofructokinase	↑ CK, ↑ uric acid,	Muscle	Available
IX	PHKA2 PHKB PHKG2	Liver phosphorylase kinase	↓ Glucose, ↑ lactic acid, ↑ serum transaminases, ↑ fasting ketone bodies, ↑ triglycerides, ↑ cholesterol	Liver, RBC	Available
0	GYS2	Glycogen synthase	↓ Glucose, ↑ lactic acid, ↑ fasting ketone bodies	Liver	Available

makes up most cases (85%); and IIIb, the hepatic form, affects only the liver and accounts for 15% of patients. Muscle symptoms become more prominent with age; however, liver symptoms improve *(10)*.

GSD IV (Andersen disease), also known as amylopectinosis or branching enzyme deficiency, can be quite heterogeneous in presentation. Presentation can range from hepatomegaly and failure to thrive in the first year of life that progresses to fatal liver cirrhosis by the fifth year of life to a mild course that includes liver disease, hypotonia, cardiomyopathy, and muscle weakness *(10)*. The disorder can be subdivided into groups on the basis of the main area of pathogenesis, with some having only liver or muscle symptomatology, whereas others have both.

GSD V (McArdle disease) is a deficiency of muscle glycogen phosphorylase and its effects are limited to muscle. Contracting muscles cannot mobilize muscle glycogen at the beginning stages of exercise, leading to fatigue *(9)*. Once the blood supply to the muscles has increased, which brings other substrates for energy generation to the muscles, symptoms disappear in what is called the "second wind" phenomenon *(9)*. Symptoms begin in childhood with muscle cramps and exercise intolerance. Acute renal failure can also be caused by transient rhabdomyolysis after exercise.

GSD VI (Hers disease) is a deficiency in liver glycogen phosphorylase, which is found only in the liver *(10)*. It has a very mild course, with hepatomegaly and fasting hypoglycemia. Patients with GSD VI are clinically identical to patients with GSD IX, phosphorylase B kinase deficiency, because the genes mutated in both disorders are involved in hepatic phosphorylase activity *(8)*. The prognosis for both disorders is good.

GSD VII (Tarui disease) is a deficiency of muscle phosphofructokinase. It is similar to GSD V in that it is divided into two forms, a severe infantile form with respiratory distress and a mild adult form with exercise intolerance *(12)*. Most patients present with muscle cramps and exercise-induced myoglobinuria. It can be distinguished from GSD V in that symptoms appear earlier in childhood and can be more severe. Nausea and vomiting, hemolytic anemia, and hyperuricemia are also present *(9)*.

X-linked GSD IX (GSD IXa or phosphorylase B kinase deficiency) is usually a mild disease, with symptoms abating during puberty. Symptoms include mild growth retardation, hepatomegaly, moderate hyperlipidemia, and fasting hypoglycemia *(1)*. GSD IXb, an autosomal-recessive condition that is caused by a mutation in the gene encoding the hepatic isoform of the b subunit of phosphorylase B kinase, is similar to GSD IXa with improvement in symptoms over time. GSD IXc is an autosomal-recessive condition caused by a mutation in the gene for the g subunit of phosphorylase B kinase, but it has a more severe course with frequent hypoglycemia and liver fibrosis that leads to cirrhosis and adenoma. Hypoglycemia and ketosis are not usually seen except in prolonged fasting or strenuous exercise *(8)*.

Genetics and Pathogenesis

The overall incidence of autosomal-recessive GSD is estimated at 1 in 20,000 to 1 in 40,000 *(1)*. GSD I is due to defective glucose-6-phosphate metabolism and can be subdivided into two disease entities based on the enzymatic defect. GSD Ia (von Gierke disease) results from mutations in the gene for glucose-6-phosphatase (*G6PC*) on chromosome 17q21.3, which is expressed in liver, kidney, and intestine. GSD Ib is caused by mutations in the *SLC37A4* gene on chromosome 11q23.3 that encodes glucose-6-phosphate translocase, which is expressed ubiquitously *(8)*. Because glucose-6-phosphate cannot be converted to glucose, release of glucose from gluconeogenesis and glycogenolysis are diminished. Catabolism of glycogen to pyruvate is not affected; thus, there is increased production of pyruvate and lactic acids. The conversion of lactic and pyruvic acids to acetyl-CoA results in increased concentrations of malonyl-CoA, which inhibits fatty acid oxidation and stimulates liponeogenesis. The net result is hypoglycemia, lactic acidemia, hyperlipidemia, and hyperuricemia and glycogen accumulation in affected organs. Patients with GSD Ib also have dysfunctional neutrophils and symptoms consistent with inflammatory bowel disease *(1)*.

GSD II is due to mutations in the *GAA* gene, which encodes lysosomal α-1,4-glucosidase located on chromosome 17q21.2-q23 *(3)*. Although this enzyme is necessary for the lysosomal degradation of glycogen to glucose, the pathogenesis of this disorder is more complicated than strictly a defect in glycogen degradation and accumulation. Recent studies point toward a problem with energy generation and autophagy as the pathogenic mechanism of cellular damage in the disorder *(13)*.

GSD III, a deficiency of glycogen debrancher enzyme, is the result of mutations *AGL* gene on chromosome 1p21.2 *(8)*. Deficiency of this enzyme, also known as amylo-1,6-glucosidase, results in massive accumulation of abnormal glycogen with shortened chains (limit dextrin) in hepatocytes *(1)*. GSD III is subdivided into four different forms based on enzyme location (a and b) and enzyme activity (c and d). Most patients have GSD IIIa, which affects liver and muscle whereas GSD IIIb only affects the liver. The glycogen debrancher enzyme has two separate catalytic activities: GSD IIIc is lacking the glucosidase activity and GSD IIId the transferase activity *(1)*.

GSD IV, also known as amylopectinosis, results from mutations in the *GBE1* gene, which encodes glycogen branching enzyme. Deficiency of this enzyme leads to accumulation of glycogen with long unbranched outer chains (amylopectin) in liver and muscle *(1)*. The gene is located on chromosome 3p12.2 *(3)*.

Myophosphorylase deficiency (GSD V) is caused by mutations in the *PYGM* gene located on chromosome 11q13.1 and it is inherited in an autosomal-recessive manner *(3)*. Muscle glycogen phosphorylase catalyzes and regulates the breakdown of glycogen to glucose-1-phosphate in the muscle; thus, symptoms are related to muscle breakdown and rhabdomyolysis secondary to energy deficiency.

GSD VI, or hepatic glycogen phosphorylase deficiency, is caused by mutations in the *PYGL* gene found on chromosome 14q22.1 *(3)*. This enzyme removes glycosyl units from the terminal branches of glycogen, forming glucose-1-phosphate, which directly enters glycolysis by conversion to glucose-6-phosphate. Although systemic hypoglycemia results from insufficient enzyme activity, the hepatic localization of this enzyme results in accumulation of glycogen in the liver with subsequent pronounced hepatomegaly.

GSD VII is caused by deficiency of muscle phosphofructokinase, which is encoded by the *PFKM* gene located on chromosome 12q13.11 *(3)*. This enzyme plays a key regulatory role in glycolysis by catalyzing the irreversible conversion of fructose-6-phosphate to fructose-1,6-bisphosphate (FBP). It is postulated that some of the observed pathogenic responses are related to increased shunting of fructose-6-phosphate through the hexose monophosphate shunt, resulting in increased hexose monophosphates, decreased 2,3-diphosphoglycerate, and increased oxygen affinity in erythrocytes *(14)*.

GSD IX is caused by multiple mutations in the phosphorylase B kinase (PHK) complex, the genes for which are found on chromosomes Xp22.1-22.2, 16q12-13, and 16p11-12 *(3, 8)*. Phosphorylase kinase activates glycogen phosphorylase, the enzyme that is deficient in GSD VI. As expected with a complex containing separate gene products, GSD IX can be divided into subtypes. The X-linked recessive form of GSD IX (XLG or IXa) is the most common form and is caused by mutations in the *PHKA2* gene. The autosomal-recessive form of GSD IX is caused by mutation in the *PHKB* gene (GSD IXb) or the *PHKG2* gene (GSD IXc) *(1)*.

GSD 0, which is really a disorder of hypoglycogenosis, is caused by mutations in the *GYS2* gene localized to chromosomal locus 12p12.1. This disorder, although included in the GSDs because of the similar clinical presentation of fasting hypoglycemia and ketosis followed by postprandial hyperlacticacidemia, actually results from decreased glycogen synthesis because of a deficiency of glycogen synthase rather than decreased glycogen catabolism and storage *(3)*.

Laboratory Diagnosis

Clinical laboratory findings seen in many of the GSDs include hypoglycemia, lactic acidemia, elevated transaminases, hyperlipidemia, hypothyroidism, prolonged bleeding time, iron refractory anemia, and hyperuricemia. These vary significantly among different forms of GSDs, although certain patterns of abnormalities may point toward a specific diagnosis. Most clinical testing used for the diagnosis of the GSDs is available as routine laboratory tests. Confirmation of diagnosis is generally accomplished by assessment of enzyme activity in erythrocytes, liver, and/or muscle. Glycogen content and structure, as identified on biopsy samples, are also used in the differential diagnosis of GSD. Glycogen content can be measured by digestion of the tissue in strong alkali and reaction of glycogen with anthrone *(15)*. Glycogen structure can be evaluated by reaction of glycogen with iodine; the wavelength of the absorption maximum increases with an increase in glycogen chain length. Table 6-1 describes commonly identified laboratory abnormalities as well as indicating appropriate tissues for enzymatic and histologic analyses.

A brief mention should be made of the nonischemic forearm test, which can be used in the evaluation if GSD V (McArdle disease) is suspected. This test relies on sampling plasma lactic acid and plasma ammonia concentrations before and immediately (within 2 min) after exercise, which consists of repeated maximal 1-second handgrips every other second for 1 min (30 contractions). Individuals with glycogenoses have exaggerated responses of plasma ammonia concentrations to exercise. In normal individuals, the lactic acid concentrations increase 5–6 times above basal concentrations whereas in individuals with GSD V, the lactic curve remains flat. The postexercise lactate/ammonia peak ratios are decreased *(16)*.

Treatment and Prognosis

Prevention of hypoglycemia is the main goal in most forms of GSD, and this can be accomplished through frequent meals of balanced carbohydrates and nocturnal continuous tube feeding or ingestion of uncooked cornstarch (8). Liver transplantation is performed in some cases of GSD (types I, III, IV), and it cures the liver disease by supplying the correct enzyme. This treatment should only be considered in cases of hepatocellular carcinoma or progressive liver failure (1).

GSD 0 can be managed by feeding the patient frequent meals that contain an increased amount of protein and fewer carbohydrates. Fasting hypoglycemia is also prevented by feeding patients uncooked cornstarch in milk at bedtime (8, 10).

Dietary control has improved the prognosis of patients with GSD I, but extended hypoglycemia can lead to mental retardation (1). Other long-term concerns for patients with GSD I are osteoporosis and fractures, gout, pancreatitis, renal complications, iron refractory anemia, and hypothyroidism (11). Most patients with GSD I have detectable hepatic adenomas by the time they reach adulthood. Progression of adenomas to hepatocellular carcinoma is a complication of GSD I and usually occurs after puberty (1). In patients with GSD Ib, granulocyte-colony stimulating factor (G-CSF) can be given to patients with neutropenia along with antibiotic prophylaxis (11). Treatment for GSD II is similar, and some patients are helped by a low-carbohydrate diet, but it is not universally successful (10).

The dietary treatment for GSD III is less intensive, with a meal of complex carbohydrates before bed being sufficient to prevent hypoglycemia. Continuous feeding of cornstarch can aid in attaining normal growth velocity for those patients who have significant growth delay (8, 10). Symptoms of patients with GSD III disappear after puberty, such as hepatomegaly, hypoglycemia, and growth retardation, but they still have a risk of developing liver cirrhosis and hepatocellular carcinoma. Once they are adults, they might experience muscle weakness that is not treatable (1).

No specific treatment exists for GSD V, but dietary modification can be helpful. It can reduce liver size and prevent hypoglycemia. Ingestion of sucrose before exercise could help ameliorate exercise intolerance (10). As in GSD V, there is no specific treatment for GSD VII, but patients can alter their physical activity and avoid strenuous exercise or stop and take breaks, resuming activity when pain and fatigue subside (9).

The prognosis for most patients with the classic, severe liver form of GSD IV is not good, with liver cirrhosis and death before the age of 5 if no transplant is received. Patients with a severe neuromuscular form also do not survive long, with severe hypotonia and muscular atrophy leading to death shortly after birth. Patients who have a rare, mild liver form can reach adulthood with no liver pathology, and patients with a juvenile muscular form have mainly myopathy (12).

GSD VI, GSD IXa (XLG), and GSD IXb all have a typically mild course, with patients' symptoms decreasing as they get older. Patients should avoid prolonged fasting and should snack before bedtime to prevent morning hypoglycemia (8). This is in contrast to patients with GSD IXc, in which liver fibrosis develops into cirrhosis and adenomas. A high-protein diet may provide increased muscle function and slow disease progression in GSD VI, but patients do not require other dietary restrictions (10).

DISORDERS OF FRUCTOSE METABOLISM

Disorders of fructose metabolism are rare with presentations ranging from benign and asymptomatic to potentially fatal. Fructose is a monosaccharide that is present in fruit, fruit juices, and honey. It is also one component of the disaccharide sucrose and is a metabolite of sorbitol. Fructose enters glycolysis after phosphorylation by fructokinase and subsequent metabolism to dihydroxyacetone phosphate and glyceraldehyde. Glucose-6-phosphate, an intermediate in glycolysis and gluconeogenesis, also undergoes isomerization to fructose-6-phosphate, which is then phosphorylated to fructose bisphosphatase. This compound is also a precursor for glyceraldehyde-3-phosphate and dihydroxyacetone phosphate and is an integral compound in glycolysis, gluconeogenesis, glyconeogenesis, and glycogenolysis. Disorders in this catabolic pathway include essential fructosuria (fructokinase deficiency), hereditary fructose intolerance (aldolase B deficiency), and fructose bisphosphatase deficiency.

Clinical Presentation

Fructokinase deficiency leads to a benign condition called essential fructosuria, which is an asymptomatic elevation of fructose in serum and urine. This condition is diagnosed accidentally when nonglucose reducing substances are identified during urine screening. The serum fructose concentration of zero in a normal individual increases to approximately 0.5 mM after an oral dose of fructose and then decreases over the next 90 min. The fructose concentration after the same dose of fructose in a fructokinase-deficient individual is closer to 3 mM and remains elevated for several hours *(17)*.

In hereditary fructose intolerance (HFI), a deficiency of the enzyme aldolase B results in an accumulation of fructose-1-phosphate and inhibition of hepatic glycogenolysis and gluconeogenesis *(1)*. HFI is the most common inborn error of fructose metabolism. Infants and children with this disorder have no symptoms until they consume fructose, sucrose, or sorbitol, which usually occurs when they are introduced to sucrose-containing formula, solid foods with added sugars, or fruits and vegetables *(18, 19)*. Breastfed infants are asymptomatic until weaning because breast milk contains lactose. Clinical symptoms include hypoglycemia, poor feeding, nausea, vomiting, pallor, abdominal pain, sweating, restlessness, lethargy, coagulation disturbances, metabolic acidosis, convulsions, and coma *(17, 18, 20)*. If fructose is not eliminated from the diet, the clinical course becomes chronic including failure to thrive, liver disease (with hepatomegaly, jaundice, steatosis, edema, and ascites), growth failure, and proximal renal tubular dysfunction *(19, 20)*. Acute hypoglycemia after fructose ingestion is short-lived and can be masked by accompanying glucose ingestion. Some older children develop an aversion to food containing fructose before a diagnosis after experiencing abdominal pain and nausea after consumption *(18, 20)*.

Fructose bisphosphatase is required for formation of glucose from gluconeogenic precursors, and deficiency leads to fasting hypoglycemia, ketosis, and acidosis. Hypotonia and hepatomegaly are often present as well *(17)*. Neonates often present in the first few days of life with hyperventilation due to severe lactic acidosis because their glycogen reserves are limited. Other fasting episodes, such as during an illness or after an overload of fructose after a fasting period, can also produce symptomatic episodes. Other clinical symptoms include irritability, somnolence, moderate hepatomegaly, muscular hypotonia, dyspnea, tachycardia, and coma *(1)*.

Genetics and Pathogenesis

Fructokinase is encoded by the *KHK* gene localized to chromosome 2p23. Fructokinase phosphorylates fructose to yield fructose-1-phosphate, which is the first step in fructose metabolism. Inheritance of essential fructosuria is autosomal recessive and has an incidence of 1 in 130,000, although this is difficult to ascertain because of the lack of identification of most affected individuals *(17)*. This is a benign condition.

Inheritance of HFI is autosomal recessive and has an incidence of 1 in 20,000 *(18)*. The aldolase B enzyme cleaves fructose-1-phosphate and FBP into dihydroxyacetone phosphate, glyceraldehydes, and glyceraldehyde-3-phosphate and converts the triose phosphates into glucose and lactate. The gene for aldolase B (*ALDOB*) is on chromosome 9q22.3 *(18)*. Hypoglycemia results from the accumulation of fructose-1-phosphate, which inhibits hepatic glycogenolysis and gluconeogenesis and depletes adenosine triphosphate. Many mutations in the aldolase B gene have been described that lead to loss of function. Approximately 50% of affected individuals of European descent have been found to have a G-to-C transversion that replaces an alanine with a proline *(19)*. A cost-effective approach to identifying molecular disorders involves screening for the most common alleles followed by complete sequencing if necessary. Approximately 84% of the mutations in the aldolase B gene found in Europeans are represented by three alleles, A149P, A174D, and N334K *(20)*.

Fructose bisphosphatase deficiency is autosomal recessive and has an unknown incidence, projected to be approximately 1 in 350,000. FBP, encoded by *FBP1* on 9q22.32, is a critical enzyme in gluconeogenesis, and when absent results in impaired formation of glucose from all gluconeogenic precursors. FBP dephosphorylates fructose-1,6-diphosphate to form fructose-6-phosphate, and when it is deficient, it disrupts the balance between glycolysis and gluconeogenesis *(17)*.

Laboratory Diagnosis

Patients with fructose metabolism disorders will have a positive test for reducing sugars but a negative test for glucose oxidase. Fructose can be identified by thin layer chromatography and be quantified by enzymatic or chromatographic methods. Patients with essential fructosuria do not show an increase in glucose with a fructose-loading test as would be seen in normal subjects, nor do these patients exhibit hypoglycemia as in HFI or FBP deficiency.

Laboratory data in HFI can include signs of acute liver failure, such as elevated serum transaminases, hyperbilirubinemia, and blood clotting factor abnormalities. Proteinuria, hyperaminoaciduria, and metabolic acidosis can also be seen, indicating proximal renal tubular dysfunction *(17, 20)*. Other metabolic abnormalities include hypoglycemia, hypophosphatemia (due to inorganic phosphate trapping), renal bicarbonate loss, and hyperuricemia (due to inhibition of adenosine monophosphate deaminase) *(20)*.

Molecular testing using either targeted mutational analysis or complete gene sequencing of the aldolase B gene is available for confirmation of HFI. If a causative mutation is not identified, aldolase B enzymatic activity can be determined from a liver biopsy. Isoenzyme activity of aldolase A is present in blood cells, muscle, and skin fibroblasts, so these specimens are not appropriate for diagnosis *(1)*. DNA analysis can be used to make the diagnosis of FBP, but if inconclusive, determination of FBP enzymatic activity from a liver biopsy sample can be done. Leukocytes may also be used to assess enzymatic activity, but normal activity in leukocytes does not rule out an abnormality in the liver activity *(17)*. Patients also show a massive lactic acidosis, with lactate of 15–25 mM and a lactate/pyruvate ratio up to 30 *(1)*. Urinary organic acid excretion is similar to that seen in tyrosinemia type 1, but with the absence of succinylacetone. Other intermediates seen include lactate; pyruvate; ketone bodies; adipic, suberic, and sebacic acids; and glycerol-3-phosphate. Glycerol is also seen on urine organic acid analysis and can be important diagnostically because the process that usually converts excess glycerol generated during fasting to glucose is nonfunctional *(17)*. Although once commonly used to make the diagnosis, intravenous or oral fructose-loading testing is no longer recommended for the diagnosis of these disorders.

Treatment and Prognosis

Disorders of fructose metabolism span the gamut of prognoses. Fructosuria is completely benign, has an excellent prognosis, and needs no treatment.

Treatment for HFI consists of elimination of fructose, sucrose, and sorbitol from the diet, including foods sweetened with high-fructose corn syrup *(20)*. This elimination resolves clinical symptoms and laboratory abnormalities. Careful examination of medications and infant formulas must be undertaken because these products often contain fructose, sucrose, or sorbitol. Parenteral infusions containing fructose or sorbitol are life-threatening *(1, 17, 18)*. With dietary treatment, the prognosis for HFI is excellent. Hepatomegaly might persist, but with unknown clinical relevance. Patients typically have no cavities throughout their life. Tolerance for fructose increases slightly with age, but multivitamins should be prescribed because of the lack of fruits and vegetables in the diet *(1)*.

Treatment for an acute metabolic decompensation related to FBP includes oral glucose or intravenous dextrose and bicarbonate to control the acidosis. After diagnosis, patients have a fairly benign course without growth or psychomotor impairment, and the tolerance of fasting improves with age *(1)*. In between attacks, patients have mild acidosis but are generally well. To avoid acute incidents, it is recommended that fasting be avoided by feeding frequently, which can be accomplished with slow-absorbing carbohydrates such as uncooked cornstarch or a gastric drip *(17)*. Additionally, it is recommended that small children restrict fructose, sucrose, sorbitol, and fat. Patients do have a tendency toward obesity because of their need for continual feeding to avoid metabolic decompensation. Similar to patients with HFI, patients with FBP deficiency should avoid infusions that contain fructose or sorbitol *(17)*.

REFERENCES

1. Mayatepek E, Hoffmann B, Meissner T. Inborn errors of carbohydrate metabolism. Best Pract Res Clin Gastroenterol 2010;24:607–18.
2. Leslie ND. Insights into the pathogenesis of galactosemia. Annu Rev Nutr 2003;23:59–80.
3. Haack Ka, Bennett MJ. Genetic metabolic disorders. In: Dietzen DJ, Bennett MJ, Wong ECC, eds. Biochemical and Molecular Basis of Pediatric Disease, 4th ed. Washington, DC: AACC Press, 2010:235–60.
4. Fridovich-Keil JL. Galactosemia: the good, the bad, and the unknown. J Cell Physiol 2006;209:701–5.
5. Bosch AM, Bakker HD, van Gennip AH, van Kempen JV, Wanders RJ, Wijburg FA. Clinical features of galactokinase deficiency: a review of the literature. J Inherit Metab Dis 2002;25:629–34.
6. Bosch AM. Classical galactosaemia revisited. J Inherit Metab Dis 2006;29:516–25.
7. Ridel KR, Leslie ND, Gilbert DL. An updated review of the long-term neurological effects of galactosemia. Pediatr Neurol 2005;33:153–61.
8. Wolfsdorf JI, Weinstein DA. Glycogen storage diseases. Rev Endocr Metab Disord 2003;4:95–102.
9. Das AM, Steuerwald U, Illsinger S. Inborn errors of energy metabolism associated with myopathies. J Biomed Biotechnol 2010; article 340849.
10. Heller S, Worona L, Consuelo A. Nutritional therapy for glycogen storage diseases. J Pediatr Gastroenterol Nutr 2008;47 Suppl 1:S15–21.
11. Koeberl DD, Kishnani PS, Bali D, Chen YT. Emerging therapies for glycogen storage disease type I. Trends Endocrinol Metab 2009;20:252–8.
12. Shin YS. Glycogen storage disease: clinical, biochemical, and molecular heterogeneity. Semin Pediatr Neurol 2006;13:115–20.
13. Raben N, Roberts A, Plotz PH. Role of autophagy in the pathogenesis of Pompe disease. Acta Myol 2007;26:45–8.
14. Vora S, Davidson M, Seaman C, Miranda AF, Noble NA, Tanaka KR, et al. Heterogeneity of the molecular lesions in inherited phosphofructokinase deficiency. J Clin Invest 1983;72:1995–2006.
15. Seifter S, Dayton S, et al. The estimation of glycogen with the anthrone reagent. Arch Biochem 1950;25:191–200.
16. Kazemi-Esfarjani P, Skomorowska E, Jensen TD, Haller RG, Vissing J. A nonischemic forearm exercise test for McArdle disease. Ann Neurol 2002;52:153–9.
17. Hommes FA. Inborn errors of fructose metabolism. Am J Clin Nutr 1993;58:788S–795S.
18. Ali M, Rellos P, Cox TM. Hereditary fructose intolerance. J Med Genet 1998;35:353–65.
19. Bouteldja N, Timson DJ. The biochemical basis of hereditary fructose intolerance. J Inherit Metab Dis 2010;33:105–12.
20. Wong D. Hereditary fructose intolerance. Mol Genet Metab 2005;85:165–7.

Chapter 7

Lysosomal Storage Disorders: Mucopolysaccharidoses and Mucolipidoses

Andrea M. Atherton, Laurie D. Smith, Bryce A. Heese, and Uttam Garg

Lysosomes are intracellular organelles that contain hydrolytic enzymes essential for the degradation and recycling of macromolecules including glycosaminoglycans, oligosaccharides, glycoproteins, and lipids. Lysosomal storage diseases include defects in specific enzymes within the lysosome as well as in the transport of enzymes into the lysosome. Over 50 inherited lysosomal storage diseases have been identified. These defects lead to an accumulation or "storage" of macromolecules within the lysosome, resulting in accumulation or increase in lysosomal size. Abnormally functioning lysosomes lead to cellular, tissue, and organ dysfunction and a clinical phenotype that typically results in multisystem involvement. Although there may be phenotypic similarities among the different disorders, the diagnoses are distinct. Also, specific lysosomal storage disorders also have marked phenotypic variability within the same disorder. Efforts have been made to identify genotype-phenotype correlations. Some mutations, such as whole gene deletions, frameshift mutations, or premature stop codons, may produce more severe phenotypes than single point mutations. The genetics of these conditions are further confounded by the presence of compound heterozygosity. This chapter will focus on the mucopolysaccharidoses, multiple sulfatase deficiency, and the mucolipidoses.

MUCOPOLYSACCHARIDOSES

Mucopolysaccharidoses (MPS) are a group of lysosomal storage disorders caused by the deficiency of enzyme(s) that break down glycosaminoglycans (GAGs). Accumulation of GAGs within the lysosomes causes multisystem cellular and organ dysfunction. All individuals with MPS disorders generally have high excretion of urine GAGs. The clinically significant GAGs are dermatan sulfate (DS), heparan sulfate (HS), keratan sulfate (KS), and chondroitin sulfate (CS). Seven types of MPS disorders have been identified (Table 7-1). There is allelic and locus heterogeneity such that different defects in the same or different genes may produce similar phenotypes. MPS disorders are chronic, progressive disorders that affect multiple organ systems. Most infants with MPS disorders appear normal at birth, developing characteristics of the disorder over time. However, coarse facial features may be present at birth in some cases.

The MPS, although differing in the enzymatic defect, characteristically present with very similar clinical features. These features include poor linear growth (short stature), macrocephaly, gingival hypertrophy, macroglossia, periorbital fullness, short neck, enlarged tonsils and adenoids, sleep apnea, hearing loss, hepatosplenomegaly, inguinal and umbilical hernias, frequent upper and lower respiratory infections and ear infections, cardiac valve disease, corneal clouding, bone dysplasia (dysostosis multiplex), scoliosis, gibbus deformity, kyphosis, hip dysplasia, cervical spine stenosis, cord compression, carpal tunnel syndrome, and cognitive impairment. Those with attenuated MPS I may have normal growth and development and typically live a normal lifespan but can develop joint disease and cardiac valve disease. Corneal clouding, although a feature of most MPS disorders, is not considered a primary characteristic of either Hunter syndrome (MPS-II) or Sanfilippo syndrome (MPS-III) *(1)*. Clinical features of various MPS are shown in Table 7-1.

Table 7-1 Clinical Features in Various MPS

MPS Type	Coarse facial features	Mental retardation	Corneal clouding	Hepatomegaly	Dysostosis multiplex	Other clinical features
Type I, Hurler	+++	+++	+++	+++	+++	Cardiac disease, motor weakness, hernia
Type I, Scheie	+	-	+	-	+	Stiff joints
Type I, Hurler/Scheie	++	±	++	+	++	Phenotype intermediate
Type II, Hunter	++	+++	-	++	++	Weakness, aggressive behavior
Type IIIA, Sanfilippo	+	+++	-	+	++	Mild somatic features, aggressive behavior
Type IIIB, Sanfilippo	+	+++	-	+	++	Mild somatic features, aggressive behavior
Type IIIC, Sanfilippo	+	+++	-	+	++	Mild somatic features, aggressive behavior
Type IIID, Sanfilippo	+	+++	-	+	++	Mild somatic features, aggressive behavior
Type IVA, Morquio	+	-	+	-	++	Hypoplastic odontoid, thin enamel
Type IVB, Morquio	+	-	+	+	+	Hypoplastic odontoid
Type VI, Maroteaux-Lamy	++	-	++	+	++	Valvular cardiac disease
Type VII, Sly	±	+	±	+	+	

The pathogenesis of the MPS disorders is caused by the accumulation of intermediates specific to the individual disorder that results in lysosomal swelling and dysfunction, ultimately disrupting normal cellular and organ functions.

Mucopolysaccharidosis Type I (Hurler Syndrome, Hurler-Scheie Syndrome, Scheie Syndrome)

Clinical Presentation. Mucopolysaccharidosis type I (MPS-I) is a chronic, progressive lysosomal storage disorder caused by a deficiency of the enzyme α-L-iduronidase *(1–3)*. Historically, the diagnosis of MPS-I has been categorized into three subgroups, Hurler syndrome, Hurler-Scheie syndrome and Scheie syndrome, on the basis of the severity of disease. There are no clear criteria that define these subgroups, and enzymatically these patients are indistinguishable from one another. The current recommendation is to use the nomenclature of severe MPS-I and attenuated MPS-I to denote those with MPS-I who have cognitive deficits and those without.

The major causes of morbidity in individuals with MPS-I include airway disease, respiratory infection, and heart disease. Lifespan is variable and dependent on the level of severity and effectiveness of interventions. Without treatment, a child with severe MPS-I may only live until the age of 5. With treatment, death may occur in the second or third decade of life secondary to cardiac disease. Individuals with mild MPS-I may live well into adulthood.

Genetics and Pathogenesis. The MPS-I spectrum is an autosomal-recessive genetic disorder caused by a mutation in the *IDUA* gene on chromosome 4p16.3, which encodes the enzyme α-L-iduronidase that removes l-iduronic acid from the nonreducing terminus of polysaccharide chains, particularly HS and DS (Figure 7-1). The enzyme deficiency causes an accumulation of DS and HS within the lysosome. The former primarily affects bones and cartilage whereas the latter is toxic to the brain. These GAGs can easily be identified in the urine.

Treatment. Individuals diagnosed with the severe form of MPS-I before 2.5–3 years of age may be offered bone marrow or stem cell transplantation as a treatment option *(3)*. Bone marrow transplantation (BMT) is not typically recommended for the milder attenuated forms of MPS-I. Bone marrow and stem cell transplantation (SCT) does not cure MPS-I. However, it does delay the progression of some of the symptoms commonly seen in this disorder *(4, 5)*. Combined therapy with enzyme replacement therapy (ERT) and BMT/SCT is currently being studied. Therapy with laronidase (Aldurazyme®), a genetically engineered enzyme, is the standard of care for the treatment of MPS-I. Overall, treatment with ERT has been shown to decrease urine GAG excretion, decrease hepatosplenomegaly, and improve pulmonary function tests and performance on a 5-min walk test *(6)*. It does not completely ameliorate the deposition of HS and DS systemically and does not cure the disease *(7)*. Other treatments are palliative and system-specific *(2)*.

Mucopolysaccharidosis Type II (Hunter Syndrome)

Clinical Presentation. Mucopolysaccharidosis type II (MPS-II or Hunter syndrome) is a chronic and progressive lysosomal storage disorder with variable age of onset, presentation of symptoms, and rate of progression, affecting multiple organ systems *(1, 3, 8)*. Given the variation in MPS-II, patients are often classified as severe MPS-II or a more mild attenuated form (attenuated MPS-II). Individuals with MPS-II are usually asymptomatic at birth, developing features over time. The more severe form of MPS-II is characterized by cognitive impairment with decline, progressive airway disease, and heart disease. Death usually occurs in the first, second, or third decades of life. Those with an attenuated form of MPS-II typically have no to minimal cognitive involvement, living well into adulthood. Pebbly, cream/white-colored skin lesions (peau d'orange) are seen in some individuals with MPS-II that are not seen in any other MPS disorder and can aid in the diagnosis of MPS-II. Corneal clouding is not typically seen in MPS-II.

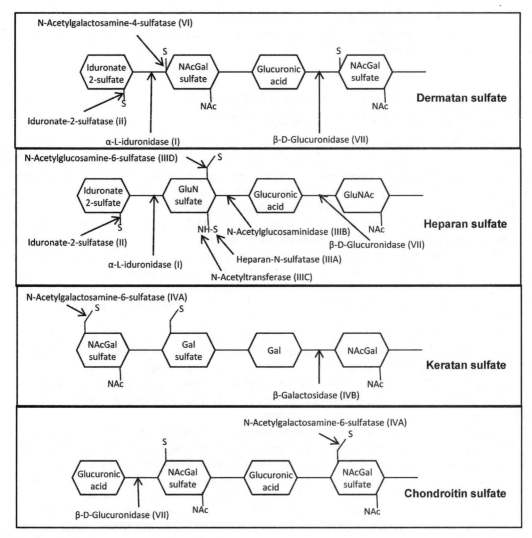

Figure 7-1 The catabolism of various GAGs. The catabolism starts from the nonreducing (left) end of GAGs. MPS types associated with different enzyme deficiencies are identified by Roman numeral in parentheses.

Genetics and Pathogenesis. MPS II is an X-linked recessive disorder that primarily affects males, although a few females have been identified because of skewed X-inactivation patterns or inheritance of another sex chromosome abnormality. Mutations in the *IDS* gene on the X-chromosome lead to a deficiency of the enzyme iduronate-2-sulfatase. This exoenzyme removes the C2 sulfate from l-iduronic acid residues at the nonreducing ends of heparin, HS, and DS. Affected individuals, similarly to those with MPS I, excrete high concentrations of urinary GAGs, HS, and DS.

Treatment. A genetically engineered ERT, idursulfase (Elaprase®) is available for the treatment of MPS II. As with Hurler syndrome, ERT slows but does not ameliorate progression of the disease and thus is not a cure. Specific effects include improvement in pulmonary function tests and performance on a 5-min walk test as well as decreasing the urinary excretion of GAGs. Phase I intrathecal delivery of iduronate-2-sulfatase is currently being investigated. BMT has not been demonstrated to be an effective treatment *(9)*. Other therapies using small molecules, substrate reduction, and gene therapy are still in preclinical development *(10)*. Other interventions are supportive and palliative.

Mucopolysaccharidosis Type III (Sanfilippo Syndrome)

Clinical Presentation. Mucopolysaccharidosis type III (MPS III or Sanfilippo syndrome) is a group of four lysosomal storage disorders that share similar clinical features but are caused by four distinct enzyme deficiencies *(1, 11)*. Collectively, MPS III is the most common MPS disorder. Unlike the other MPS disorders, features of MPS III are not typically apparent until after the first year of life with most symptoms developing between the ages of 2 and 6 years. Given the variability in the enzymes, the presentation of MPS III may be delayed well into adulthood. The hallmark features are cognitive impairment with regression, behavior abnormalities, mild coarse facial features with full lips, thick eyebrows with synophrys, diarrhea, sleep disturbances, vision loss (retinopathy), seizures, joint limitations, difficulties with ambulation, and neuropathy.

Genetics and Pathogenesis. Four enzymatic steps are required for the removal of N-sulfated or N-acetylated glucosamine residues during the degradation of HS: heparan-*N*-sulfatase (sulfamidase), *N*-acetylglucosaminidase, glucosamine-*N*-acetyltransferase, and *N*-acetylglucosamine-6-sulfatase *(12)*. Deficiency of any one of these enzymes, encoded by four different genes, leads to MPS III. All of these conditions are inherited in an autosomal-recessive manner. The brain is preferentially affected rather than somatic tissues.

MPS IIIA, the most severe form, is caused by a deficiency of heparan-*N*-sulfatase (sulfamidase), which is encoded by the *SGSH* gene on chromosome 17q25.3. Approximately 60% of individuals with MPS III have a deficiency of this enzyme deficiency.

MPS IIIB is caused by a deficiency of α-*N*-acetylglucosaminidase, which is encoded by the *NAGLU* gene on chromosome 17q21.1. MPS IIIB accounts for 30% of patients with MPS III.

MPS IIIC is caused by a deficiency of glucosamine-*N*-acetyltransferase, which is encoded by the *HGSNAT* gene on chromosome 8p11.1. MPS IIIC accounts for 5% of patients with MPS III.

MPS IIID is caused by a deficiency of *N*-acetylglucosamine-6-sulfatase, which is encoded by the *GNS* gene on chromosome 12q14. MPS IIID accounts for 5% of patients with MPS III.

Treatment. Although currently under development for MPS IIIA, ERT is not yet available for any of the subtypes of MPS III. Interventions include behavioral management and supportive and palliative measures.

Mucopolysaccharidosis Type IV (Morquio Syndrome)

Clinical Presentation. Mucopolysaccharidosis type IV (MPS IV, Morquio syndrome) is a lysosomal storage disorder with two subtypes—MPS IVA and MPS IVB—that are clinically and biochemically indistinguishable *(1, 13)*. Affected individuals, although having significant short stature in addition to clinical findings similar to the other MPS disorders, have no cognitive deficits but may have neurological involvement secondary to severe skeletal involvement and spinal cord compression. MPS IVB is allelic to GM1 gangliosidosis, but cognitive impairment is seen in the latter condition and not in MPS IVB. There can be a wide range of phenotypic variability among affected individuals. Rib cage abnormalities combined with severe scoliosis often lead to marked respiratory insufficiency *(13)*.

Genetics and Pathogenesis. MPS IV is inherited in an autosomal-recessive manner. Two genes have been identified that produce two different enzymatic defects with similar phenotypes.

MPS IVA is caused by mutations in the GALNS gene located on chromosome 16q24 that encodes the enzyme *N*-acetylgalactosamine-6-sulfatase, which is responsible for the breakdown of keratan sulfate and chondroitin-6-sulfate. Deficiency results in an accumulation of keratan sulfate within the lysosome. Keratan sulfate and chondroitan-6-sulfate are major structural molecules in the cornea, connective tissue, cartilage, and bone.

MPS IVB is caused by deficiency of the enzyme β-galactosidase encoded by the GLB1 gene located on chromosome 3p21.33. Mutations in the GLB1 gene associated with MPS IVB are different from those seen in GM1 gangliosidosis. Enzyme concentrations and turnover are normal; however, there is a decrease in affinity and catalytic activity for keratan sulfate with preservation of degradative activity for GM1 ganglioside *(14)*. An alternative splice form of β-galactosidase has been identified (S-Gai/EBP) that acts as an elastin-/laminin-binding protein. Compound heterozygotes for this splice site variant and a mutation in the *GLB1* gene present as a unique form of MPS IVB with absent catalytic activity for KS, along with functionally impaired tropoelastin secretion and elastin fiber assembly *(15)*.

Treatment. Currently, treatments are all supportive and palliative. ERT for MPS IVA, although being developed and tested, is not currently available.

Mucopolysaccharidosis Type VI (Maroteaux-Lamy Syndrome)

Clinical Presentation. Mucopolysaccharidosis type VI (MPS VI) is a chronic and progressive lysosomal storage disorder affecting multiple body systems. Cognition is typically spared in individuals with MPS VI. As with the other MPS disorders, the severity of disease status varies from mild to severe *(16)*.

Genetics and Pathogenesis. MPS VI is an autosomal-recessive genetic disorder caused by defects in the *ARSB* gene, which encodes *N*-acetylgalactosamine-4-sulfatase (arylsulfatase B) and is located on chromosome 5q14.1. The enzyme removes a 4-sulfate group from the nonreducing terminus of chondroitin-4-sulfate and DS. The enzyme deficiency results in accumulation of DS primarily in the skin, cornea, cartilage, and bones. The central nervous system is spared. It has recently been postulated that the enzyme may have a broader influence on cellular function as a regulatory protein by modifying chondroitin-4-sulfate *(17)*.

Treatment. ERT (galsulfase; Naglazyme®) is available for the treatment of MPS VI. This, along with supportive and palliative interventions, is the current standard of care for treatment of the disorder.

Mucopolysaccharidosis Type VII (Sly Syndrome)

Clinical Presentation. Mucopolysaccharidosis type VII (MPS VII or Sly disease) is a highly variable lysosomal storage disorder with a range of presentation from severe hydrops fetalis in utero to a milder form with an intermediate phenotype consisting of hepatomegaly, coarse facial features, skeletal abnormalities, cardiac valve disease, and varying degrees of cognitive impairment. It is very rare, occurring at a frequency of less than 1 in 250,000 births *(18)*.

Genetics and Pathogenesis. MPS VII is an autosomal-recessive genetic disorder caused by mutations in the *GUSB* gene located on chromosome 7q21.11, leading to a deficiency of the enzyme β-glucuronidase. The enzyme is involved in the catabolism of the glucuronic acid containing the GAGs chondroitin sulfate, DS, and HS.

Treatment. Treatment is primarily supportive and palliative. ERT is not currently under development.

Laboratory Diagnosis of MPS

Because mucopolysaccharides (GAGs) are excreted in the urine of patients with MPS, urine is a specimen of choice for initial testing. The urine testing for GAGs generally involves qualitative screening and quantification of total GAGs. Identification of GAGs is generally done through thin layer chromatography (TLC) or electrophoresis. Confirmation involves assay of specific enzyme(s) in leukocytes or cultured fibroblasts. Confirmation may also involve mutational analysis or DNA sequencing of a specific gene.

Random urine is generally used for the assay of GAGs. There is no need for preservatives if the sample is refrigerated and the testing can be done in 2–3 days. If the testing cannot be completed in 2–3 days, the sample should be frozen. For send-out laboratory studies, the sample should be frozen after collection and shipped frozen to the reference laboratory.

Common screening methods for GAGs are the Berry spot test and cetylpyridinium chloride (CPC) precipitation. Berry spot tests are based on the principle that toluidine blue, a cationic dye, reacts with GAGs to produce a pink-colored complex. The test can be performed on a filter paper or in a tube. Use of a sample spotted on filter paper is more common. The dried filter paper is dipped into a toluidine solution followed by washing the paper with acetic acid to remove excess dye. A positive test is indicated by pinkish-light blue spot. The reaction of CPC with the acidic GAGs forms a turbid solution and/or precipitate. This screening method is neither very sensitive nor specific. Therefore, the results should be interpreted with caution.

Quantification of total GAGs is also used in the laboratory diagnosis of the MPS. Because excretion of GAG varies with age and sample dilution, quantitative methods provide better results than qualitative methods. Several methods exist for the quantification of total GAGs. One method involves the use of Alcian blue dye. The dye is added to the urine sample resulting in a dye-GAG complex that forms a precipitate. The precipitate is isolated by centrifugation, dissolved in sodium dodecylsulfate, and measured at 620 nm by a spectrophotometer. Another method for quantification of GAGs is the 1,9-dimethylene blue (DMB) binding method. This method is preferred over the Alcian blue method because of higher sensitivity. DMB forms complexes with GAGs that can be measured at 520 nm.

Identification of GAGs is required to make a diagnosis of a MPS and should be performed on all positive screen samples and suspected negative samples. Electrophoresis and TLC are two commonly used methods for the identification of GAGs. After isolation of GAGs from urine by precipitation with buffered quaternary ammonium salts such as CPC, the precipitated GAGs are isolated by centrifugation and washed with ethanol and resuspended in water. Five to ten microliters of the suspension is applied to the electrophoretic or TLC plate. After separation of GAGs, the plate is dried and stained with dyes such as Alcian blue and toluidine blue. The plate is destained with acetic acid. An example of a TLC plate is shown in Figure 7-2.

Table 7-2 shows the urinary GAG excretion pattern seen in the different MPS. Confirmation of a suspected MPS requires specific enzyme analysis. Enzyme assays should be performed on all positive samples and suspected negative samples. Leukocytes or cultured fibroblasts are generally used for measuring the enzyme activities.

Techniques for measuring lysosomal enzymes in dried blood spots have recently been developed for use in newborn screening. For leukocytes, blood is collected in heparin- or ethylenediaminetetraacetic acid (EDTA)-containing tubes and sent to a reference laboratory by overnight mail in a container containing cold packs. It is important that the sample be shipped cold but not frozen. For fibroblasts, cultured cells or a skin biopsy sample is sent in an appropriate culture medium. Leukocytes or fibroblasts are isolated by density gradient centrifugation and buffered homogenates are made using sonication. Commonly used assays involve artificial 4-methylumbelliferyl substrates in acidic buffers. Cleavage of these substrates produces fluorescence that is measured by a fluorometer at an excitation wavelength of 365 nm and an emission wavelength of 450 nm and is directly proportional to the enzyme activity. Commonly used substrates are given in Table 7-3. Tandem mass spectrometric methods involving artificial substrates are also available.

Molecular testing including targeted mutation and sequence and deletion/duplication analysis is recommended for confirmation of this disorder.

MULTIPLE SULFATASE DEFICIENCY

Clinical Presentation

Multiple sulfatase deficiency (MSD) is a severe disorder that presents with combined clinical and biochemical features of the MPS and metachromatic leukodystrophy. The biochemical defect results in a deficiency of 12 sulfatases leading to rapid neurological deterioration, excessive excretion of GAGs in several tissues, and excretion of sulfatides in the urine. Coarse facial features are not usually a feature

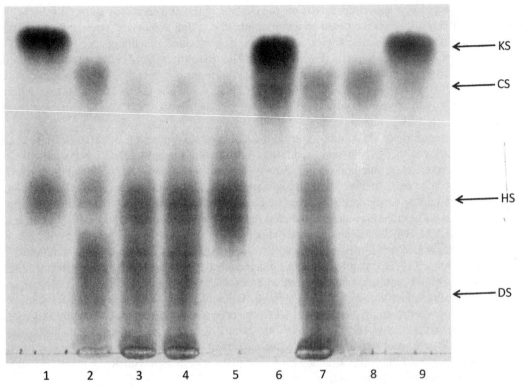

Figure 7-2 TLC for separation of various GAGs *(24)*. Urine GAGs were precipitated with CPC-citrate, washed with ethanol, and dissolved in water. Ten microliters of the solution was applied to the cellulose TLC plate. GAGs were separated using six mobile phases containing an increasing concentration of acetate buffer and a decreasing concentration of ethanol. The plate was dried, stained with toluidine blue, and destained with acetic acid. Lane 1 = keratin sulfate (KS) and HS, lane 2 = chondroitin-4-sulfate (CS4), HS, and DS, lane 3 = MPS I, lane 4 = MPS-II, lane 5 = MPS-III, lane 6 = MPS IV, lane 7 = MPS VI, lane 8 = normal, and lane 9 = chondroitin-6-sulfate (CS6) and KS.

of the disorder; however, the somatic features of dysostosis multiplex, cardiac valve disease, corneal clouding, retinopathy with vision loss, hearing loss, recurrent infections, gingival hypertrophy, joint stiffness, carpal tunnel syndrome, and neuropathy are present. Ichthyosis is also common because of steroid sulfatase deficiency. Metachromatic degeneration of myelin on peripheral nerve biopsy and elevated urinary sulfitides, which are cardinal features of metachromatic leukodystrophy, are also seen in MSD. MSD is a highly variable disorder with a wide range of clinical features. Most individuals with MSD die before the age of 10, although several individuals have been reported to have lived into the second and third decades of life *(19)*.

Table 7-2   Urinary GAG Excretion Pattern in Different Mucopolysaccharidoses

Mucopolysaccharidoses	DS	HS	CS-4	CS-6	KS
Type I, Hurler	Elevated	Elevated	Normal	Normal	Normal
Type II, Hunter	Elevated	Elevated	Normal	Normal	Normal
Type III, Sanfilippo	Normal	Elevated	Normal	Normal	Normal
Type IVA, Morquio A	Normal	Normal	Normal	Elevated	Elevated
Type IVB, Morquio B	Normal	Normal	Normal	Normal	Elevated
Type VI, Maroteaux-Lamy	Elevated	Normal	Normal	Normal	Normal
Type VII, Sly	Elevated	Elevated	Normal	Elevated	Normal

Table 7-3 Commonly Used Fluorescent Substrates for Different Enzymes in Various Mucopolysaccharidoses

Mucopolysaccharidoses	Enzyme	4-Methylumbelliferyl-β-ᴅ-glucuronide
Type I, Hurler	α-ʟ-Iduronidase	4-Methylumbelliferyl-α-ʟ-(idopyranosid)-uronic acid
Type II, Hunter	Iduronate-2-sulfatase	4-Methylumbelliferyl-α-iduronate-2-sulfate
Type IIIA, Sanfilippo	Heparan-N-sulfatase	4-Methylumbelliferyl-α-ᴅ-N-sulfoglucosamide
Type IIIB, Sanfilippo	α-N-Acetylglucosaminidase	4-Methylumbelliferyl-N-acetyl-α-ᴅ-glucosaminide
Type IIIC, Sanfilippo	Glucosamine-N-acetyltransferase	4-Methylumbelliferyl-β-ᴅ-glucosaminide
Type IIID, Sanfilippo	N-Acetylglucosamine-6-sulfatase	4-Methylumbelliferyl α-N-acetylglucosaminide-6-sulfate
Type IV-A, Morquio	N-Acetylgalactosamine-6-sulfatase	4-Methylumbelliferyl-β-ᴅ-6-sulfo-N-acetylglucosaminide
Type IV-B, Morquio	α-ᴅ-Galactosidase	4-Methylumbelliferyl-β-ᴅ-galactoside
Type VI, Maroteaux-Lamy	N-Acetylgalactosamine-4-sulfatase (arylsulfatase B)	4-Nitrocatechol
Type VII, Sly	α-ᴅ-Glucuronidase	4-Methylumbelliferyl-β-ᴅ-glucuronide

Genetics and Pathogenesis

MSD is an autosomal-recessive condition caused by defects in the *SUMF1* gene located on chromosome 3p26 that leads to a deficiency of the enzyme formylglycine-generating enzyme. This enzyme is responsible for activating a group of enzymes known as sulfatases by generating an α-formylglycine residue from an evolutionarily conserved active site cysteine residue by oxidation of the thiol group. In MSD, all sulfatase enzymes (iduronate-2-sulfatase, sulfamidase, glucosamine-6-sulfatase, *N*-acetylgalactosamine-6-sulfatase, arylsulfatase B, *N*-acetylgalactosamine-4-sulfatase, glucuronate-2-sulfatase, glucosamine-3-sulfatase, arylsulfatase A, arylsulfatase C, arylsulfatase E, and arylsulfatase F) are affected and have reduced activities toward their substrates. Deficiency of these enzymes leads to abnormal accumulation of oligosaccharides, mucopolysaccharides, and glycoproteins.

Although rare, MSD must be considered whenever a lysosomal storage disease is suspected because there is considerable clinical phenotypic overlap among the lysosomal storage disorders. Genotype/phenotype correlations have been reported with nonsense mutations being the most severe and missense mutations being less severe. Mutations can be correlated with projected enzymatic stability and residual activity *(19)*. An incorrect diagnosis can be given if a complete workup is not done. If a lysosomal storage disorder is identified involving a deficiency of one of the sulfatases and DNA testing does not confirm the disorder, additional testing for MSD may be warranted.

Laboratory Diagnosis

Laboratory diagnosis of MSD is relatively straightforward because a characteristic pattern of deficiency is observed in various cell types. Identification of abnormal urinary oligosaccharides, mucopolysaccharides, and glycoprotein profiles by TLC or matrix-assisted laser desorption–tandem time-of-flight mass spectrometry suggests the diagnosis, as well as enzymatic assay of arylsulfatase A and arylsulfatase B. Confirmation of the diagnosis is by DNA sequencing of *SUMF1*.

Treatment

Treatment is supportive and palliative.

MUCOLIPIDOSES

Sialidosis (Mucolipidosis Type 1, ML I)

Clinical Presentation.   Sialidosis, or mucolipidosis type I (ML I), is a severe condition caused by a deficiency of lysosomal α-neuraminidase *(20)*. There are two types: sialidosis type I and sialidosis type II. Sialidosis type I, the less severe form, presents in the second to third decades of life with macular cherry-red spots and generalized myoclonus. Approximately 50% of affected individuals will also have seizures, hyperreflexia, and/or ataxia. Sialidosis type I has no effect on cognitive ability or life expectancy, but it does affect multiple body and organ systems. Sialidosis type II, the more severe form, is further characterized as a congenital, infantile, or juvenile form. The congenital form of sialidosis type II is often identified prenatally with hydrops fetalis, fetal demise, stillbirth, or death shortly after birth. Features of hepatosplenomegaly and dysostosis multiplex are seen. The infantile form of this condition is a progressive disorder with an MPS-like phenotype with hepatosplenomegaly, dysostosis multiplex, myoclonus, macular cherry-red spots, hearing loss, and intellectual disability. The juvenile form presents in late childhood with a mild MPS phenotype of coarse facial features, mild dysostosis multiplex, myoclonus, macular cherry-red spots, and intellectual disability. Life expectancy is dependent on the severity of symptoms.

Genetics and Pathogenesis.   Sialidosis is an autosomal-recessive genetic disorder caused by defects in the *NEU1* gene located on chromosome 6p21.3, which leads to a deficiency of lysosomal α-neuraminidase. Neuraminidase is important for removing sialic acid from sialiated glycoproteins and oligosaccharides in the lysosomes. Lamp1 (lysosomal associated membrane protein), which provides selectins with carbohydrate ligands, is a substrate for neuraminidase activity. Abnormal desialation of Lamp1 results in dysregulation of and an increase in the calcium-dependent exocytosis of lysosomal hydrolases *(21)*. This ultimately results in lysosome dysfunction with accumulation and excretion of sialidated glycoproteins and oligosaccharides along with increased excretion of sialic acid. Unlike Salla disease, in which sialic acid accumulates in its free form, absent neuraminidase activity results in accumulation of sialic acid bound to glycoproteins and oligosaccharides.

Laboratory Diagnosis.   If sialidosis is suspected, a urine screening test evaluating urinary oligosaccharides and sialylglycoproteins should be done. Abnormal patterns of these compounds will be seen on TLC. Confirmation of a definitive diagnosis depends on direct measurement of enzyme activity, using 4-methylumbelliferyl-β-*N*-acetylneuraminic acid as the substrate, in fibroblasts, cultured amniocytes, or leucocytes. Care must be taken to avoid freezing or sonication of the tissue sample. Confirmation may also be made by determining specific mutations within the *NEU1* gene.

Treatment.   There is no definitive treatment for sialidosis, and interventions revolve around supportive care.

Mucolipidosis Type II/III (I-Cell Disease and Pseudo-Hurler Polydystrophy)

Clinical Presentation.   Mucolipidosis type II or I-cell disease (ML-II) and pseudo-Hurler polydystrophy (ML-III) result from different mutations in the enzyme *N*-acetylglucosamine-1-phsophotransferase. These disorders lead to defective targeting and transport of hydrolytic enzymes into the lysosome. ML-II has many features in common with MPS I but with an earlier presentation. Notably, there is no or minimal elevation of urine mucopolysaccharides. ML-II is a very severe and progressive disorder characterized by severe psychomotor retardation and many of the stigmata of MPS I, which are often noted at birth, if not in early infancy, with death usually occurring in early childhood. On the other hand, ML-III is milder with a later presentation and survival into adulthood *(22)*.

Genetics and Pathogenesis.   ML-II and ML-III are autosomal-recessive genetic disorders caused by defects in the *GNPTAB* gene located on chromosome 12q23.3. This gene encodes *N*-acetylglucosamine-1-phosphotransferase, an enzyme required for synthesis of mannose-6-phosphate recognition markers for enzymes transport to the lysosome. Without this recognition marker, receptor-mediated targeting of hydrolytic enzymes to the lysosomes from the Golgi apparatus does not occur and the hydrolases are secreted into the extracellular medium *(23)*. Plasma activities of β-D-hexosaminidase, β-D-glucuronidase, β-D-galactosidase, and α-L-fucosidase are most helpful in determining the diagnosis. ML-II and ML-III are considered to represent a continuum on a clinical spectrum. There is no true genotype-phenotype correlation; rather, the disorders are distinguished by age of onset and severity of clinical symptoms.

Laboratory Diagnosis.   As described above, in ML-II and ML-III, *N*-acetylglucosamine-1-phosphotransferase, an enzyme required for synthesis of mannose-6-phosphate recognition sites for enzymes transport to the lysosomes, is deficient. This results in very low intracellular enzyme activities and very high lysosomal hydrolase activities (five- to twentyfold) in the plasma and cell culture media. Diagnosis of ML-II and ML-III is made by assessment of serum lysosomal enzyme concentrations and by estimating the ratio of extracellular to intracellular enzyme activities. Assay of all of the lysosomal enzymes is not needed for the confirmation of diagnosis. Demonstration of increased activity, in plasma or cell culture media, of a few enzymes (particularly β-D-hexosaminidase, β-D-glucuronidase, β-D-galactosidase, and α-L-fucosidase) suffices to make the diagnosis. Phosphotransferase activity can also be measured. Specific activities of lysosomal hydrolases in peripheral leukocytes is normal; thus, measurement in leukocytes is of no additional diagnostic value. Mutation analysis is useful in confirming the diagnosis of a mucolipidosis but cannot distinguish between ML-II and ML-III.

Treatment.   There is currently no definitive treatment for ML-II or ML-III other than supportive interventions. BMT has not been demonstrated to be effective.

ACKNOWLEDGMENTS

The authors thank Judy Peat for Figure 7-2 in the TLC of MPS.

REFERENCES

1. Coutinho MF, Lacerda L, Alves S. Glycosaminoglycan storage disorders: a review. Biochem Res Int 2012; article 471325.
2. Beck M, Muenzer J, Scarpa M. Evaluation of disease severity in mucopolysaccharidoses. J Pediatr Rehabil Med 2010;3:39–46.
3. Neufeld E, Muenzer J. The mucopolysaccharidoses. In: Scriver CR, Beaudet AL, Sly WS, Valle D, Childs B, Kinzler KW, Vogelstein B, eds. The Metabolic and Molecular Basis of Inherited Disease, 8th ed. New York: McGraw-Hill, 2001.
4. Souillet G, Guffon N, Maire I, Pujol M, Taylor P, Sevin F, et al. Outcome of 27 patients with Hurler's syndrome transplanted from either related or unrelated haematopoietic stem cell sources. Bone Marrow Transplant 2003;31:1105–17.
5. Staba SL, Escolar ML, Poe M, Kim Y, Martin PL, Szabolcs P, et al. Cord-blood transplants from unrelated donors in patients with Hurler's syndrome. N Engl J Med 2004;350:1960–9.
6. Wraith EJ, Hopwood JJ, Fuller M, Meikle PJ, Brooks DA. Laronidase treatment of mucopolysaccharidosis I. BioDrugs 2005;19:1–7.
7. Clarke LA, Wraith JE, Beck M, Kolodny EH, Pastores GM, Muenzer J, et al. Long-term efficacy and safety of laronidase in the treatment of mucopolysaccharidosis I. Pediatrics 2009;123:229–40.
8. Muenzer J, Beck M, Eng CM, Escolar ML, Giugliani R, Guffon NH, et al. Multidisciplinary management of Hunter syndrome. Pediatrics 2009;124:e1228–39.
9. Mullen CA, Thompson JN, Richard LA, Chan KW. Unrelated umbilical cord blood transplantation in infancy for mucopolysaccharidosis type IIB (Hunter syndrome) complicated by autoimmune hemolytic anemia. Bone Marrow Transplant 2000;25:1093–7.
10. Beck M. Therapy for lysosomal storage disorders. IUBMB Life 2010;62:33–40.
11. Valstar MJ, Neijs S, Bruggenwirth HT, Olmer R, Ruijter GJ, Wevers RA, et al. Mucopolysaccharidosis type IIIA: clinical spectrum and genotype-phenotype correlations. Ann Neurol 2010;68:876–87.
12. Esposito S, Balzano N, Daniele A, Villani GR, Perkins K, Weber B, et al. Heparan N-sulfatase gene: two novel mutations and transient expression of 15 defects. Biochim Biophys Acta 2000;1501:1–11.
13. Tomatsu S, Montano AM, Oikawa H, Smith M, Barrera L, Chinen Y, et al. Mucopolysaccharidosis type IVA (Morquio A disease): clinical review and current treatment. Curr Pharm Biotechnol 2011;12:931–45.
14. van der Horst GT, Kleijer WJ, Hoogeveen AT, Huijmans JG, Blom W, van Diggelen OP. Morquio B syndrome: a primary defect in beta-galactosidase. Am J Med Genet 1983;16:261–75.
15. Hinek A, Zhang S, Smith AC, Callahan JW. Impaired elastic-fiber assembly by fibroblasts from patients with either Morquio B disease or infantile GM1-gangliosidosis is linked to deficiency in the 67-kD spliced variant of beta-galactosidase. Am J Hum Genet 2000;67:23–36.
16. Giugliani R, Federhen A, Rojas MV, Vieira T, Artigalas O, Pinto LL, et al. Mucopolysaccharidosis I, II, and VI: brief review and guidelines for treatment. Genet Mol Biol 2010;33:589–604.
17. Bhattacharyya S, Kotlo K, Shukla S, Danziger RS, Tobacman JK. Distinct effects of N-acetylgalactosamine-4-sulfatase and galactose-6-sulfatase expression on chondroitin sulfates. J Biol Chem 2008;283:9523–30.
18. Norato DJ. Mucopolysaccharidosis type VII (Sly Disease): clinical, genetic diagnosis and therapies. In: Barranger JA, Cabrera-Salazar MA, eds. Lysosomal Storage Disorders. New York: Springer, 2007.
19. Schlotawa L, Ennemann EC, Radhakrishnan K, Schmidt B, Chakrapani A, Christen HJ, et al. SUMF1 mutations affecting stability and activity of formylglycine generating enzyme predict clinical outcome in multiple sulfatase deficiency. Eur J Hum Genet 2011;19:253–61.

20. Lowden JA, O'Brien JS. Sialidosis: a review of human neuraminidase deficiency. Am J Hum Genet 1979;31:1–18.
21. Yogalingam G, Bonten EJ, van de Vlekkert D, Hu H, Moshiach S, Connell SA, et al. Neuraminidase 1 is a negative regulator of lysosomal exocytosis. Dev Cell 2008;15:74–86.
22. Otomo T, Muramatsu T, Yorifuji T, Okuyama T, Nakabayashi H, Fukao T, et al. Mucolipidosis II and III alpha/beta: mutation analysis of 40 Japanese patients showed genotype-phenotype correlation. J Hum Genet 2009;54:145–51.
23. Jornfeld S, Sly WS. I-cell disease and pseudo-Hurler polydystrophy: disorders of lysosomal enzyme phosphorylation and localization. In: Shriver DR, Beaudet AL, Sly WS, Valle D, eds. The Metabolic and Molecular Basis of Inherited Disease, 8th ed. New York: McGraw-Hill, 2001;3469–82.
24. Dembure PP, Roesel RA. Screening of mucopolysaccharidoses by analysis of urinary glycosaminoglycans. In: Hommes FA, ed. Techniques in diagnostic human biochemical genetics. New York: Wiley-Liss, 1991: 77–86.

Chapter 8

Lysosomal Storage Disorders: Sphingolipidoses and Lysosomal Transport Disorders

Andrea M. Atherton, Laurie D. Smith, Bryce A. Heese, and Uttam Garg

As noted in the previous chapter, the mucopolysaccharidoses and mucolipidoses occur because of deficiencies of lysosomal enzymes necessary for the catabolism of glycosaminoglycans, sialiated glycoproteins, and oligosaccharides. However, lysosomes also play an important role in the degradation of other molecules. The accumulation of the catabolic intermediates associated with other enzyme deficiencies also results in lysosomal dysfunction. This chapter will discuss several other inborn errors of lysosomal degradation. With the large number of known lysosomal storage disorders, an in-depth discussion of each is not possible given the scope of this book. Common sphingolipidoses and lysosomal transport defects are discussed. The metabolism of various glycosphingolipids and sphingomyelin is shown in Figure 8-1.

SPHINGOLIPIDOSES

Fabry Disease

Clinical Presentation.   Fabry disease is a highly variable and slowly progressive lysosomal storage disorder, with insidious onset of acroparesthesia of the hands and feet, often during childhood. Neuropathy and hypohydrosis are also common features. Angiokeratomas, characteristic skin lesions on the lower abdomen, buttocks, and scrotum, occur in approximately 80% of affected individuals. Ocular lesions include dilatation of conjunctival and retinal venules. Whorl-like corneal opacities may be seen as early as 6 months of age. Posterior capsule cataracts are pathognomonic for the disorder. Renal disease develops slowly with initial proteinuria progressing to end-stage renal disease. Pulmonary and cardiac involvement along with cerebral vascular disease are also known complications that often lead to premature death. Psychiatric illness (depression and bipolar disorder) is common, as is chronic pain. Males are typically more severely affected than affected females because this is an X-linked disorder. There is more clinical variability in heterozygous females secondary to random X-chromosome inactivation. Death in males usually occurs in the fifth decade from renal or heart disease *(1)*.

Genetics and Pathogenesis.   Fabry disease is an X-linked lysosomal storage disorder caused by deficiency of α-galactosidase A secondary to mutations in the *GLA* gene located on chromosome Xq22. This enzyme functions to break down glycosphingolipids such as globotriaoslyceramide (Gb3). Inability to degrade these glycosphingolipids results in intralysosomal accumulation in the nerves, vessels, tissues, and organs throughout the body. Fabry disease is the most common lysosomal storage disease after Gaucher disease, occurring in between 1 in 40,000 and 60,000 live births for males.

Laboratory Diagnosis.   Diagnosis is usually made, after the disorder is clinically suspected in males, by measuring α-galactosidase activity in plasma, leukocytes, or cultured cells. Diagnosis can be

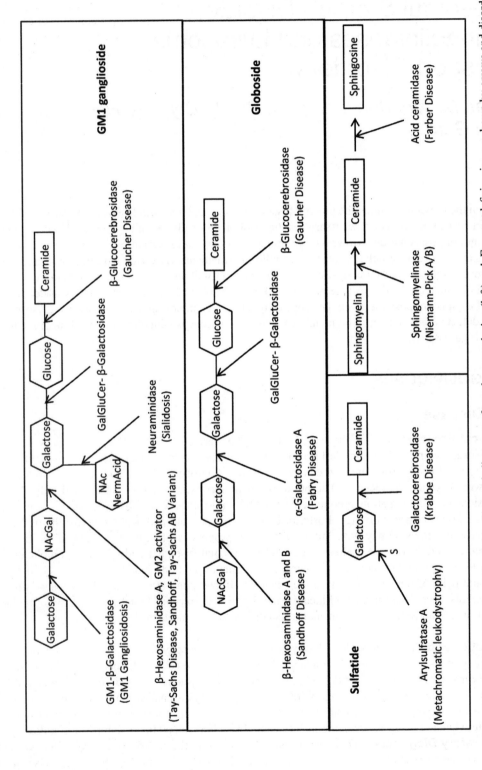

Figure 8-1 The catabolism of various glycolipids. The catabolism starts from the nonreducing (left) end. Enzyme deficiencies are shown by arrows and disorders are shown in parentheses.

made using dried blood spots, but confirmation in leukocytes and/or plasma is recommended. Certain pathologic mutations such as p.Asn215Ser affect intracellular trafficking, packaging, and secretion of the enzyme. To demonstrate reduced enzyme activity due to these mutations, plasma is a better specimen than leukocytes. Because enzyme concentrations may be normal in heterozygous females, enzyme assay is not considered a reliable method to assess carrier status. The α-galactosidase assay is a fluorometric method that uses 4-methylumbelliferyl-α-D-galactopyranoside as substrate. Fluorescence is measured at an excitation wavelength of 366 nm and an emission wavelength of 442 nm.

Urinary Gb3 can also be used as a marker for diagnosis and treatment monitoring of Fabry disease. This may be the most reliable biochemical screening test because urinary Gb3 is elevated in untreated hemizygous males and heterozygous females. Plasma Gb3 is elevated in males but not in heterozygous females. Gb3 can be measured by incubating a urine sample with the enzyme agalsidase-a and subsequently determining the amount of galactose produced. Gb3 can also be measured by mass spectrometry.

Molecular testing involving targeted mutational or sequence analysis of *GLA* is available. Molecular testing is particularly useful in the confirmation of diagnosis of heterozygous females with a related affected male. Without a related male, molecular testing can be difficult to interpret given the many polymorphisms in the gene.

Treatment.   Enzyme replacement therapy (ERT) with agalsidase-β and agalsidase-α (Fabrazyme® and Replagal®) is available for the treatment of Fabry disease. ERT has been demonstrated to reduce the risks of the renal and cardiac disease associated with Fabry disease. It has not been shown to ameliorate pain, thus additional treatment is supportive *(2)*.

Gaucher Disease

Clinical Presentation.   Gaucher disease (GD), another highly variable lysosomal storage disorder, has been subdivided into five subgroups: type I, type II, type III, perinatal-lethal, and cardiovascular.

GD type I is the most common form of GD, particularly in the Ashkenazi Jewish population. It is a non-neuronopathic condition that presents with anemia, thrombocytopenia, hepatosplenomegaly, fatigue, pulmonary disease, and bony problems (osteoporosis, lytic lesions, and avascular necrosis). Cognition is not affected *(3)*. With the advent of enzyme replacement and substrate reduction therapies, the lifespan of affected individuals can be normal.

Types II and III, in addition to having the typical systemic features of type I, also have primary neurological dysfunction *(4)*. Type II is a more severe, progressive disorder with earlier onset than type III. Neurologic abnormalities include oculomotor apraxia, cognitive impairment, psychomotor impairment, and seizures. Death usually occurs between 2 and 4 years of age. GD type III is more slowly progressive with death occurring in the third to fourth decade of life: This can be variable and is dependent on the rate of progression of disease. Although ERT or substrate reduction therapy is designed to ameliorate the systemic features of GD, ERT does not cross the blood brain barrier and therefore has no effect on the neurological features of the more severe forms of GD. Substrate reduction therapy may cross the blood brain barrier, but it has not yet been studied in patients with type II and III GD.

The perinatal-lethal form of GD often presents with nonimmune hydrops fetalis, collodion membrane defects, and ichthyoids in utero. These babies are stillborn or die shortly after birth.

The cardiovascular form of GD presents with calcification of the heart valves, splenomegaly, supranuclear ophthalmoplegia, and corneal opacities. The varying levels of heart disease (age of onset and severity) that have been described in all subtypes of GD should be monitored accordingly.

Genetics and Pathogenesis.   All forms of GD are inherited in an autosomal-recessive fashion and are caused by mutations in the *GBA* gene located on chromosome 1q21, which encodes acid β-glucocerebrosidase, the enzyme for the breakdown of glucosylcerebroside. Accumulation of glycosylcerebroside affects mononuclear phagocytosis and results in the presence of "Gaucher cells" *(5)*.

There is some genotype-phenotype correlation. Homozygosity for the N370S mutation may lead to a milder form of GD type I, although variability exists. Compound heterozygosity for N370S and another mutation results in GD type I but with earlier onset of clinical symptoms. Homozygosity for the L444P mutation has been associated with neurological symptoms and GD type III. The L444P mutation in association with a more severe mutation, such as a recombinant allele, produces a phenotype of GD type II. Homozygosity for the recombinant allele produces a perinatal-lethal phenotype. Additional mutations in the GBA gene have been classified and are associated with specific genotype-phenotype correlations, but additional discussion on this topic is beyond the scope of this book.

Laboratory Diagnosis. Laboratory diagnosis of GD is made by demonstration of reduced acid β-glucocerebrosidase activity in leukocytes or cultured fibroblasts using fluorometric methods. Enzyme activity is not reliable for identifying carrier status. The method uses 4-methylumbelliferyl-β-D-glucopyranoside as substrate and measurement of fluorescence at an excitation wavelength of 366 nm and emission wavelength of 442 nm.

Molecular testing of the *GBA* gene is used for the confirmation of biochemical findings of GD or carrier detection. Molecular testing involving targeted mutational or sequence analysis of *GBA* gene is available. Four mutations, N370S, L444P, 84GG, and IVS2+1, account for approximately 90% of the disease-causing alleles in the Ashkenazi Jewish population. In non-Jewish populations, these four alleles account for approximately 50–60% of disease-causing alleles.

Treatment. ERT (Cerezyme® and VPRIV®) and a substrate reduction therapy (Zavesca®) are clinically available treatment modalities that have led to improvement and stabilization of biochemical markers, stabilization of anemia and thrombocytopenia, normalization of splenomegaly, reduction in liver size, and decreased frequency of bone crises.

Acid-Sphingomyelinase Deficiency (Niemann-Pick Disease Type A and B)

Clinical Presentation. Acid sphingomyelinase deficiency has historically been classified into two categories: neuronopathic and non-neuronopathic. The former is known as Niemann-Pick type A (NPD-A) and the latter as Niemann-Pick type B (NPD-B). NPD-A presents with progressive hepatosplenomegaly before 3 months of age, jaundice, psychomotor and cognitive impairment with regression, failure to thrive, macular cherry-red spots, and interstitial lung disease. Death usually occurs by the age of 3. NPD-B has similar systemic features but slower progression and disease severity than NPD-A. Cognition is often normal in these patients who may live well into adulthood. Hyperlipidemia and thrombocytopenia are also observed in NPD-B *(6)*.

Genetics and Pathogenesis. Acid sphingomyelinase deficiency is an autosomal-recessive genetic condition caused by defects in the *SMPD1* gene located on chromosome 11p15.4-p15.1. This enzyme is responsible for breakdown of sphingomyelin. Accumulation of sphingomyelin occurs in the reticuloendothelial and other cell types within the body. Ganglion cells in the brain are also affected. Founder effects have been identified in the Ashkenazi Jewish population for NPD-A and in the African population for NPD-B *(6)*.

Laboratory Diagnosis. Diagnosis of NPD-A/NPD-B is made by demonstrating acid sphingomyelinase deficiency in blood lymphocytes or cultured fibroblasts. Enzyme activity in affected individuals is typically <10% of controls. Enzyme assays using artificial fluorogenic substrates or radioactive natural substrates have been described. It is important to note that individuals with the *SMPD1* mutation p.Gln294Lys may have apparently normal enzymatic activity when using artificial fluorogenic substrates.

Molecular testing involving targeted mutational or sequence analysis of the *SMPD1* gene is available. Three mutations, p.Arg498Leu, p.Leu304Pro, and p.Phe333SerfsX52, account for approximately 90% of NPD-A disease-causing alleles in the Ashkenazi Jewish population. The p.Arg610del is a major mutation in NPD-B disease. It may account for almost 90% of mutant alleles in individuals from the Maghreb region of North Africa (i.e., Tunisia, Algeria, and Morocco), 100% of alleles in Gran Canaria Island, and 20–30% of NPD-B mutant alleles in persons of North African descent in the United States *(7)*. Analysis of other disease-causing mutations and sequence analysis of *SMPD1* is used to detect mutations in affected individuals and carriers.

Treatment. Treatment for NPD-A and NPD-B is generally supportive. Bone marrow transplantation has been tried for the treatment of NPD-B, but it does not affect the neurologic deterioration, limiting its effectiveness given the morbidity and mortality associated with the procedure. ERT for NPD-B is in development.

GM1 Gangliosidosis

Clinical Presentation. GM1 gangliosidosis, a variable and progressive lysosomal storage disorder, can present as an infantile form (type I), a late infantile/juvenile form (type II), or an adult/chronic form (type III). Type I is associated with onset of symptoms within the first 6 months of life with dysmorphic facial features, hepatosplenomegaly, skeletal involvement (dysostosis multiplex), cherry-red macular changes, and rapid neurologic and psychomotor regression. Death usually occurs early in life. Type II disease, which presents with neurocognitive and psychomotor regression but lacks hepatic and splenic involvement and cherry-red macular changes, usually presents between 7 months of age and 3 years of life with death occurring in the late first decade or second decade of life. Type III GM1 gangliosidosis is characterized by onset of disease between the ages of 3 and 30 years with localized central nervous system (CNS) involvement (dystonia, ataxia, or speech disturbances), muscle atrophy, angiokeratomas, and/or corneal opacities. As with type II, hepatosplenomegaly and macular cherry-red spots are not generally present in type III GM1 gangliosidosis *(8)*.

Genetics and Pathogenesis. GM1 gangliosidosis is an autosomal-recessive genetic condition caused by defects in the *GLB1* gene located on chromosome 3p21.33 that result in a deficiency of β-galactosidase. This lysosomal enzyme is important in the breakdown of ganglioside substrates. Accumulation of gangliosides is toxic to the CNS system and there is an inverse correlation between disease severity and residual enzyme activity *(8)*. A founder effect for this disorder exists in the Ashkenazi Jewish, French Canadian, and Louisiana Cajun populations with a carrier frequency of 1 in 27.

Laboratory Diagnosis. Laboratory diagnosis of GM1 gangliosidosis involves the measurement of β-galactosidase activity in leukocytes or cultured fibroblasts with affected individuals having enzyme activity of <0.1% of normal. Low β-galactosidase activity is not a specific finding in GM1 gangliosidosis because it is also low in Morquio syndrome B and galactosialidosis, clinically distinct disorders. Other clinical and laboratory findings must be used to distinguish these disorders: In galactosialidosis, neuraminidase activity will also be low whereas in Morquio syndrome B there will be increased excretion of keratan sulfate in urine. Enzyme activity does not reliably detect carriers. "Pseudodeficient enzyme activity," a situation in which an individual shows greatly reduced enzyme activity without pathologic or clinical features, has been reported for β-galactosidase.

Measurement of β-galactosidase activity involves the use of fluorescent substrate 4-methylumbelliferyl-β-D-galactoside and measurement of fluorescence at an excitation wavelength of 365 nm and an emission wavelength of 450 nm.

Treatment. Treatment is currently limited to supportive and symptomatic treatment.

GM2 Gangliosidosis (Tay-Sachs Disease, Sandhoff Disease, and GM2-Activator Deficiency)

Clinical Presentation. The GM2 gangliosidoses are a group of autosomal-recessive disorders that affect the expression of β-*N*-acetyl-hexoaminidase A (Hex A), β-*N*-acetyl-hexoaminidase B (Hex B), and/or GM2-activator protein, resulting in neuronal accumulation of GM2-ganglioside and several other related glycolipids *(9)*. All present with progressive cerebral degeneration, blindness, hyperacusis, and cherry-red macular spots with onset of symptoms typically beginning at approximately 6 months of age.

Tay-Sachs disease, a deficiency of Hex A, presents with infantile cerebral and retinal degeneration that initially becomes clinically apparent at approximately 6 months of age. Accumulation of GM2-ganglioside begins in utero. The disease is rapidly progressive with blindness, rigidity, and decerebrate posturing universally present by 12–18 months followed by death, usually from aspiration and pneumonia, by 2–4 years of age.

Sandhoff disease, a deficiency of both Hex A and Hex B, is difficult to clinically distinguish from Tay-Sachs disease. Hepatosplenomegaly is often present in Sandhoff disease and absent in Tay-Sachs disease. The age and progression of presentation is also very similar to Tay-Sachs disease. Later-onset forms have been described. Those with the most severe forms die by age 4 from aspiration or pneumonia. Those with less severe forms of the disorder have been reported to present between 2 and 10 years of age with blindness and decerebrate posturing by 10–15 years and death soon thereafter. Adult patients presenting with psychiatric symptoms have been described.

GM2-activator deficiency is nearly identical in its presentation and course to Tay-Sachs disease, although onset and progression may be slightly slower. GM2-activator acts as a protein cofactor for Hex A. There is no obvious storage of GM2-ganglioside in the viscera, as can be seen with Hex B deficiency. Death usually occurs between 1 and 4 years of age.

Genetics and Pathogenesis. Tay-Sachs disease is caused by mutations in the *HEXA* gene on chromosome 15 and subsequent dysfunction of the α subunit of Hex A. Sandhoff disease is caused by mutations in the *HEXB* gene on chromosome 5 that produce defective β subunits, affecting Hex A and Hex B activity *(10)*. GM2-activator deficiency is caused by mutations in the *GM2A* gene on chromosome 5. GM2A encodes a protein that acts as a cofactor that stimulates Hex A activity. Its effects are related to the inability of Hex A to degrade GM2-ganglioside. A pseudodeficiency state has also been identified with no activity against artificial in vitro substrates with functional in vivo Hex A activity. All result from the interruption of the metabolic pathway of glycosphingolipid metabolism and the accumulation of GM2-ganglioside. All disorders have lipid-laden histiocytes along with membranous cytoplasmic bodies on electron microscopy. Conjunctival biopsy will also show vacuolated cells and lamellar inclusions.

Laboratory Diagnosis. Diagnosis of Tay-Sachs disease relies on demonstration of an isolated deficiency of the enzyme Hex A with normal or increased activity of Hex B, typically using leukocytes. Serum and cultured fibroblasts can also be used. Figure 8-2 shows the graphic representation of correlation between HEX A activity and degradation of GM2-ganglioside in fibroblasts from normal individuals; heterozygous parents; and patients with severe, juvenile, and adult forms of Tay-Sachs disease. Affected individuals have <10% enzyme activity. Obligate heterozygotes have enzyme activities between affected and normal individuals *(11)*. The Hex A fluorescent assay involves 4-methylumbelliferyl-6-sulfo-2-acetamido-2-deoxy-β-D-glucopyranoside as a substrate. Enzyme activity is estimated by measuring the fluorescence at an excitation wavelength 366 nm and an emission wavelength of 442 nm. Tandem mass spectrometric assays are also available for the assay of Hex A. Confirmation is done by DNA mutation analysis. Molecular testing may also be helpful in distinguishing pseudodeficiency alleles from disease-causing mutations.

Lack of both Hex A and Hex B activity in leukocytes, serum, or cultured fibroblasts is used to diagnose Sandhoff disease with confirmation by DNA mutational analysis. The combined activity of Hex A and Hex B can be measured using 4-methylumbelliferyl-6-sulfo-2-acetamido-2-deoxy-β-D-glucopyranoside as a substrate. Because Hex A is heat labile, the activity of Hex B can be measured by heating the homogenate at 51.5 °C for 1 h to inactivate Hex B *(12)*. Patients with Sandhoff disease may have *N*-acetylglucosamine-containing oligosaccharides in their urines.

GM2-activator deficiency is suspected when in vitro assays for Hex A and Hex B are normal or elevated with artificial substrates but the patient clinically appears to have Tay-Sachs disease. GM2-activator deficiency is often diagnosed by demonstration of GM2-ganglioside in

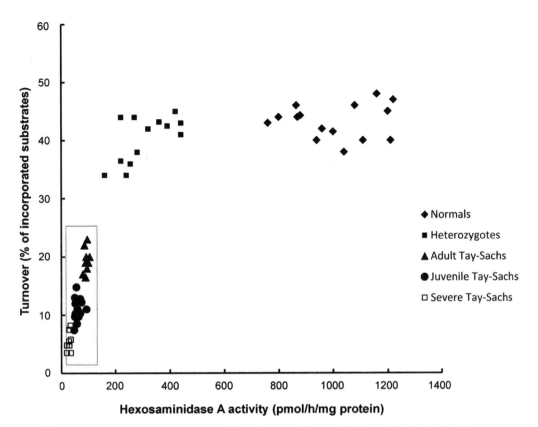

Figure 8-2 Correlation between HEXA activity and degradation of GM2-ganglioside in fibroblasts from normal individuals; heterozygous parents; and patients with severe, juvenile, and adult forms of Tay-Sachs disease. Affected individuals have <10% enzyme activity (dashed square). Obligate heterozygotes have enzyme activities between that of affected and normal individuals. Modified and adapted with permission from *(11)*.

cerebrospinal fluid, urinary oligosaccharide/glycan screening of urine by matrix-assisted laser desorption/ionization–tandem time-of-flight mass spectrometry (MALDI-TOF/TOF), or by DNA sequence analysis. The deficiency can also be diagnosed by decreased metabolism of GM2-ganglioside in fibroblasts with a ganglioside-loading test or by mutation analysis of the GM2-activator protein gene.

Treatment.   Treatment of the GM2 gangliosidoses is supportive.

Krabbe Disease (Globoid Cell Leukodystrophy)

Clinical Presentation.   Krabbe disease, a chronic and progressive lysosomal storage disorder, is classified as infantile-onset or later-onset "classic" disease. The more common infantile form (85–90% of diagnosed patients) presents with irritability, spasticity, and hypertonia in the first months of life with rapid neurologic regression. White matter disease with progressive cerebellar atrophy is identified by magnetic resonance imaging (MRI). Death usually occurs before age 2. Approximately 10–15% of patients present between the first year of life and the fifth decade of life with a variable onset of vision disturbance/loss, weakness, and cognitive decline *(13)*.

Genetics and Pathogenesis.   Krabbe disease is an autosomal-recessive genetic condition caused by defects in the *GALC* gene (chromosome 14q31), which encodes the enzyme galactocerebrosidase (GALC) *(13)*. GALC deficiency causes accumulation of galactolipids within the lysosome with subsequent defective myelin production, affecting the CNS white matter and myelination of peripheral nerves. A genotype-phenotype correlation has been reported for homozygosity for a 30-kbp deletion and for homozygosity for the c.857G>A mutation: The former correlates with the infantile form and the latter correlates with late-onset disease. Compound heterozygosity complicates prediction of genotype-phenotype correlations given the variability of disease in individuals with different mutations. No evidence supports a correlation between age of onset and residual enzyme activity.

Laboratory Diagnosis. Diagnosis of Krabbe disease is based on the demonstration of deficiency of the enzyme GALC in leukocytes or cultured fibroblasts. The enzyme activity is measured by the use of radiolabeled natural substrate galactosylceramide or synthetic fluorescent substrate 6-hexadecanoylamino-4-metylumbelliferyl-β-D-galactopyranoside. Methods using other substrates and tandem mass spectrometry (MS/MS) are also available. The use of natural substrate is preferred to avoid problems because certain mutations may render the enzyme less or more active on artificial substrate. Carrier detection with enzyme assay is not reliable. Spectrophotometry and MS/MS methods using dried blood spots have recently been developed. Targeted mutational analysis and DNA sequencing of the entire coding region, intron-exon boundaries, and 5′-untranslated region of *GALC* can essentially identify 100% of the disease-causing mutations.

Treatment. Hematopoietic stem cell transplantation (HSCT) is recommended in children with the infantile form of Krabbe disease before evidence of the disease is present or in individuals with the late-onset form and few symptoms for improved outcome over palliative care alone *(14)*. Long-term data demonstrate that even with HSCT there is progression of the disease, even if cognition remains intact.

Metachromatic Leukodystrophy

Clinical Presentation. As with many of the other lysosomal storage diseases, metachromatic leukodystrophy (MLD) may present as any of several clinical subtypes *(15)*. The late-infantile form accounts for 50–60% of cases of MLD with onset between the ages of 1 and 2 years. Presenting symptoms include hypotonia, weakness, clumsiness, toe walking, and slurred speech. Regression of neurocognitive and psychomotor skills ensues (rigidity, hypertonia, hearing and vision loss, pain, peripheral neuropathy, and seizures). Affected individuals eventually progress to posturing, tonic spasms, and loss of awareness with death by age 5 years. The juvenile form accounts for 20–30% of cases of MLD and presents with behavioral problems, decline in school performance, gait disturbances, clumsiness, slurred speech, and incontinence between the ages of 4 and 14 years. Seizures may be seen in the juvenile form of MLD. Progression and features of juvenile MLD are similar to, but more slowly progressive than, the late-infantile form, with death usually occurring approximately 20 years after the onset of symptoms. Adult-onset MLD accounts for 15–20% of cases of MLD. It often presents from the ages of 14 into the fifth decade of life with personality changes, decline in ability to function in a professional setting, and emotional issues progressing to loss of coordination, peripheral neuropathy, and seizures. Disease progression is highly variable. Death, resulting from pneumonia or another related illness, usually occurs approximately 20 years after the onset of symptoms.

Genetics and Pathogenesis. MLD is an autosomal-recessive genetic condition caused by defects in the *ARSA* gene located on chromosome 22q13.31-q13.33, which encodes the enzyme arylsulfatase A. Arylsulfatase A functions in the breakdown of sulfatides or sulfate-containing lipids. These lipids make up approximately 5% of myelin production in the body. Accumulation of these lipids results in CNS and peripheral nervous system involvement with leukodystrophy noted on MRI.

Laboratory Diagnosis. Diagnosis of MLD is based on the demonstration of deficiency of the enzyme arylsulfatase A in leukocytes or cultured fibroblasts. Activity is measured using the chromogenic substrate *p*-nitrocatecholsulfate and measurement of the product *p*-nitrocatechol at 515 nm. If there is deficiency of arylsulfatase A, at least one other sulfatase should be measured to rule out multiple sulfatase deficiency. Pseudodeficiency (very low concentrations of arylsulfatase enzyme activity in an otherwise healthy individual) has been reported and should be suspected when arylsulfatase A enzyme activity in leukocytes is 5–20% that of normal controls. Pseudodeficiency is difficult to distinguish from true arylsulfatase A enzyme deficiency by biochemical testing alone. Other means such as increased excretion of urinary sulfatides, molecular testing, and finding of metachromatic lipid deposits in nervous system tissue are used to establish diagnosis of MLD. Urine sulfatides can be measured by thin layer chromatography, high-performance liquid chromatography, or MS/MS. DNA testing for the arylsulfatase A gene is clinically available.

 Treatment. Treatment is palliative. Bone marrow transplantation, which may slow progression but has significant morbidity and mortality, remains controversial and is used to primarily treat the CNS manifestations of the disease. It may be more useful in individuals with later-onset disease or in presymptomatic patients *(16)*. ERT is under development (rhARSA; metazyme) and is undergoing clinical trials in Europe.

LYSOSOMAL TRANSPORT DISORDERS

Pompe Disease (Acid Maltase Deficiency, Glycogen Storage Disease Type II)

 Clinical Presentation. Pompe disease, although a lysosomal storage disease, has historically been classified as a glycogen storage disease because of the identification of glycogen deposition on muscle biopsy. There are three recognized subtypes: classical infantile, nonclassical infantile, and late-onset Pompe disease. The classic infantile form is characterized by early-onset cardiac involvement (cardiomegaly/hypertrophic cardiomyopathy) and profound hypotonia. Without ERT, these children usually die before their first birthday. The nonclassical infantile form usually presents with onset of symptoms, ranging from hypertrophic cardiomyopathy in the first year of life to progressive muscle weakness and respiratory failure during early childhood. Without treatment with ERT, death usually occurs in early childhood because of respiratory failure. The late-onset form, classified as the adult-onset form, primarily affects respiratory function and ambulation. Proximal muscle weakness with or without an elevation of creatine phosphokinase can be seen. Survival can be well into adulthood, but dependence on mechanical ventilation and ambulatory devices is common *(17)*.

 Genetics and Pathogenesis. All forms of Pompe disease are due to mutations in the *GAA* gene resulting in a deficiency of the enzyme acid α-glucosidase. The *GAA* gene is located on chromosome 17q25.2-q25.3 and is inherited in an autosomal-recessive manner.

 Laboratory Diagnosis. The diagnosis of Pompe disease is established by measuring the activity of α-glucosidase in cultured fibroblasts. Patients with classic infantile-onset Pompe disease have no detectable activity of α-glucosidase (<1% of normal controls). Patients with nonclassic infantile-onset and the late-onset forms have some activity of α-glucosidase (2–40% of normal controls). Because fibroblast testing may take 4–6 weeks, assays may be performed in liver or muscle tissue or leukocytes. However, muscle and liver testing is invasive, and leukocytes may show interference from maltase-glucoamylase. For newborn screening, α-glucosidase enzyme activity analysis can be performed on dried blood spots. Targeted mutational analysis, DNA sequencing, and deletion/duplication analysis of the *GAA* gene can be performed for diagnosis and confirmation of Pompe disease.

 Measurement of urinary tetrasaccharide can serve as sensitive marker for the detection of Pompe disease because it is elevated in nearly 100% of individuals with infantile Pompe disease. However, the test is not very specific because elevated tetrasaccharide concentrations are seen in other glycogen storage diseases. Creatine kinase is also highly elevated in infantile-onset Pompe disease.

 Treatment. ERT with alglucosidase alfa, along with supportive interventions and monitoring, is the treatment for all forms of Pompe disease *(18)*. Additional investigations of other possible therapies for the treatment of Pompe disease are currently underway.

Mucolipidosis Type IV

Clinical Presentation. Mucolipidosis type IV (ML IV) is a progressive neurological lysosomal storage disorder characterized by psychomotor delay, little to no speech, progressive corneal clouding, and retinal degeneration. Facial features are not coarse and hepatosplenomegaly is not present in this disorder. Asymptomatic achlorhydria secondary to dysfunction of the acid-secreting $H^+K^+ATPase$ in stomach parietal cells may be present. Elevated plasma gastrin concentration is typical. Poor gastric iron absorption results in iron-deficiency anemia. Onset of symptoms is variable but typically occurs in early childhood. An atypical form of ML IV has been described that is less severe with a later age of onset and slower progression of the disease. The neurologic abnormalities tend to be relatively static, thus any individual with the diagnosis of cerebral palsy should probably be evaluated for possible ML IV (19, 20).

Genetics and Pathogenesis. Originally described as a lysosomal storage disease because of the observed accumulation of lipids and water-soluble substances within the lysosome, it is now known that the disorder results from mutation in the *MCOLN1* gene. Mucolipin-1, the affected protein, is a member of the transient receptor potential family and appears to function as a cation channel in the membranes of lysosomes and endosomes. Mutations in the protein lead to defective trafficking of lipids and proteins between the two intracellular compartments. The disorder is inherited in an autosomal-recessive manner. The gene is located on chromosome 19p13.3-p13.2. It is thought that lack of the cation channel function results in defective white matter organization in the CNS and affects maintenance of retinal and optic nerve cells (21).

Laboratory Diagnosis. The diagnosis can be established by measuring the plasma gastrin concentrations followed by molecular genetic testing. Virtually all affected individuals have elevated plasma gastrin concentrations. Skin or conjunctival biopsies have been used to confirm the diagnosis with demonstration of accumulation of abnormal lamellar membrane structures and amorphous cytoplasmic inclusions without cell type specificity (22). Periodic-acid–Schiff-stained conjunctival cells obtained by swab rather than biopsy can also be used to identify the typical vacuolation associated with the disorder.

Treatment. Treatment is supportive and symptomatic. Topical ocular lubricants are recommended, as is surgical correction of strabismus. Corneal transplantation is not successful. Iron supplementation to prevent anemia is recommended. Permanent joint contractures may be prevented by physical therapy.

Niemann-Pick Disease Type C

Clinical Presentation. Niemann-Pick disease type C (NPC) is a highly variable lipid storage trafficking disorder that can present in infancy, childhood, or adulthood. Classically, NPC presents in mid- to late childhood with vertical supranuclear gaze palsy, ataxia, dementia, and psychiatric disturbances. Seizures, dystonia, dysarthria, loss of learned speech, and dysphagia may also be present. Death occurs in the second or third decade of life, usually from aspiration pneumonia. Infants can present with liver disease, ascites, or lung disease or may simply present with hypotonia and developmental delay. Adults typically present with the classical features later in life and are more likely to present with a psychotic episode or dementia (23).

Genetics and Pathogenesis. NPC is an autosomal-recessive genetic condition caused by defects in two different genes: *NPC1* and *NPC2* (24). The primary defect in NPC relates to abnormal trafficking of lipids. Defective trafficking essentially traps cholesterol and lipid molecules in the membrane of the endosome and lysosome. Cholesterol is necessary for membrane integrity and function. Abnormal amounts of cholesterol in the cell membrane lead to dysfunction and cell apoptosis. *NPC1* encodes a large protein that resides in the membrane of endosomes and lysosomes that functions to allow for appropriate transport of cholesterol and lipids across cell membranes. *NPC2* encodes a protein that binds to cholesterol and transports it out of the luminal space of the late endosome/lysosome into the delimiting membrane. Most patients with NPC have defects in *NPC1* (95%) and only 5% of patients have defects in *NPC2*.

Laboratory Diagnosis.   The diagnosis can be suspected with the identification of foamy macrophages in blood smears or other tissue samples (liver, tonsil). Diagnosis of NPC relies on demonstration of impaired cholesterol esterification followed by filipin staining in cultured skin or rectal fibroblasts. Cholesterol esterification is usually <10% of controls. Molecular genetic testing is used to confirm the diagnosis, especially in cases in which biochemical tests are inconclusive.

Treatment.   Treatment is generally symptomatic and supportive. There is evidence that *N*-butyldeoxynojirimycin (miglustat; Zavesca®) may lead to stabilization of symptoms in some individuals. Small-molecule therapies are being investigated but are not clinically available.

Cystinosis

Clinical Presentation.   Cystinosis is a lysosomal storage disease that results from accumulation of cystine secondary to a defect in the membrane cystine transporter protein, cystinosin. Accumulation of cystine from impaired cystine efflux results in cellular dysfunction in multiple organ systems and specifically in a renal Fanconi syndrome. The exact pathogenic mechanism of damage remains unclear. Three clinical phenotypes have been described: the nephropathic or infantile form, an intermediate or juvenile form, and a benign or adult form *(25)*.

The nephropathic form is the most common form with onset of symptoms at approximately 6 months of age. Symptoms represent the development of a Fanconi proximal renal tubulopathy with failure to thrive, photophobia, anorexia, and polyuria. Polyuria can be dramatic with excretion of between 2 and 5 L of pale, cloudy urine with an unusual odor daily. End-stage renal disease ensues between 6 and 12 years of age. Early treatment with cysteamine delays the onset of renal insufficiency. Hemodialysis and peritoneal dialysis are effective for renal replacement therapy. Kidney transplantation for end-stage renal disease is the treatment of choice. Notably, although crystals can be observed in the graft, the disease does not recur in the transplanted kidney.

The juvenile form is diagnosed in approximately 5% of patients. Presentation can range from a milder proximal tubulopathy to nephrotic syndrome with slower progression of renal disease along with photophobia secondary to crystal deposition in the cornea of the eye.

The adult, or non-nephropathic, form presents with photophobia. This is due to deposition of cystine in the cornea; other organ systems are not affected.

Genetics and Pathogenesis.   All forms of cystinosis are inherited in an autosomal-recessive manner and are caused by mutations in the *CTNS* gene, which is localized to 17p13 and encodes the lysosomal cystine carrier cystinosin. Although point mutations are common, >76% of patients of European descent carry a 57-kbp deletion *(26)*. The disorder is thought to occur in approximately 1 in 180,000 live births.

Although the function of cystinosin has been known for many years, the exact mechanism of pathogenesis has not been elucidated. Animal models exist for the study of the disorder. As of yet, although hypotheses exist as to why cystine accumulation results in cell dysfunction and renal Fanconi syndrome, no definitive mechanism has been identified. One hypothesis suggests that there are decreased concentrations of ATP in cystinotic cells *(25)*, possibly related to abnormal mitochondrial complex I activity. This hypothesis has not stood up to rigorous scientific testing. A second hypothesis invokes increased cellular apoptosis secondary to leaky lysosomal membranes secondary to cystine accumulation. It is hypothesized that cytosolic cystine binds to PKC-δ (proapoptotic protein kinase), which then stimulates apoptosis. Increased expression of caspase-4, a cysteine protease important in programmed cell death, in areas of cystinotic renal tissues with decreased numbers of proximal tubules supports this hypothesis. As with Pompe disease, an increased number of autophagosomes and autophagocytic vacuoles have also been observed, suggesting a problem with autophagy in cystinosis. The third hypothesis invokes sequestration of cystine within the lysosome, resulting in depletion of the cytosolic pool of cysteine, which has a negative effect on glutathione metabolism and the response to oxidative stress. Results from experimental models are inconclusive *(25)*.

Laboratory Diagnosis.   Diagnosis of cystinosis depends first and foremost on clinical suspicion. Urine and serum biochemical parameters should be evaluated. Hypokalemia, hypophosphatemia, metabolic acidosis, low serum uric acid, glucose wasting, and proteinuria are commonly seen. Renal Fanconi syndrome can be identified on urine amino acid profile. Diagnosis is made by measuring free cystine content in leukocytes. Leukocytes are separated from the whole blood using ACD-Dextran solution. The whole blood (~5 mL) is mixed with an equal volume of ACD-Dextran solution. The mixture is left at room temperature for approximately 40 min. The leukocyte-rich solution, approximately 5 mL, is taken and centrifuged to obtain leukocytes. The pellet is suspended in hypotonic saline to remove erythrocyte contamination. Purified leukocytes are suspended in water and undergo several freeze-thaw cycles to rupture them. Cystine in the homogenate is measured using an amino acid analyzer or MS/MS. Proteins are also measured in the homogenate to express the results in units of cystine per milligram of protein. Cystine concentrations in healthy individuals range from 0.04 to 0.16 nmol cystine/mg protein, in heterozygous carriers from 0.14 to 0.57 nmol/mg protein, and in affected individuals concentrations are typically >1 nmol/mg protein. Concentrations are often expressed as ½ cystine/mg protein, in which ½ cystine/mg protein is 2 times cystine/mg protein. Ophthalmologic examination, looking for corneal crystals, is an integral part of diagnosis. Confirmation of the disorder is by molecular analysis of the CTNS gene *(27)*.

Treatment.   Treatment includes supportive and medical interventions *(25, 27)*. Even with treatment, extrarenal involvement of the thyroid, pancreas, and gonadal function is seen by the end of the first decade. Access to water is critical in the treatment because polyuria and polydipsia are quite pronounced. Because of the risks of dehydration secondary to impaired sweating, prolonged exposure to heat should be avoided. Growth hormone treatment has been used to help with growth. Most children require nasogastric or gastronomy treatment secondary to oral motor dysfunction, anorexia, and vomiting. Treatment of hypothyroidism, hypogonadism, and diabetes mellitus is indicated as these complications develop.

Treatment of cystinosis was revolutionized with the discovery that the compound cysteamine combines with cystine via a disulfide exchange, resulting in cysteine-cysteamine mixed disulfide and cysteine. Efflux of the mixed disulfide by a lysine porter and cysteine by a cysteine carrier results in intralysosomal cystine depletion. Doses range from 1.3 to 1.9 g/m^2, and medication should be started as soon as the diagnosis is made because treatment can delay or prevent renal disease and extrarenal complications. The major side effects of cysteamine include gastric upset along with halitosis and an unusual body odor related to the cysteamine metabolites dimethylsulfide and methanethiol.

Hemodialysis and peritoneal dialysis are effective in treating renal failure, followed by renal transplantation. As noted above, disease does not recur in the kidney graft. Transplantation does not prevent extrarenal complications.

REFERENCES

1. Mehta A, Beck M, Eyskens F, Feliciani C, Kantola I, Ramaswami U, et al. Fabry disease: a review of current management strategies. QJM 2010;103:641–59.
2. Eng CM, Germain DP, Banikazemi M, Warnock DG, Wanner C, Hopkin RJ, et al. Fabry disease: guidelines for the evaluation and management of multi-organ system involvement. Genet Med 2006;8:539–48.
3. Chen M, Wang J. Gaucher disease: review of the literature. Arch Pathol Lab Med 2008;132:851–3.
4. Pastores GM. Neuropathic Gaucher disease. Wien Med Wochenschr 2010;160:605–8.
5. Hughes DA, Pastores GM. The pathophysiology of GD—current understanding and rationale for existing and emerging therapeutic approaches. Wien Med Wochenschr 2010;160:594–9.
6. Schuchman EH. The pathogenesis and treatment of acid sphingomyelinase-deficient Niemann-Pick disease. Int J Clin Pharmacol Ther 2009;47 Suppl 1:S48–57.

7. McGovern MM, Schuchman EH. Acid sphingomyelinase deficiency. 2006 Dec 7 [updated 2009 Jun 25]. In: Pagon RA, Bird TD, Dolan CR, Stephens K. GeneReviews [Internet]. Seattle: University of Washington, 2009.

8. Suzuki Y, Oshima A, Namba E. β-Galactosidase deficiency (β-galactosidosis) GM1 gangliosidosis and Morquio B disease. In: Shriver CR; Beaudet AL, Sly WS, Valle, D, eds. The Metabolic and Molecular Basis of Inherited Diseases, 8th ed. New York: McGraw-Hill, 2001:3775–809.

9. Gravel RA, Kaback MM, Proia RL, Sandhoff K, Suzuki K, Suzuki K. The GM2 gangliosidoses. In: Shriver CR, Beaudet AL, Sly WS, Valle, D, eds. The Metabolic and Molecular Basis of Inherited Diseases, 8th ed. New York, McGraw-Hill, 2001:3827–76.

10. Gilbert F, Kucherlapati R, Creagan RP, Murnane MJ, Darlington GJ, Ruddle FH. Tay-Sachs' and Sandhoff's diseases: the assignment of genes for hexosaminidase A and B to individual human chromosomes. Proc Natl Acad Sci U S A 1975;72:263–7.

11. Leinekugel P, Michel S, Conzelmann E, Sandhoff K. Quantitative correlation between the residual activity of beta-hexosaminidase A and arylsulfatase A and the severity of the resulting lysosomal storage disease. Hum Genet 1992;88:513–23.

12. O'Brien JS, Okada S, Chen A, Fillerup DL. Tay-sachs disease. Detection of heterozygotes and homozygotes by serum hexosaminidase assay. N Engl J Med 1970;283:15–20.

13. Wenger DA, Suzuki K, Suzuki Y, Suzuki K. Galactosylceramide lipidosis. Globoid cell leukodystrophy (Krabbe disease). In: Scriver CR, Beaudet AL, Sly WS, Valle D, Childs B, Vogelstein B, eds. The Metabolic and Molecular Bases of Inherited Disease, 8th ed. New York: McGraw-Hill, 2001:3669–94

14. Escolar ML, Poe MD, Provenzale JM, Richards KC, Allison J, Wood S, et al. Transplantation of umbilical-cord blood in babies with infantile Krabbe's disease. N Engl J Med 2005;352:2069–81.

15. Gieselmann V, Krageloh-Mann I. Metachromatic leukodystrophy—an update. Neuropediatrics 2010;41:1–6.

16. Biffi A, Lucchini G, Rovelli A, Sessa M. Metachromatic leukodystrophy: an overview of current and prospective treatments. Bone Marrow Transplant 2008;42 Suppl 2:S2–6.

17. Fukuda T, Roberts A, Plotz PH, Raben N. Acid alpha-glucosidase deficiency (Pompe disease). Curr Neurol Neurosci Rep 2007;7:71–7.

18. Kishnani PS, Steiner RD, Bali D, Berger K, Byrne BJ, Case LE, et al. Pompe disease diagnosis and management guideline. Genet Med 2006;8:267–88.

19. Bach G. Mucolipidosis type IV. Mol Genet Metab 2001;73:197–203.

20. Altarescu G, Sun M, Moore DF, Smith JA, Wiggs EA, Solomon BI, et al. The neurogenetics of mucolipidosis type IV. Neurology 2002;59:306–13.

21. Slaugenhaupt SA. The molecular basis of mucolipidosis type IV. Curr Mol Med 2002;2:445–50.

22. Bargal R, Avidan N, Ben-Asher E, Olender Z, Zeigler M, Frumkin A, et al. Identification of the gene causing mucolipidosis type IV. Nat Genet 2000;26:118–23.

23. Rosenbaum AI, Maxfield FR. Niemann-Pick type C disease: molecular mechanisms and potential therapeutic approaches. J Neurochem 2011;116:789–95.

24. Ory DS. The Niemann-Pick disease genes; regulators of cellular cholesterol homeostasis. Trends Cardiovasc Med 2004;14:66–72.

25. Wilmer MJ, Emma F, Levtchenko EN. The pathogenesis of cystinosis: mechanisms beyond cystine accumulation. Am J Physiol Renal Physiol 2010;299:F905–16.

26. Bendavid C, Kleta R, Long R, Ouspenskaia M, Muenke M, Haddad BR, Gahl WA. FISH diagnosis of the common 57-kb deletion in CTNS causing cystinosis. Hum Genet 2004;115:510–4.

27. Wilmer MJ, Schoeber JP, van den Heuvel LP, Levtchenko EN. Cystinosis: practical tools for diagnosis and treatment. Pediatr Nephrol 2011;26:205–15.

Chapter 9

Peroxisomal Disorders

Laurie D. Smith and Uttam Garg

Peroxisomes are unique intracellular organelles that perform catabolic and anabolic functions. They are involved in the degradation of very-long-chain fatty acids and polyunsaturated fatty acids by β-oxidation, the degradation of phytanic acid and α-hydroxylated fatty acids by α-oxidation, and in the generation of bile salts and plasmalogens *(1)*. In addition, they play a role in purine, polyamine, glyoxalate, amino acid, and reactive oxygen metabolism. Major metabolic functions of peroxisomes are depicted in Figure 9-1. Human disorders associated with aberrant peroxisomal biogenesis were first described by Goldfischer et al. *(2)* in 1973 when electron microscopic studies on biopsy and autopsy specimens from two infants diagnosed with cerebro-hepato-renal syndrome pointed to the absence of peroxisomes in renal proximal tubules and hepatocytes. At the time, the functional role of the peroxisome had not yet been elucidated. It is now known that, in addition to Zellweger spectrum and rhizomelic chondrodysplasia punctata type 1, which constitute the peroxisomal biogenesis disorders, there are at least nine other human conditions linked to impaired peroxisomal dysfunction *(1, 3)*. After the suspicion arises for a peroxisomal disorder, diagnosis depends on biochemical, functional, and molecular testing.

CLINICAL PRESENTATION

Peroxisomal disorders can be divided into essentially two distinct classes of disorders: those that present as metabolic disorders associated with single gene defects and specific enzyme deficiencies and those that present as disorders of peroxisome biogenesis. The latter can further be subdivided into conditions that lead to a complete lack of the intracellular organelle and rhizomelic chondrodysplasia punctata type 1, which involves a subset of three matrix proteins that depend on the peroxisome targeting signal 2 *(1, 3)*.

Zellweger spectrum forms a continuum of disorders that were previously known as Zellweger syndrome, neonatal adrenoleukodystrophy, and infantile Refsum disease *(4)*. The former is considered the most severe of the three whereas infantile Refsum disease is considered the least severe on the continuum. The diagnosis is usually made in the neonatal period. Hallmark features include hypotonia, poor feeding, hepatomegaly with liver dysfunction, and jaundice. Infants usually have a very characteristic facial appearance with a high forehead, shallow supraorbital ridges, and very large fontanelles. Cataracts or corneal clouding may also be present. Bony stippling of the patella and long bones may be radiographically evident if the diagnosis is suspected early. Growth deficiency, mental deficiency, and seizures are also present. Hypomyelination, gyral cortical malformations, and subependymal cysts are commonly seen on magnetic resonance imaging (MRI) along with frontal and perisylvian cortex microgyria and periolandic and occipital pachygyria. Increased fatty acid resonance and decreased *N*-acetylaspartate are observed on magnetic resonance spectroscopy (MRS) *(5)*.

Rhizomelic chondrodysplasia punctata type 1 (RCDP1) classic type has a somewhat different presentation than classic Zellweger spectrum. Proximal shortening of the humeri and femurs, along with epiphyseal and metaphyseal punctate calcifications of cartilage, are common findings. Coronal clefts

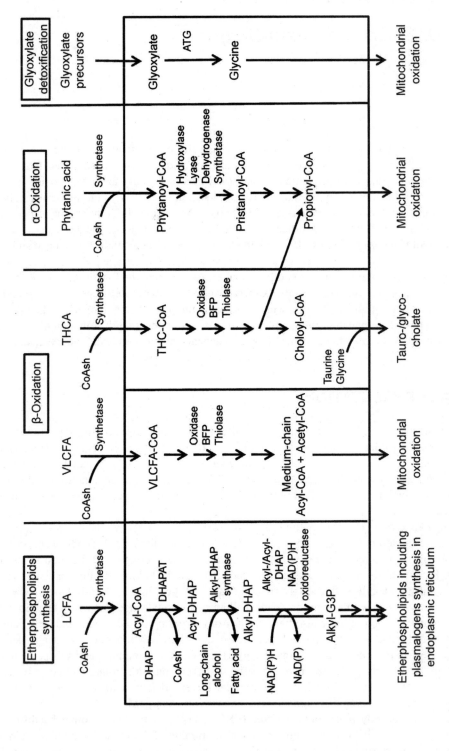

Figure 9-1 Simplified schematic depiction of main functions of peroxisomes.

of vertebral bodies are also characteristic. Cataracts may be present at birth or develop over the first several months of life. Profound postnatal growth deficiency is the rule as is severe mental deficiency and seizures *(6)*. MRI findings include delayed myelination, hypomyelination, and symmetric cerebellar dentate nuclei signal abnormalities. Elevated choline and lipids and decreased *N*-acetylaspartate are characteristic MRS findings *(5)*. There is variability in presentation and severity, although all are considered to be severe disorders.

Metabolic disorders affecting peroxisomal function are variable in presentation. The most well known of these disorders is X-linked adrenoleukodystrophy (ALD) and its later-onset counterpart adrenomyeloneuropathy (AMN) *(7)*. Presentation can be variable, even within the same family. Affected males classically present in the preteen years with hearing, behavioral, and learning difficulties that progress to gait abnormalities, ultimately resulting in spastic quadriparesis, blindness, deafness, and death. The diagnoses may be preceded by a diagnosis of Addison disease or adrenal insufficiency. This presentation occurs in approximately 35–50% of affected males whereas approximately 25% present with AMN. The spinal cord is more highly affected than the brain in this condition, which presents with onset of ambulation difficulties between the ages of 14 and 60 years. Others with ALD may be identified before the onset of symptoms because of family history. Between 20 and 25% of female carriers present with milder, later onset of AMN-like symptoms because of skewed X-inactivation *(8)*.

Other metabolic disorders of peroxisomal dysfunction include acyl-CoA oxidase deficiency (pseudoneonatal adrenoleukodystrophy), racemase deficiency, bile acid CoA:amino acid *N*-acyltransferase deficiency (familial hypercholanemia), D-bifunctional protein deficiency, Refsum disease, sterol carrier protein X deficiency, peroxisomal thiolase deficiency (pseudo-Zellweger syndrome), dihydroacetone phosphate acyltransferase deficiency (rhizomelic chondrodysplasia type 2), and primary hyperoxaluria type 1. Key features of these disorders are found in Table 9-1.

GENETICS AND PATHOGENESIS

All of the peroxisomal disorders, except for X-linked ALD/AMP, are inherited in an autosomal-recessive fashion. Specific genes have been identified in the single-gene metabolic disorders (Table 9-1) whereas 13 genes have been identified through complementation assays to be involved in the biogenesis disorders.

The single-gene disorders exert their influence on peroxisomal function via the absence of functioning enzyme. The biogenesis disorders result from an intrinsic inability of cells to generate the peroxisome membrane, to undergo fission, or to import proteins into the peroxisome to form functioning organelles. Twelve of these genes encode proteins called peroxins. *PEX5* plays an important role in the biosynthetic pathway because it encodes the peroxisomal targeting signal 1 receptor. Most of the *PEX* gene products are transported into the peroxisome via a C-terminal targeting sequence that is recognized by this receptor. Peroxisomes are histologically absent if there is a mutation in any one of three *PEX* genes: *PEX3*, *PEX16*, or *PEX19*, whereas the remainder of the PEX gene products are required for import of matrix proteins. The gene responsible for RCDP1 results from a mutation in a specific peroxisomal targeting signal 2 receptor (*PEX7*) that functions in the transport of three proteins with N-terminal transport signals (alkyl-dihydroxyacetone phosphate synthetase, phytanoyl-CoA hydroxylase, and peroxisomal 3-ketoacyl-CoA thiolase). Isolated deficiencies of each of these enzymes have also been reported.

LABORATORY DIAGNOSIS

Peroxisomal disorders are not associated with acute metabolic derangements. Common laboratory tests such as basic metabolic panel, complete blood counts, and renal function tests are normal. Liver function tests may be normal or elevated. The laboratory diagnosis of the peroxisomal biosynthesis

Table 9-1 Clinical and Laboratory Features in Peroxisomal Disorders

Disorder	Gene (chromosome location)	Clinical symptoms	VLCFA (plasma)	Pristanic acid (plasma)	Phytanic acid (plasma)	Plasmalogens (erythrocyte)	C27 Bile acids	Other laboratory tests
Zellweger spectrum	PEX1 (7q21.2), PEX2 (PXMP3) (8q21.11), PEX3 (6q24.2), PEX5 (12p13.31), PEX6 (6p21.1), PEX10 (1p36.32), PEX12 (17q12), PEX13 (2p16.1), PEX14 (1p36.22), PEX16 (11p11.2), PEX19 (1q23.2), PEX26 (22q11.21),	Hypotonia, poor feeding, dysmorphic facial features (especially large fontanelles), hepatomegaly, renal abnormalities, cataracts, corneal clouding, delayed psychomotor development, seizures. Variability in presentation ranging from severe with death before age 1 to milder with survival into the teens.	Increased	Increased	Increased	Decreased	Increased	Hyperbilirubinemia, abnormal liver function tests, normal-increased pipecolic acid, decreased docossahexa- noic acid. Confirmation of biochemi- cal findings in plasma using fibroblasts is recom- mended. DNA sequence analysis is clinically available for all 12 genes.
Rhizomelic chondro- dysplasia punctata type 1	PEX7 (6q23.3)	Rhizomelia, microcephaly, dysmorphic facial features (frontal bossing, flat face, upslanting palpebral fissures, low nasal bridge), sensorineural deafness, cataracts, cleft palate, calcific stippling of infantile cartilagi- nous skeleton, joint contractures, splayed metaphyses, coronal clefts of vertebrae, ichthyosis, alopecia, spasticity, seizures, severely delayed myelination, death before age 2.	Normal	Decreased	Normal- Increased	Decreased	Normal	Acyl-CoA:dihydroxyacetone- phosphate deficiency. Unprocessed 3-oxoacyl CoA thiolase. DNA sequence analysis is clinically available.
Rhizomelic chon- drodysplasia punctata type 2 (dihydroxyac- etone phosphate acyltransferase deficiency)	GNPAT (1q42.2)	Disproportionate short stature, failure to thrive, dysmorphic facial features (large fontanelles, high forehead, low nasal bridge, high arched pal- ate, microcephaly), cataracts, rhi- zomelia, stippled proximal humeral epiphyses, contractures, scoliosis, hypotonia, mental deficiency.	Normal	Normal	Normal	Decreased		Decreased dihydroxyaceto- nephosphate acyltransfer- ase activity in fibroblasts. DNA sequence analysis is not clinically available in the United States.
Rhizomelic chondro- dysplasia punc- tata type 3 (alkyl- dihydroxyacetone phosphate syn- thase deficiency)	AGPS (2q31.2)	Disproportionate short limbs and short stature with severe rhizomelic short- ening of the humeri and femurs. Stippled epiphyses. Failure to thrive.	Normal	Normal	Normal	Decreased		DNA sequence analysis is not clinically available in the United States.

Disorder	Gene (locus)	Clinical features						Diagnostic tests
X-linked adrenoleukodystrophy, adrenomyeloneuropathy (VLCFA-CoA synthase transport defect)	ABCD1 (Xq28)	Degenerative neurologic disorder: limb/truncal ataxia, slurred speech, peripheral neuropathy, spastic paraplegia, incontinence, blindness, hearing loss, primary adrenal insufficiency, hypogonadism.	Increased	Normal	Normal	Normal	Normal	VLCFA analyses specifically look at C26:0, C24:0/C22:0, and C26:0/C22:0. Diagnostic parameters are available (9). DNA sequence analysis is clinically available. Pontine and cerebellar atrophy on MRI.
Phytanoyl-CoA-α-hydroxylase deficiency (Refsum disease)	PHYH (10p13)	Progressive sensorineural deafness, anosmia, cardiac involvement, multiple epiphyseal dysplasia, short metacarpals and metatarsals, ichthyosis, peripheral sensorimotor neuropathy, limb weakness/atrophy, nerve hypertrophy, insidious presentation in late first through third decades of life.	Normal	Decreased	Increased	Normal	Normal	Increased CSF protein with normal cell count. DNA sequence analysis is not clinically available in the United States. >90% are associated with mutations in PHYH whereas <10% are associated with mutations in PEX7.
Acyl-CoA oxidase deficiency (pseudoneonatal adrenoleukodystrophy)	ACOX1 (17q25.1)	Dysmorphic features (frontal bossing, low-set ears, broad/depressed nasal bridge), sensorineural hearing loss, visual findings (nystagmus, strabismus, optic atrophy, tapetoretinal degeneration, pigmentary retinopathy), hepatomegaly, diffuse hepatic steatosis, delayed psychomotor development with neurologic deterioration after age 2, dystonia, seizures.	Increased	Normal	Normal	Normal	Normal	Normal-increased pipecolic acid. Flattened or absent electroretinogram. Absence of flash-evoked visual responses. Abnormal liver function tests. Liver biopsy with normal number of enlarged peroxisomes. White matter hypodensities and demyelination on MRI.
2-Methylacyl-CoA racemase deficiency	AMACR (5p13.2-q11.2)	Failure to thrive, liver dysfunction (intrahepatic cholestasis, jaundice, hepatomegaly, liver failure), coagulopathy, fat-soluble vitamin malabsorption.	Normal	Increased	Mildly increased	Normal	Increased	Abnormal liver function tests. Hyperbilirubinemia. Decreased serum cholesterol. Increased bile, urine, and serum THCA. Liver biopsy: giant cell hepatitis, nonspecific inflammation, necrotic hepatocytes, decreased numbers of peroxisomes. Enzyme assay and DNA sequence analyses are not clinically available in the United States.

(Continued)

137

Table 9-1   Clinical and Laboratory Features in Peroxisomal Disorders (Continued)

Disorder	Gene (chromosome location)	Clinical symptoms	VLCFA (plasma)	Pristanic acid (plasma)	Phytanic acid (plasma)	Plasmalogens (erythrocyte)	C27 Bile acids	Other laboratory tests
Bile acid CoA: amino acid N-acyltransferase deficiency (familial hypercholanemia)	BAAT (9q22.3) Liver specific	Failure to thrive, vitamin-K-dependent coagulopathy, rickets, pruritis, and fat malabsorption. Identified in the Amish population.	Normal	Normal	Normal	Normal	Normal	Increased serum bile acids. DNA sequence analysis is not clinically available in the United States.
D-Bifunctional protein deficiency	17HSD4 (5q21) High expression in liver, adipose, spleen, brain	Failure to thrive, macrocephaly with large fontanelles, dysmorphic facial features (frontal bossing, high forehead, micrognathia, long philtrum, low-set ears, upslanting palpebral fissures, epicanthal folds, depressed nasal bridge, high arched palate), hearing loss, vision problems (nystagmus, strabismus, inability to fixate, vision loss, abolished electroretinogram), funnel chest, hepatomegaly, cholestasis, renal abnormalities (renal cysts, adrenal cortex atrophy), generalized osteopenia, delayed bone maturation, calcific stippling, claw hand deformity, decreased muscle mass, neonatal hypotonia, seizures, severe psychomotor developmental delay, adrenal insufficiency. Death before 2 years.	Increased	Increased	Increased	Normal	Increased	Increased plasma bile acid intermediates. Liver biopsy: abnormal peroxisomes, fibrosis, hemosiderosis, bile cananiculi proliferation, steatosis. MRI with polymicrogyria, ventricular dilatation, white matter dysmyelination, neocortical dysplasia, generalized cerebral/cerebellar hypoplasia/atrophy. Enzyme assay on fibroblasts is available. DNA sequence analysis is not clinically available in the United States.
Sterol carrier protein X deficiency	SCP2 (1p32)	Leukoencephalopathy with dystonia and motor neuropathy, dystonic head tremor, spasmodic torticollis, hyosmia, saccadic eye movements, hypoacusis, intention tremor, hypergonadotrophic hypogonadism, adult onset.	Mildly increased	Increased	Mildly increased	Normal	Increased	Abnormal urinary bile alcohol glucuronides. Enzymatic testing and DNA sequence analysis is not clinically available.

Disorder	Gene (locus)	Clinical features						Diagnosis
Alanine:glyoxalate-aminotransferase deficiency (primary hyperoxaluria type 1)	AGXT (2q37.3)	Vision involvement with mild visual impairment (optic atrophy, retinopathy, choroidal neovascularization), dental abnormalities (root resorption, tooth mobility), heart block, calcium oxalate urolithiasis, renal failure, peripheral vascular insufficiency with arterial spasm/occlusion, Raynaud phenomenon, acrocyanosis, peripheral neuropathy, diffuse calcium oxalate deposition in various tissues/organs, variable age of onset, death from renal failure in adulthood.	N/A	N/A	N/A	N/A	N/A	Increased urine oxalate:creatinine ratio. Increased plasma oxalate concentration. DNA sequence analysis is clinically available. If DNA testing is negative, enzymatic analysis of liver tissue is recommended.
Acatalasemia	CAT (11p13)	Progressive oral gangrene, diabetes, total or near-total loss of catalase activity in erythrocytes.	N/A	N/A	N/A	N/A	N/A	No frothing with hydrogen peroxide application to gums. Biochemical identification of catalase activity.
Glutaric aciduria III	C7orf10 (7p14.1)	Failure to thrive; may be asymptomatic.	N/A	N/A	N/A	N/A	N/A	Increased glutaric acid on urine organic acid profile. Increased glutaric acid excretion with lysine loading.

N/A = not applicable, THCA = $3\alpha,7\alpha,12\alpha$-trihydroxy-5-β-choestanoic acid, VLCFA = very-long-chain fatty acids.

disorders depends on the measurement of plasma very-long-chain fatty acids, plasma pristanic acid, plasma phytanic acid, plasma bile acids, serum/urinary pipecolic acid, erythrocyte plasmalogens, and enzyme activities (Tables 9-1 and 9-2). Specific patterns of increased and decreased analytes guide the biochemical diagnosis. For example, in Zellweger spectrum, very-long-chain fatty acids, pristanic acid, phytanic acid, and bile acids are increased whereas erythrocyte plasmalogens are decreased. In X-linked ALD/AMP, plasma C26:0 and the C24:0/C22:0 and C26:0/C22:0 ratios are elevated. The diagnosis of the biogenesis disorders is confirmed by biochemical assays on fibroblasts. Mutational analyses are also becoming more readily available. Dihydroxyacetonephosphate acyltransferase activity and C26:0 β-oxidation in fibroblasts have been shown to be useful in predicting life expectancy in the biogenesis disorders *(10)*.

TREATMENT

Treatment of most of these disorders remains symptomatic and supportive. Limitation of dietary phytanic acid by limiting cow milk consumption may be of some minimal benefit in the Zellweger spectrum disorders and Refsum disease. There is no evidence for the efficacy of Lorenzo's oil in X-linked ALD *(11)*. Management revolves around provision of corticosteroids if adrenal insufficiency is present. Bone marrow transplantation has been successful in the treatment of boys in the early stages with evidence of brain involvement on MRI but with minimal neuropsychologic involvement and a normal neurologic exam. Bile acid binders can be used in the case of elevated plasma bile acids.

The treatment of hyperoxaluria type I revolves around increasing fluid intake to minimize stone formation. Some individuals are responsive to treatment with pyridoxine. Thiazide diuretics and potassium citrate have also been reported to decrease calcium oxalate deposition. Liver or combined liver/kidney transplantation may be indicated. Foods high in oxalates (rhubarb, chocolate), high doses of vitamin C, and loop diuretics should be avoided *(12)*.

Table 9-2 Laboratory Tests for the Diagnosis of Peroxisomal Disorders

Analyte/assay	Patient preparation	Specimen type	Specimen handling	Common method
Very-long-chain fatty acids	Fasting	EDTA plasma or serum	Freeze	Gas chromatography–mass spectrometry
Bile acids	Fasting preferred	Serum	Room temperature	Liquid chromatography–tandem mass spectrometry
Phytanic/pristanic acid	Fasting	Serum	Freeze	Gas chromatography–mass spectrometry
Pipecolic acid	Fasting	Serum or urine	Freeze	Gas chromatography–mass spectrometry
Polyunsaturated fatty acids	Fasting	Serum	Freeze	Gas chromatography–mass spectrometry
Erythrocyte plasmalogens	None	EDTA blood	Room temperature	Gas chromatography–mass spectrometry
Glutaric/oxalic/mevalonic acids	None	Urine	Freeze if send out	Gas chromatography–mass spectrometry
Peroxisomal plasmalogen synthesis	None	Fibroblasts	In culture medium	Dual isotope labeling
Phytanic/pristanic acid oxidase	None	Fibroblasts	In culture medium	Measurement of enzyme activities through metabolism of radiolabeled substrates

EDTA = ethylenediaminetetraacetic acid.

No treatment recommendations have been made for glutaric aciduria III, other than good nutrition practices, because asymptomatic individuals have been described. Good dental hygiene is recommended for catalase-deficient individuals.

PROGNOSIS

The overall prognosis for the peroxisomal biosynthesis disorders is relatively poor with severe disability and increased morbidity and mortality being the rule rather than the exception. The prognosis for the metabolic disorders associated with single-gene defects and specific enzyme deficiencies is somewhat dependent on the specific defect, but, in general, the prognosis for these disorders is also poor. Individuals with hyperoxaluria type I typically require dialysis with the development of end-stage renal disease in their mid-twenties to forties. Liver transplantation decreases oxalate production (which may be curative) and kidney transplantation restores renal function.

REFERENCES

1. Van Veldhoven PP. Biochemistry and genetics of inherited disorders of peroxisomal fatty acid metabolism. J Lipid Res 2010;51:2863–95.
2. Goldfischer S, Moore CL, Johnson AB, Spiro AJ, Valsamis MP, Wisniewski HK, et al. Peroxisomal and mitochondrial defects in the cerebro-hepato-renal syndrome. Science 1973;182:62–4.
3. Ma C, Agrawal G, Subramani S. Peroxisome assembly: matrix and membrane protein biogenesis. J Cell Biol 2011;193:7–16.
4. Ebberink MS, Mooijer PA, Gootjes J, Koster J, Wanders RJ, Waterham HR. Genetic classification and mutational spectrum of more than 600 patients with a Zellweger syndrome spectrum disorder. Hum Mutat 2011;32:59–69.
5. Cakir B, Teksam M, Kosehan D, Akin K, Koktener A. Inborn errors of metabolism presenting in childhood. J Neuroimaging 2011;21:e117–33.
6. Braverman N, Chen L, Lin P, Obie C, Steel G, Douglas P, et al. Mutation analysis of PEX7 in 60 probands with rhizomelic chondrodysplasia punctata and functional correlations of genotype with phenotype. Hum Mutat 2002;20:84–97.
7. Moser HW. Adrenoleukodystrophy: phenotype, genetics, pathogenesis and therapy. Brain 1997;120:1485–1508.
8. Jangouk P, Zackowski KM, Naidu S, Raymond GV. Adrenoleukodystrophy in female heterozygotes: underrecognized and undertreated. Mol Gen Med 2012;105:180–5.
9. Steinberg S, Jones R, Tiffany C, Moser A. Investigational methods for peroxisomal disorders. Curr Protoc Hum Genet 2008; Chapter 17: Unit 17.6.
10. Gootjes J, Mooijer PA, Dekker C, Barth PG, Poll-The BT, Waterham HR, Wanders RJ. Biochemical markers predicting survival in peroxisome biogenesis disorders. Neurology 2002;59:1746–9.
11. Semmler A, Köhler W, Jung HH, Weller M, Linnebank M. Therapy of X-linked adrenoleukodystrophy. Expert Rev Neurother 2008;8:1367–79.
12. Harambat J, Fargue S, Bacchetta J, Acquaviva C, Cochat P. Primary hyperoxaluria. Int J Nephrol 2011;2011:864580. Epub 2011 Jun 16. doi: 10.4061/2011/864580.

Chapter 10

Disorders of Purine and Pyrimidine Metabolism

Bryce A. Heese

Over 12 known defects involving purine and pyrimidine metabolism have been described. Individually, most of these conditions are rare; for some, only a handful of cases have been described. These disorders constitute a clinically diverse group of inherited diseases that may affect any number of systems. Purines and pyrimidine metabolites are the building blocks of DNA and RNA. They are also important in energy metabolism, formation of phospholipids and glycolipids, signal transduction, and drug metabolism. Table 10-1 lists the known inherited disorders of purine and pyrimidine metabolism.

PURINES

Inherited disorders of purine metabolism include defects in the de novo synthesis of purines, purine catabolism, or the purine salvage pathway. The nucleotides, inosine monophosphate (IMP), guanosine monophosphate (GMP), and adenosine monophosphate (AMP), are formed by de novo purine biosynthesis and are further converted to their respective di- and triphosphate nucleotides (e.g., ATP) and to corresponding deoxyribonucleotides. Uric acid is the end product of purine degradation. Purine bases, such as guanine, hypoxanthine, and adenine, are recovered from the turnover of nucleotide bases or obtained from the diet. These bases may be (re-)converted into their respective nucleotide monophosphates by a separate salvage pathway. The following are descriptions of known defects of purine metabolism (see metabolism of purines, Figure 10-1).

PHOSPHORIBOSYLPYROPHOSPHATE SYNTHETASE SUPERACTIVITY (INCLUDING ARTS SYNDROME)

Phosphoribosylpyrophosphate synthetase (PRPS) overactivity is a disorder of purine nucleotide synthesis. It is typically associated with adult early-onset hyperuricemia. A more severe, infantile-onset form of the disease has been described with hyperuricemia, sensorineural deafness, hypotonia, motor incoordination, and developmental delay *(1)*. Arts syndrome, reported in two families, includes PRPS superactivity (hyperuricemia), X-linked Charcot-Marie-Tooth type 5, and nonsyndromic hearing loss and has been linked to defects within this same gene, PRPS1 *(2)*. PRPS1-related disorders are all inherited in an X-linked manner. PRPS functions as the initial step in the de novo synthesis of purines. A defect in this gene leads to a structural alteration that increases the enzymes activity to produce excess purine nucleotides, which ultimately leads to overproduction of uric acid. Allopurinol, which inhibits xanthine oxidase, is used to reduce uric acid production. Uricosuric agents are contraindicated for disorders causing overproduction of uric acid and can lead to acute renal failure. Management includes increased fluid intake and avoidance of dietary sources of purine such as shellfish or beer. For renal stones, lithotripsy and typical management may be considered. Hearing aids and typical supportive management is used for hearing loss.

Table 10-1 Inherited Metabolic Disorders of Purine and Pyrimidine Metabolism

Disorder	Genetics	Clinical findings	Laboratory findings
Defects in purine synthesis			
Phosphoribosylpyrophosphate synthetase superactivity	PRPS1, Xq22.3	Hyperuricemia, renal stones	High uric acid (B,U), hypoxanthine (U)
Adenylosuccinase deficiency	ADSL, 22q13.1	Psychomotor delay, seizures	Succinyladenosine (U, CSF), SAICAR (U, CSF)
AICA-ribosiduria	ATIC, 2q35	Psychomotor delay, seizures	Succinyladenosine (U, CSF), SAICAR (U, CSF)
Defects in purine catabolism			
Myoadenylate deaminase deficiency	AMPD1, 1p13.2	Muscle pain and fatigue	CPK (B), myoglobin (U)
Adenosine deaminase deficiency	ADA, 20q13.12	Severe combined immunodeficiency	Lymphopenia (B), hypogammaglobulinemia (B), deoxyadenosine (U), deoxyATP (RBC)
Purine nucleoside phosphorylase deficiency	PNP, 14q11.2	Severe combined immunodeficiency	Lymphopenia (B), hypogammaglobulinemia (B), guanosine (U), inosine (U), deoxyguanosine (U), deoxyinosine (U)
Xanthine oxidase deficiency	XDH, 2p23.1	Asymptomatic, renal stones	Low uric acid (B,U), xanthine (U), hypoxanthine (U)
Defects in purine salvage			
Hypoxanthine-guanine-phosphoribosyltransferase deficiency	HPRT1, Xq26.2-q26.3	Psychomotor delay, self-mutilation, hyperuricemia, renal stones	Uric acid (B,U), hypoxanthine (U), xanthine (U)
Adenine phosphoribosyltransferase deficiency	APRT, 16q24.3	Hyperuricemia, renal stones	2,8-Dihydroxyadenine (U), adenine (U)
Deoxyguanosine kinase deficiency	DGUOK, 2p13.1	Psychomotor delay, seizures, liver disease	Reduced mtDNA content
Other defects associated with purine metabolism			
Thiopurine methyltransferase deficiency	TPMT, 6p22.3	Defect in drug metabolism	

144

	Gene, locus	Clinical features	Metabolites
Defects in pyrimidine synthesis			
UMP synthase deficiency	UMPS, 3q21.2	Psychomotor delay, megaloblastic anemia	Orotic (U)
Defects in pyrimidine catabolism			
Dihydropyrimidine dehydrogenase deficiency	DPYD, 1p21.3	Psychomotor delay, seizures, defect in drug metabolism	Uracil (U), thymine (U)
Dihydropyrimidinase deficiency	DPYS, 8q22.3	Psychomotor delay	Uracil (U), thymine (U), dehydrouracil (U), dehydrothymine (U)
Ureidopropionase deficiency	UPB1, 22q11.23	Psychomotor delay	Dihydrouracil (U), dihydrothymine (U), ureidopropionic (U), ureidoisobutyric (U)
Pyrimidine 5'-nucleotidase deficiency	NT5C3, 7p14.3	Hemolytic anemia	Basophilic stippling (RBC), increased pyrimidines (RBC), elevated glutathione (RBC)
Pyrimidine nucleotide depletion syndrome	?	Psychomotor delay, seizures, infections	Low uric acid (B,U)
Thymidine phosphorylase deficiency	TYMP, 22q13.33	Myopathy, neuropathy, gastrointestinal	Thymidine (P), deoxyuridine (P)
Defects in pyrimidine salvage			
Thymidine kinase deficiency	TK2, 16q21	Myopathy	Reduced mtDNA content

AICA = 5-phosphoribosyl-5-amino-4-imidazole-carboxamide, B = blood, CSF = cerebrospinal fluid, mtDNA = mitochondrial DNA, RBC = erythrocytes, SAICAR = 5-phosphoribosyl-5-amino-4-imidazole-succinocarboxamide riboside, U = urine, UMP = uridine-5-monophosphate.

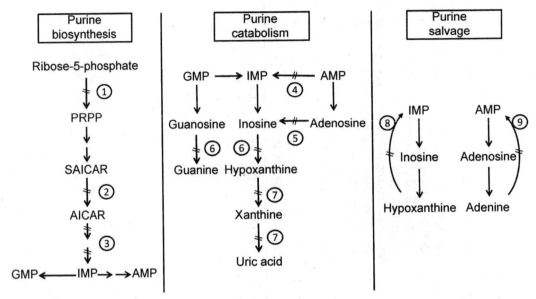

Figure 10-1.   Metabolism of purines. 1 = Phosphoribosyl pyrophosphate synthetase, 2 = adenylosuccinase, 3 = AICAR transformylase and IMP cyclohydrolase (bifunctional enzyme), 4 = myoadenylate deaminase, 5 = adenosine deaminase, 6 = purine nucleoside phosphorylase, 7 = xanthine oxidase, 8 = hypoxanthine-guanine phosphoribosyltransferase, and 9 = adenine phosphoribosyltransferase.

Laboratory Diagnosis

The clinical findings with hyperuricemia should be differentiated from that of hypoxanthine-guanine-phosphoribosyltransferase deficiency. Serum uric acid and urinary excretion of uric acid will be elevated. Urinary excretion of hypoxanthine may be elevated, but this is not a consistent finding (see Table 10-2). Enzyme activity can be analyzed in fibroblasts, lymphoblasts, and erythrocytes, but this testing is not currently available clinically. Genetic testing for PRPS1 is available, but with a reportedly poor detection rate in milder, adult-onset PRPS deficiency (100% in the two families with Arts syndrome).

ADENYLOSUCCINASE DEFICIENCY (OR ADENYLOSUCCINATE LYASE DEFICIENCY)

Adenylosuccinase deficiency is a disorder of purine synthesis. It has been described as a clinically heterogeneous disorder marked by a variable degree of psychomotor delay, autistic features, seizures, and hypotonia (3). The enzyme, which catalyzes the conversion of 5-phosphoribosyl-5-amino-4-imidazole-succinocarboxamide (SAICA) to 5-phosphoribosyl-5-amino-4-imidazole-carboxamide (AICA), is involved in de novo purine synthesis. Treatment is supportive.

Laboratory Diagnosis

Succinyladenosine and SAICA-riboside will be elevated in the urine and cerebrospinal fluid (CSF) from patients with adenylosuccinate lyase (ADSL; see Table 10-2). A screen called the Bratton-Marshall test utilizing a diazo reaction with N-(1-naphthyl)ethylendiamine can also detect SAICAR, but it can lead to false-positive results in patients on sulfonamide medication (4). Gene sequencing is clinically available for the ADSL gene.

5-AMINO-4-IMIDAZOLECARBOXAMIDE-RIBOSIDURIA

A single case report of AICA-ribosiduria describes a child with severe intellectual disability, seizures, congenital blindness, and dysmorphic features (5). AICAR transformylase is part of de novo purine synthesis. The enzyme, AICAR transformylase, is responsible for converting AICAR to formyl-AICAR. Treatment is supportive.

Laboratory Diagnosis

As in the condition ADSL deficiency, succinyladenosine and SAICA-riboside are expected to be elevated in urine as well as in CSF from a patient with AICA-ribosiduria (see Table 10-2). In addition, the Bratton-Marshall screen, described under *Adenylosuccinase Deficiency* (or *Adenylosuccinate Lyase Deficiency*), is expected to be positive.

MYOADENYLATE DEAMINASE DEFICIENCY (OR MUSCLE AMP DEAMINASE DEFICIENCY)

Most individuals with myoadenylate deaminase are asymptomatic. Some experience muscle cramps, pain, or fatigue with exercise associated with elevated plasma creatine kinase (CK) concentrations. This condition is inherited in an autosomal-recessive fashion. Myoadenylate deaminase is an enzyme within the purine catabolism pathway. It has been proposed to be important in muscle function during exercise by recycling excess AMP and by anaplerotic effects on the tricyclic acid cycle. However, this process has not been proven, and further evidence suggests that this enzyme may not cause muscle disease (6). In a study of enzyme activity in muscle from a general Caucasian population, myoadenylate deficiency was reported in 2% of individuals. Acute rhabdomyolysis requires immediate attention for management. Caution is warranted with prolonged isometric exercise that can lead to symptoms. The administration of ribose has been suggested to increase PRPS synthesis with reported improvement of symptoms.

Laboratory Diagnosis

Plasma CK is elevated in most patients, but typically seen only after exercise. Urine myoglobin is rarely detected. A modified forearm ischemic exercise test can show an abnormal response of venous ammonia after exercise. In patients with myoadenylate deaminase deficiency, ammonia does not increase with exercise (7). Enzyme activity can be measured in a muscle specimen. Sequencing of the gene AMPD1 is available clinically.

ADENOSINE DEAMINASE DEFICIENCY

Adenosine deaminase (ADA) deficiency is a severe combined immunodeficiency (SCID) disorder that causes defective humoral and cellular immunity. Most patients present in early infancy with failure to thrive and multiple severe bacterial and viral infections. Neurological findings such as tremor, spasticity, nystagmus, and hypotonia rarely accompany the presentation. Left untreated, survival past the first year of life is unlikely. A milder, later-onset form has been described. ADA deficiency is an autosomal-recessive disorder of purine catabolism. The enzyme catalyzes the conversion of adenosine to inosine, resulting in accumulation of deoxyadenosine triphosphate (dATP), which is thought to inhibit ribonucleotide reductase, important in cell division. Therapy includes aggressive treatment of infections. Bone marrow transplantation, ideally from human leukocyte antigen (HLA)-matched siblings, is the treatment of choice. Enzyme replacement using PEGylated bovine ADA is used.

Laboratory Diagnosis

Evaluation of blood cells shows profound lymphopenia, typically from birth. All lymphocyte cell lines are depleted by flow cytometry. Lymphocyte response to mitogens and antigens is low or absent. Serum immunoglobulins are low. Urine deoxyadenosine excretion is significantly elevated (see Table 10-2). Erythrocyte dATP is elevated. Enzyme activity is measured in erythrocytes or fibroblasts. Sequencing of the ADA gene, as well as deletion/duplication analysis, is available. Newborn screening has been recently implemented in certain states for the detection of SCID from a blood spot on a filter paper card, which involves measurement of T-cell receptor excision circles (TRECs).

PURINE NUCLEOSIDE PHOSPHORYLASE DEFICIENCY

Purine nucleoside phosphorylase (PNP) deficiency is a SCID disorder that causes defective humoral and cellular immunity. However, the onset of symptoms typically presents later in childhood. Some patients have neurological findings, such as spasticity, tremor, and ataxia. Inherited as an autosomal-recessive disorder of purine catabolism, a defect in PNP leads to accumulation of guanosine, inosine, deoxyguanosine, and deoxyinosine. The accumulation of these metabolites, namely deoxyguanosine triphosphate, is thought to inhibit ribonucleotide reductase, which is important in cell division. Aggressive treatment of infections, and, as in ADA deficiency, early bone marrow transplantation is the definitive treatment for PNP deficiency.

Laboratory Diagnosis

Severe lymphopenia and low immunoglobulins are seen in patients with PNP deficiency. Individuals may also have significantly reduced serum and urinary excretion of uric acid. Urine studies show increased excretion of guanosine, inosine, deoxyguanosine, and deoxyinosine (see Table 10-2). Enzyme activity can be measured from erythrocytes or from fibroblasts. Newborn screening has been recently implemented in many states for the detection of SCID from a blood spot on a filter paper card that involves measurement of TRECs.

XANTHINE OXIDASE DEFICIENCY (HEREDITARY XANTHINURIA)

Most individuals with isolated xanthine oxidase deficiency are asymptomatic with laboratory findings of hypouricemia. Some individuals develop renal stones (i.e., xanthine calculi). This autosomal-recessive condition is a defect in purine catabolism. The enzyme, xanthine oxidase, catalyzes the final steps in purine degradation with the conversion of hypoxanthine to xanthine and the conversion of xanthine to uric acid leading to an accumulation of xanthine and hypoxanthine. Supportive management of renal stones is indicated.

Laboratory Diagnosis

Serum and urinary excretion of uric acid is abnormally low. Excretion of xanthine and hypoxanthine are elevated in urine (see Table 10-2).

MOLYBDENUM COFACTOR DEFICIENCY (COMBINED XANTHINE OXIDASE DEFICIENCY AND SULFITE OXIDASE DEFICIENCY)

Individuals with molybdenum cofactor deficiency (as with isolated sulfite oxidase deficiency) classically present shortly after birth with profound seizures, axial hypotonia with peripheral hypertonicity, and global developmental delay. Ocular lens dislocation, cortical blindness, and facial dysmorphism have been described. Molybdenum cofactor deficiency is not specifically a defect in purine catabolism, but rather a defect in the synthesis of a molybdenum containing cofactor that is important in the function of several enzymes, including xanthine oxidase. The disruption in xanthine oxidase leads to the finding of hypouricemia and xanthine calculi. Molybdenum cofactor is synthesized by several steps, the most common genes associated with molybdenum cofactor deficiency are *MOCS1* on chromosome 6p21.2 and *MOCS2* on chromosome 5q11.2. *GPHN*, on chromosome 14q23.3, has also been associated with this condition *(8)*. All forms of molybdenum cofactor deficiency are inherited in an autosomal-recessive manner. No specific treatment exists for this condition. Symptomatic treatment for seizures and other manifestations is per standard of care.

Laboratory Diagnosis

The primary manifestation of this condition is related to a dysfunction of sulfite oxidase, which is not a function of purine metabolism. Sulfite oxidase deficiency leads to elevated urinary excretion of sulfite, which should be measured in a fresh urine given rapid spontaneous oxidation. Many laboratories still use urine sulfite dipsticks for this reason. *S*-Sulfocysteine and taurine may be markedly elevated in the urine and plasma amino acid profile. Molybdenum cofactor disease also affects xanthine oxidase, in which serum and urinary excretion of uric acid is abnormally low. Excretion of xanthine and hypoxanthine are elevated in urine (see Table 10-2). Molecular sequencing of *MOCS1* and *MOCS2* are clinically available.

HYPOXANTHINE-GUANINE-PHOSPHORIBOSYLTRANSFERASE DEFICIENCY

Patients, typically males, with profound hypoxanthine-guanine-phosphoribosyltransferase (HGPRT) deficiency present with the classic findings of Lesch-Nyhan disease, which typically includes seemingly normal early development followed by psychomotor delay, choreo-athetoid movements, spasticity, hyperreflexia, and severe behavioral problems including aggressive striking as well as self-injurious behaviors such as biting fingers and lips. Patients with Lesch-Nyhan disease have hyperuricemia with deposition of urate crystals in joints leading to gouty arthritis and in soft tissues resulting in tophaceous gout as well as formation of uric acid stones in the kidney. HGPRT is part of the purine salvage responsible for reusing hypoxanthine or guanine that leads to the increased formation of uric acid. The exact mechanism of neurological symptoms is unclear. HGPRT deficiency is transmitted in an X-linked recessive manner. Uricosuric agents are contraindicated for disorders causing overproduction of uric acid and may lead to acute renal failure. Unfortunately, allopurinol does not improve behavioral or neurological manifestations of Lesch-Nyhan syndrome. For renal-formed renal stones, lithotripsy may be considered. Patients with Lesch-Nyhan syndrome may benefit from a muscle relaxant such as valium or baclofen. Patients with uncontrollable self-injurious behavior, teeth removal, or physical restraints may be required to prevent severe tissue damage.

Laboratory Diagnosis

High serum and urinary excretion of uric acid is typically seen. Excretion of hypoxanthine and xanthine may be elevated in urine studies, but this is not a consistent finding (see Table 10-2). HGPRT activity can be measured in erythrocytes, the "gold-standard" diagnostic test. It can also be measured in fibroblasts. Patients with Lesch-Nyhan syndrome have essentially no detectable activity in contrast to individuals with partial HGPRT activity *(9)*. HGPRT activity in erythrocytes is not appropriate for determining carrier status in females. Sequencing of the HPRT1 gene is clinically available for confirmation.

ADENINE PHOSPHORIBOSYLTRANSFERASE DEFICIENCY

Individuals with adenine phosphoribosyl transferase (APRT) deficiency typically manifest in childhood with renal stones. Partial deficiency is common in the Japanese population. The enzyme, APRT, is part of the purine salvage pathway converting adenine to AMP. Excess adenine is converted to 2,8-dihydroxyadenine with the help of xanthine oxidase. 2,8-Dihydroxyadenine is precipitated in the urine. These renal stones are not easily distinguished from uric acid stones by typical chemical and radiologic testing. APRT deficiency is inherited in an autosomal-recessive manner. The gene responsible for this condition, APRT, is on chromosome 16q24.3. Low purine diet and allopurinol is effective in reducing the amount of 2,8-dihydroxyadenine formation. Alkalization of the urine is not effective; otherwise, treatment includes the standard management of renal stones.

Laboratory Diagnosis

Although macroscopic analysis of renal stones may differentiate 2,8-dihydroxyadenine stones from other types of stones, the compound itself is chemically analogous to uric acid and therefore may be mistakenly identified as uric acid in routine chemical analysis. Special techniques, beyond routine analysis, using ultraviolet, infrared, mass spectrometry, X-ray crystallography, high-performance liquid chromatography (HPLC), or capillary electrophoresis is needed to chemically identify this compound *(10)*. Adenine may be elevated in urine (see Table 10-2). Measurement of enzyme activity in erythrocytes is diagnostic and confirmation is by molecular analysis.

DEOXYGUANOSINE KINASE DEFICIENCY

Individuals with deoxyguanosine kinase (DGUOK) deficiency typically present in infancy or early childhood with progressive multisystem disease including liver disease (cholestasis), psychomotor delay, and hypotonia. The enzyme, DGUOK, is involved in purine salvage converting deoxyguanosine into deoxyguanosine monophosphate. This reduced enzyme activity causes an imbalance of the mitochondrial deoxynucleotide pools. Because the mitochondria depend heavily on the salvage pathway for the supply of deoxynucleotides, DGUOK deficiency results in mitochondrial DNA depletion. No specific treatment exists for this condition. Symptomatic treatment is indicated for liver disease. Patients should avoid sodium valproate.

Laboratory Diagnosis

Because DGUOK is considered a mitochondrial disorder, a thorough discussion of laboratory diagnosis will not be discussed in this chapter. Reduced mitochondrial DNA content can be measured by quantitative polymerase chain reaction (PCR) analysis; this is typically done in affected tissues such as liver or muscle *(11)*. Molecular genetic testing of the DGUOK gene is available.

THIOPURINE METHYLTRANSFERASE DEFICIENCY

Individuals with thiopurine methyltransferase (TPMT) deficiency are generally asymptomatic; however, they do have reduced ability to metabolize thiopurine medications that are commonly used in chronic inflammatory disease. Toxic effects of these medications include myelosuppression, hepatotoxicity, and pancreatitis. TPMT is not specifically a disorder of the purine pathway, but it is involved in methylating thioinosine monophosphate. It also catalyzes the methylation of and inactivation of the thiopurine-based drugs such as azathioprine and 6-mercaptopurine. It is commonplace to pretest TPMT activity or TPMT genotyping in patients with chronic inflammatory disease before thiopurine

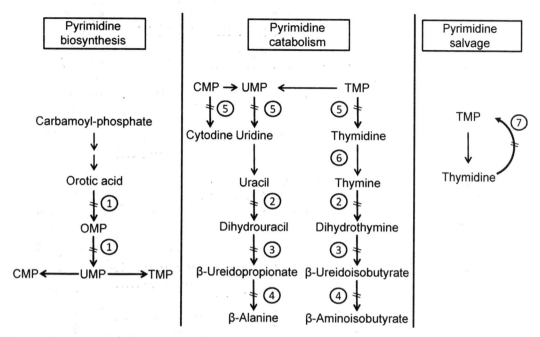

Figure 10-2. Metabolism of pyrimidines. 1 = Uridine-5-monophosphate synthase (bifunctional enzyme), 2 = dihydropyrimidine dehydrogenase, 3 = dihydropyrimidinase, 4 = ureidopropionase, 5 = pyrimidine 5′-nucleotidase, 6 = thymidine phosphorylase, 7 = thymidine kinase.

therapy to reduce the risk of toxicity; however, there is insufficient evidence that shows reduced harm compared with appropriate complete blood count monitoring *(12)*.

Laboratory Diagnosis

Enzyme activity can be measured by various methods including HPLC and tandem mass spectrometry. Alternatively, genotyping has been used to determine TPMT deficiency. There are limited data on the sensitivity of molecular testing using different methods *(12)*.

PYRIMIDINES

Inherited disorders of pyrimidines involve defects in the synthesis, catabolism, or salvage pathway of pyrmidine metabolism. The de novo synthesis of pyrimidines involves the formation of orotic acid from carbamoylphosphate and subsequently to uridine-5-monophosphate (UMP). From UMP, cytidine monophosphate (CMP) and thymidine monophosphate (TMP) are formed. From these nucleotides their corresponding di- and triphosphates (e.g., CTP) and deoxyribonucleotides are formed. Degradation of pyrimidines leads to the formation of the end products, β-alanine and β-aminoisobutyrate. Pyrimidines may be salvaged from pyrimidine nucleosides back into their corresponding nucleotides by pyrimidine kinases (see Figure 10-2 on the metabolism of pyrimidines).

URIDINE-5-MONOPHOSPHATE (UMP) SYNTHASE DEFICIENCY (OROTIC ACIDURIA)

Patients with UMP synthase deficiency typically present with megaloblastic anemia within the first months of life. Untreated, this may lead to failure to thrive and psychomotor delay. Immunodeficiency has been reported. Orate crystalluria has also been reported. UMP synthase is an enzyme involved in pyrimidine nucleotide synthesis. It catalyzes two steps: the conversion of orotic acid into orotidine monophosphate (OMP) and OMP to UMP. It is believed that the deficiency of pyrimidine nucleotides leads to impaired cell division and to symptoms. Administration of uridine is effective in reversing anemia and improving growth and development by replacing missing pyrimidines. Orotic acid is elevated in the urine. Confirmation is by molecular testing.

DIHYDROPYRIMIDINE DEHYDROGENASE DEFICIENCY

Profound dihydropyrimidine dehydrogenase deficiency may present with developmental delay and seizures in childhood. Variability in symptoms from asymptomatic to hypertonia, hyperreflexia, growth delay, and dysmorphic features have been reported. Individuals with dihydropyrimidine dehydrogenase receiving the medication 5-fluorouracil, in the treatment of certain cancers, may develop a toxic reaction potentially resulting in severe neurological dysfunction with loss of speech, paralysis, demyelination, and neutropenia. The enzyme is responsible for the first step in pyrimidine catabolism, catalyzing the conversion of uracil and thymine to dehydrouracil and dehydrothymine, respectively. The specific etiology of neurological symptoms is uncertain, which is likely related to accumulation of uracil and thymine. The enzyme is also important in the metabolism of 5-fluorouracil leading to excessive accumulation of the active compound and ultimately to its toxicity. A common mutation, IVS14+1G>A, accounts for many of the mutations found in a European population and is found in the heterozygous state in approximately 25% of patients with 5-fluorouracil toxicity *(13)*. For profound infantile-onset dihydropyrimidine dehydrogenase deficiency, no specific treatment exists and management is based on symptomatic care. In patients receiving 5-fluorouracil medication, avoidance or prompt discontinuation of this medication is indicated.

Laboratory Diagnosis

Elevated amounts of uracil and thymine are seen in urine (see Table 10-2). Enzyme activity can be measured in erythrocytes. Individuals with profound dihydropyrimidine dehydrogenase activity will have no (or near zero) activity, as opposed to patients at risk for 5-fluorouracil toxicity with some residual activity up to 30% *(14)*. Sequencing of the gene is available. In addition, molecular testing specifically for the common mutation IVS14+1G>A is available, but it should be interpreted with caution because it accounts for only about half of known mutations.

DIHYDROPYRIMIDINASE DEFICIENCY (DIHYDROPYRIMIDINURIA)

This is a rare condition with a variable presentation from asymptomatic to psychomotor delay, seizures, dysmorphic features, and microcephaly *(15)*. As in the deficiency of the previously described enzyme dihydropyrimidine dehydrogenase, individuals with dihydropyrimidinase deficiency may be at risk for toxicity to the medication 5-fluorouracil. Dihydropyrimidinase is the second step in pyrimidine catabolism that breaks down dihydrouracil and dihydrothymine to ureidopropionic acid and ureidobutyric acid, respectively. This condition is inherited in an autosomal-recessive manner. No specific treatment exists and management is based on symptomatic care.

Laboratory Diagnosis

In addition to elevated excretion of uracil and thymine, dehydrouracil and dehydrothymine are elevated in urine (see Table 10-2). Enzyme activity must be measured in liver cells.

UREIDOPROPIONASE DEFICIENCY (β-ALANINE SYNTHASE DEFICIENCY)

This is a rare condition that may present with severe psychomotor delay and seizures. Asymptomatic patients have been reported *(16)*. This enzyme is responsible for the third step of pyrimidine catabolism converting ureidopropionic and ureidobutyric acids to β-alanine and β-aminoisobutyric acid, respectively. No specific treatment exists and management is based on symptomatic care.

Laboratory Diagnosis

Analysis of the urine shows elevation of dihydrouracil and dihydrothymine (metabolites involved in the previous step of pyrimidine catabolism) as well as elevated ureidopropionic acid (also referred to as *N*-carbamyl-β-alanine) and ureidoisobutyric acid (also referred to as carbamyl-β-aminoisobutyric acid; see Table 10-2 and discussion of urinary excretion of purine and pyrimidines).

PYRIMIDINE 5′-NUCLEOTIDASE DEFICIENCY (URIDINE 5′-MONOPHOSPHATE HYDROLASE-1 DEFICIENCY)

Patients with this pyrimidine 5′-nucleotidase deficiency present in infancy or early childhood with unconjugated hyperbilirubinemia and anemia. Severe hemolytic anemia crises have been reported. Splenomegaly may be observed. This is an autosomal-recessive inborn error of pyrimidine catabolism leading to the accumulation of pyrimidine nucleotides, specifically in the erythrocytes. The enzyme is responsible for converting CMP and UMP into cytidine and uridine, respectively. Elevated pyrimidine nucleotides are believed to impair the ATP-requiring oxidized glutathione transport as a possible etiology of hemolytic anemia. Specific therapy does not exist for this condition. Standard management of hemolytic anemia is indicated.

Laboratory Diagnosis

Erythrocytes may have basophilic stippling on a peripheral blood smear. Erythrocyte glutathione is increased. Accumulation of excess pyrimidine nucleotides in deproteinated erythrocytes may be detected by an alteration in ultraviolet absorption or quantified by HPLC or other methods *(17)*.

PYRIMIDINE NUCLEOTIDE DEPLETION SYNDROME (CYTOSOLIC 5′-NUCLEOTIDASE SUPERACTIVITY)

Pyrimidine nucleotide depletion syndrome is a rare condition that presents with psychomotor delay, seizures, ataxia, alopecia, behavior problems, and mild immunodeficiency. Decreased excretion of uric acid in the urine has been reported. Fewer than 10 patients have been described. The disorder is believed to be due to increased degradation of pyrimidine nucleotides caused by overactivity of cytosolic 5′-nucleotidase activity. The disease is believed to be autosomal recessive. A molecular defect has not been discovered. Treatment with uridine showed improved development and decrease in seizures and infections *(18)*.

THYMIDINE PHOSPHORYLASE DEFICIENCY (MITOCHONDRIAL NEUROGASTROINTESTINAL ENCEPHALOMYOPATHY DISEASE)

Patients with mitochondrial neurogastrointestinal encephalomyopathy (MNGIE) typically present in the first 2 decades of life with progressive gastrointestinal and neurological symptoms. Patients manifest with gastrointestinal dysmotility, cachexia, ptosis, external ophthalmoplegia, sensorimotor neuropathy, and asymptomatic leukoencephalopathy. This condition is an autosomal-recessive disorder of pyrimidine catabolism. A defect in the enzyme thymidine phosphorylase leads to accumulation of thymidine, which presumably causes an imbalance of mitochondrial nucleotides and disruption of mitochondrial DNA replication. No specific treatment exists.

Laboratory Diagnosis

Plasma thymidine and plasma deoxyuridine are elevated as measured by HPLC. Thymidine phosphorylase enzyme activity in leukocytes will be decreased. Individuals with MNGIE may also have findings suggestive of mitochondrial DNA depletion or other mitochondrial DNA mutations. Gene testing for thymidine phosphorylase is available.

THYMIDINE KINASE DEFICIENCY

This condition typically presents in childhood with variable muscle weakness from slowly progressive myopathy to a rapidly progressive course and profound respiratory compromise *(19)*. Thymidine kinase enzyme is important in the pyrimidine salvage pathway converting deoxythymidine back to deoxythymidine monophosphate. A defect in this enzyme leads to an imbalance of the mitochondrial deoxynucleotide pools. Because the mitochondria depend heavily on the salvage pathway for the supply of deoxynucleotides, thymidine kinase deficiency results in mitochondrial DNA depletion.

Laboratory Diagnosis

Because thymidine kinase deficiency is considered a mitochondrial disorder, a thorough discussion of laboratory diagnosis will not be discussed in this chapter. Reduced mitochondrial DNA content can be measured by quantitative PCR analysis; this is typically done in affected muscle tissue. Molecular genetic testing of the TK2 gene is available.

URINARY EXCRETION OF PURINE AND PYRIMIDINE METABOLITES

Many of the defects in the purine and the pyrimidine pathway can be differentiated by analysis of urine using HPLC followed by ultraviolet detection or by mass spectrometry detection (see Table 10-2 for a list of disorders detected and the corresponding analytes). A random urine sample is collected and stored at 4 °C if analyzed within a week or frozen and stored at −20 °C if stored longer. A frozen sample should be shipped on dry ice. On the other hand, filter paper can be dipped into a fresh urine sample and fully dried at room temperature *(20)*. Important pitfalls to consider in the analysis of urine purines and pyrimidines include bacterial contamination, which can lead to increased excretion of uracil. Bacterial contamination in the presence of alkaline urine may also lead to hydrolysis of deoxynucleosides to corresponding nucleoside bases. Increased tissue breakdown can lead to elevated thymine and uracil excretion. Patients with certain urea cycle defects may exhibit increased excretion of orotidine, uridine, and uracil as a consequence of accumulation of carbamylphosphate *(21)*.

Table 10-2   Patterns of Urinary Excretion of Purines and Pyrimidines in Metabolic Disorders and Correlation of Uric Acid Concentration in Blood and/or Urine

Disorder	Elevated urine purine/ pyrimidine	Uric acid (B,U)
Phosphoribosylpyrophosphate synthetase super-activity	Hypoxanthine	High
Adenylosuccinase deficiency	Succinyladenosine SAICAR	
AICA-ribosiduria	Succinyladenosine SAICAR	
Adenosine deaminase deficiency	Deoxyadenosine	
Purine nucleoside phosphorylase deficiency	Guanosine Inosine Deoxyguanosine Deoxyinosine	Low
Xanthine oxidase deficiency (and molybdenum cofactor deficiency)	Hypoxanthine Xanthine	Low
Hypoxanthine-guanine-phosphoribosyltransferase deficiency	Hypoxanthine Xanthine	High
Adenine phosphoribosyltransferase deficiency	Adenine Dihydroxyadenine	Normal
UMP synthase deficiency	Orotic acid	
Dihydropyrimidine dehydrogenase deficiency	Uracil Thymine	
Dihydropyrimidinase deficiency	Uracil Thymine Dehydrouracil Dehydrothymine	
Ureidopropionase deficiency	Uracil Thymine Dehydrouracil Dehydrothymine Ureidopropionic Ureidoisobutyric	
Pyrimidine nucleotide depletion syndrome	Psychomotor delay, seizures, infections	Low

SAICAR = 5-phosphoribosyl-5-amino-4-imidazole-succinocarboxamide riboside.

REFERENCES

1. Becker MA, Puig JG, Mateos FA, Jimenez ML, Kim M, Simmonds HA. Inherited super activity of phosphoribosylpyrophosphate synthetase: association of uric acid overproduction and sensorineural deafness. Am J Med 1988;85:385–90.
2. Brouwer A, Duley JA, Christodoulou J. Updated March 29, 2011. Arts syndrome. In: GeneReviews at GeneTests: Medical Genetics Information Resource (database online). Copyright, University of Washington, Seattle, 1997-2012. http://www.genetest.org (Accessed January 2012).
3. Kohler M, Assmann B, Bräutigam C, Storm W, Marie S, Vincent MF, et al. Adenylosuccinase deficiency: possibly underdiagnosed encephalopathy with variable clinical features. Eur J Paediatr Neurol 1999;3:3–6.
4. Laikind PK, Seegmiller JE, Gruber HE. Detection of 5'-phosphoribosyl-4-N-succinylcarboxamide-5-aminoimidazole in urine by use of the Bratton-Marshall reaction: identification of patients deficient in adenylosuccinate lyase activity. Anal Biochem 1986;156:81–90.

5. Marie S, Heron B, Bitoun P, Timmerman T, Van Den Berghe G, Vincent MF. AICA-ribosiduria: a novel, neurologically devastating inborn error of purine biosynthesis caused by mutation of ATIC. Am J Hum Genet 2004;74:1276–81.

6. Tarnopolsky MA, Parise G, Gibala MJ, Graham TE, Rush JW. Myoadenylate deaminase deficiency does not affect muscle anaplerosis during exhaustive exercise in humans. J Physiol 2001;533(Pt 3):881–9.

7. Tarnopolsky M, Stevens L, MacDonald JR, Rodriguez C, Mahoney D, Rush J, Maguire J. Diagnostic utility of a modified forearm ischemic exercise test and technical issues relevant to exercise testing. Muscle Nerve 2003;27:359–66.

8. Reiss J, Gross-Hardt S, Christensen E, Schmidt P, Mendel RR, Schwarz G. A mutation in the gene for the neurotransmitter clustering protein gephyrin causes a novel form of molybdenum cofactor deficiency. Am J Hum Genet 2001;68:208–13.

9. Page T, Bakay B, Nissinen E, Nyhan WL. Hypoxanthine-guanine phosphoribosyltransferase variants: correlation of clinical phenotype with enzyme activity. J Inherit Metab Dis 1981;4:203–6.

10. Sahota AS, Tischfield JA, Kamatani N, Simmonds NA. Chapter 108. Adenine phosphoribosyltransferase deficiency and 2,8-dihydroxyadenine lithiasis. In: Valle D, Beaudet AL, Vogelstein B, Kinzler KW, Antonarakis SE, Ballabio A, eds. Scriver's Online Metabolic & Molecular Bases of Inherited Disease. New York: McGraw-Hill. http://www.ommbid.com (Accessed January 2012).

11. Dimmock DP, Zhang Q, Dionisi-Vici C. Clinical and molecular features of mitochondrial DNA depletion due to mutations in deoxyguanosine kinase. Hum Mutat 2008;29:330–1.

12. Booth RA, Ansari MT, Loit E, Tricco AC, Weeks L, Doucette S, et al. Assessment of thiopurine S-methyltransferase activity in patients prescribed thiopurines: a systematic review. Ann Intern Med 2011;154:814–23.

13. Van Kuilenberg A. Dihydropyrimidine dehydrogenase and the efficacy and toxicity of 5-fluorouracil. Eur J Can 2004;40:939–50.

14. Harris B, Carpenter J, Diasio R. Severe 5′-fluorouracil toxicity secondary to dihydropyrimidine dehydrogenase deficiency: a potentially more common pharmacogenetic syndrome. Cancer 1991;68:499–501.

15. Van Gennip AH, Abeling NG, Vreken P, van Kuilenburg AB. Inborn errors of pyrimidine degradation: clinical, biochemical and molecular aspects. J Inherit Metab Dis 1997;20:203–13.

16. Yaplito-Lee J, Pitt J, Meijer J. Beta-ureidopropionase deficiency presenting with congenital anomalies of the urogenital and colorectal systems. Molec Genet Metab 2008;93:190–4.

17. Simmonds HA, Duley JA, Davies PM. Analysis of purines and pyrimidines in blood, urine and other physiological fluids. In: Hommes FA, ed. Techniques in Diagnostic Human Biochemical Genetics: A Laboratory Manual. New York: Wiley-Liss, 1991.

18. Page T, Yu A, Fontanesi J, Nyhan WL. Developmental disorder associated with increased cellular nucleotides activity. Proc Natl Acad Sci USA 1997;94:11601–6.

19. Oskoui M, Davidzon G, Pascual J, Erazo R, Gurgel-Giannetti J, Krishna S, et al. Clinical spectrum of mitochondrial DNA depletion due to mutations in the thymidine kinase 2 gene. Arch Neurol 2006;63:1122–6.

20. Ito T, van Kuilenburg AB, Bootsma AH, Haasnoot AJ, van Cruchten A, Wada Y, van Gennip AH. Rapid screening of high-risk patients for disorders of purine and pyridine metabolism using HPLC-electrospray tandem mass spectrometry of liquid urine or urine-soaked filter paper strips. Clin Chem 2000;46:445–52.

21. van Kuilenburg AB, van Lenthe H, Löffler M, van Gennip AH. Analysis of pyrimidine synthesis "de novo" intermediates in urine and dried urine filter paper strips with HPLC-electrospray tandem mass spectrometry. Clin Chem 2004;50:2117–24.

Chapter 11

Laboratory Diagnosis of Serotonin and Catecholamine Disorders

Keith Hyland and Lauren A. Hyland

The disorders of neurotransmitter metabolism are varied and include, but are not limited to, those affecting the amino acids glutamate, glycine, and γ-aminobutyric acid (GABA), as well as the monoamines, including serotonin and the catecholamines, which include dopamine, norepinephrine, and epinephrine. This chapter will only concentrate on the laboratory diagnosis of the identified defects that affect serotonin and catecholamine metabolism. These neurotransmitters affect motor, perceptual, cognitive, and emotional brain functions. The pathways involved in their synthesis and catabolism are shown in Figure 11-1. Known defects of monoamine neurotransmitter metabolism include those affecting the cofactors required for their synthesis, enzymes required for synthesis and catabolism, and those affecting other regulatory mechanisms (1). The cofactors required for synthesis are tetrahydrobiopterin (BH_4) and pyridoxal 5′-phosphate (PLP or vitamin B6). BH_4 is synthesized from guanosine triphosphate (GTP) in a three-step reaction involving GTP cyclohydrolase (GTPCH), 6-pyruvoyltetrahydropterin synthase (PTS), and sepiapterin reductase (SR). It is an obligatory cofactor for tyrosine hydroxylase (TH) and tryptophan hydroxylase (TPH). These enzymes convert tyrosine to L-dopa and tryptophan to 5-hydroxytryptophan, and they are the rate-limiting enzymes required for the synthesis of the catecholamines and serotonin, respectively. After its oxidation in the hydroxylase reactions, BH_4 is reduced back to the active cofactor via the actions of pterin 4-α-carbinolamine dehydratase (PCD) and dihydropteridine reductase (DHPR). BH_4 is also required in the liver for the conversion of phenylalanine to tyrosine in a reaction catalyzed by phenylalanine hydroxylase (PAH), and several defects affecting BH_4 metabolism lead to hyperphenylalaninemia. These include autosomal recessively inherited GTPCH deficiency, 6PTS deficiency, PCD deficiency, and DHPR deficiency.

Defects affecting monoamine biosynthesis include the deficiencies of TH, aromatic L-amino acid decarboxylase (AADC), and dopamine β-hydroxylase (DBH). AADC catalyzes the decarboxylation of L-dopa to dopamine and 5-hydroxytryptophan to serotonin. It is a PLP-requiring enzyme, and mutations in the *AADC* gene and in pyridoxamine phosphate oxidase (PNPO), which is required for PLP synthesis, can lead to decreased AADC activity. In noradrenergic neurons, dopamine can be converted to norepinephrine by DBH.

Catabolism of the monoamine neurotransmitters requires the action of monoamine oxidase (MAO) and aldehyde dehydrogenase for serotonin, and MAO, aldehyde dehydrogenase, and catechol-*O*-methyltransferase (COMT) for the catecholamines. The end products of catabolism are 5-hydroxyindoleacetic acid (5HIAA) for serotonin, homovanillic acid (HVA) for dopamine, and 3-methoxy-4-hydroxyphenylglycol (MHPG) for norepinephrine. It is the profile of these metabolites in cerebrospinal fluid (CSF) that can provide evidence for the presence and location of a disturbance of neurotransmitter metabolism. It should be noted that the measurement of MHPG is generally not necessary for diagnosis.

Of the three degradation enzymes, only defects of MAO have currently been described.

Recently, mutations in the dopamine transporter (*DAT1*) were recognized (2). This protein removes dopamine from the synaptic cleft, therefore terminating its action on post- and presynaptic receptors. It is certain that in the near future other defects of monoamine metabolism will be discovered involving

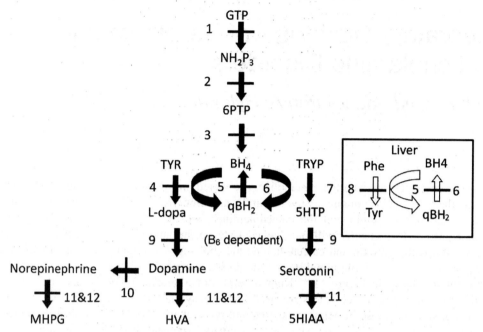

Figure 11-1   Synthesis and catabolism of serotonin, dopamine, and norepinephrine. 1 = GTP cyclohydrolase, 2 = 6-pyruvoyltetrahydropterin synthase, 3 = sepiapterin reductase, 4 = tyrosine hydroxylase, 5 = dihydropteridine reductase, 6 = pterin-4α-carbinolamine dehydratase, 7 = tryptophan hydroxylase, 8 = phenylalanine hydroxylase, 9 = aromatic L-amino acid decarboxylase, 10 = dopamine β-hydroxylase, 11 = monoamine oxidase, 12 = catechol-O-methyltransferase. BH_4 = tetrahydrobiopterin, GTP = guanosine triphosphate, 5HIAA = 5-hydroxyindoleacetic acid, 5HTP = 5-hydroxytryptophan, HVA = homovanillic acid, MHPG = 3-methoxy-4-hydroxyphenylglycol, NH_2P_3 = dihydroneopterin triphosphate, Phe = phenylalanine, 6PTP = 6-pyruvoyltetrahydropterin, qBH_2 = quinonoid dihydrobiopterin, TRYP = tryptophan, Tyr = tyrosine, — = site of a known defect.

COMT together with those affecting the myriad of serotonin and catecholamine pre- and postsynaptic receptors and other proteins that are involved in controlling the delicate balance required for maintenance of the homeostasis of neurotransmission.

DISORDERS OF BH$_4$ METABOLISM

Disorders of BH_4 metabolism can be divided into those with and those without the presence of hyperphenylalaninemia. In addition to having a role in monoamine neurotransmitter biosynthesis, BH_4 is also required for the activity of all forms of nitric oxide synthase (NOS) and, in the liver, for the metabolism of phenylalanine to tyrosine *(3)*. In the absence of BH_4, phenylalanine accumulates and the elevated concentrations can be detected by analysis of phenylalanine in blood. Autosomal-dominant GTPCH deficiency (also known as Segawa disease or dopa-responsive dystonia), a few cases of compound heterozygous autosomal-recessive GTPCH deficiency, and SR deficiency do not lead to hyperphenylalaninemia and, in general, are not considered until the onset of symptoms, which can occur at any age from early infancy into adulthood. In these conditions, diagnosis often relies on neurotransmitter metabolite analysis in CSF.

Clinical Presentation

Most of the defects in BH_4 metabolism in which there is associated hyperphenylalaninemia have a similar clinical presentation *(4)*. Patients present in infancy with symptoms typical of combined serotonin and dopamine deficiency. Obvious neurologic signs appear after 2 months of age and include hypersalivation and temperature disturbance, sweating, pinpoint pupils, oculogyric crises, hypokinesis, distal chorea, truncal hypotonia, swallowing difficulties, tremors, drowsiness, irritability, myoclonus, and brisk tendon jerks. In addition, there may be microcephaly, progressive neurologic deterioration, developmental delay, and convulsions (grand mal or myoclonic), the latter being more frequent in DHPR deficiency. Patients with SR deficiency can have excessive somnolence. There is a mild "peripheral" form of PTS deficiency in which central neurotransmitter metabolism is unaffected. Clinical presentation in this disorder relates only to the presence of hyperphenylalaninemia, and once this is corrected clinical signs are minor or absent. Clinical presentation in the autosomal-dominant form of GTPCH deficiency is different. This classically presents as a dystonic gait disorder with diurnal variation of symptoms at approximately 5–6 years of age. However, the clinical manifestations can be broad and may include a total absence of symptoms, minor muscle cramps, infantile or adult onset, an early non-progressive course, delayed attainment of motor milestones, spastic diplegia, and the occurrence of Parkinsonian-like features in later life.

Genetics and Pathogenesis

Except for the autosomal-dominant form of GTPCH deficiency, all of the primary defects of BH_4 metabolism are inherited in an autosomal-recessive fashion.

GTP Cyclohydrolase Deficiency. GTPCH deficiency can lead to different biochemical perturbations depending on whether it is inherited in the autosomal-dominant or recessive form. It is caused by mutations in the *GCH1* gene located at 14q22.1-q22.2. Severe BH_4 deficiency (as seen in the autosomal-recessive disorder) leads to inactivation of TH, TPH, PAH, and all forms of NOS. This leads to decreased synthesis of serotonin and the catecholamines, to the presence of hyperphenylalaninemia, and to perturbation of nitric oxide metabolism. In the dominantly inherited form there is sufficient BH_4 in the liver to metabolize a normal intake of phenylalanine because hyperphenylalaninemia is generally not seen. Within the brain BH_4 concentrations are reduced but the major effect appears to be on dopamine synthesis. BH_4 acts as a protective chaperone, and in its absence the concentrations of TH protein diminish *(5)*. It is presumed that it does not have a chaperone function for TPH because 5HIAA concentrations in CSF are not as severely affected.

6-Pyruvoyltetrahydropterin Synthase Deficiency. PTS deficiency is caused by mutations in the *PTS* gene, which is located at 11q22.3-q23.3. Severe and mild phenotypes are found. The severe form leads to hyperphenylalaninemia and neurotransmitter deficiency, whereas in the mild form the deficiency seems to be localized to the periphery because hyperphenylalaninemia is present but there is little effect on neurotransmitter metabolism.

SR Deficiency. SR deficiency is caused by mutations in the *SPR* gene located at 2p14-p12. In this disorder, hyperphenylalaninemia is not present because other enzymes are found in the liver that can take the place of the enzyme. These enzymes are not present in the brain, so SR deficiency leads to a profound decrease in serotonin and catecholamine biosynthesis. The lack of SR activity also leads to the accumulation of 7,8-dihydrobiopterin (BH_2), which is an inhibitor of TH, TPH, and NOS. This likely exacerbates the neurotransmitter deficiency and leads to altered nitric oxide metabolism.

Pterin 4-α Carbinolamine Dehydratase. PCD deficiency is caused by mutations in the *PCBD1* gene located at 10q22. Deficiency of this enzyme leads to transient hyperphenylalaninemia but does not affect central neurotransmitter metabolism. Clinical symptoms are minimal if present at all.

Dihydropteridine Reductase. DHPR deficiency is caused by mutations in the *qDPR* gene located at 4p15.31. Deficiency leads to hyperphenylalaninemia and decreased neurotransmitter synthesis. As in SR deficiency, BH_2 also accumulates and likely accentuates the deleterious effect on neurotransmitter biosynthesis. In DHPR deficiency, quinonoid dihydrobiopterin also accumulates. This is thought to be a competitive inhibitor of 5,10-methylenetetrahydrofolate reductase (6). Inhibition of this enzyme leads to a central nervous system (CNS) deficiency of 5-methyltetrahydrofolate (5MTHF) and to the development of periventricular calcifications and demyelination.

Laboratory Diagnosis

Methods used for the laboratory diagnosis of the disorders of BH$_4$ metabolism that lead to hyperphenyl-alaninemia using peripheral fluids have been described in Chapter 2 and will not be explained in detail here. All of the BH$_4$ metabolism defects that affect neurotransmitter metabolism can be diagnosed by the measurement of HVA and 5HIAA and the different oxidation states of biopterin and neopterin in CSF (7). The oxidation states of biopterin include the fully reduced BH$_4$, the partially oxidized BH$_2$, and the fully oxidized biopterin. Neopterin in CSF is found in the 7,8-dihydroneopterin form and as fully oxidized neopterin.

The method of CSF collection is critical if useful data are to be collected (7). There is a rostrocaudal gradient for the pterins and neurotransmitter metabolites in CSF, with values becoming increasingly elevated with the more spinal fluid that is collected. It is therefore important that reference ranges be based on a particular fraction of CSF and that this fraction be used for the analysis of clinical samples. In our laboratory we use the first 0.5 mL collected for the analysis of neurotransmitter metabolites. A second 0.5 mL is collected as a backup, and then the next milliliter collected is used for the analysis of BH$_4$, BH$_2$, and neopterins. BH$_4$ is particularly sensitive to oxidation, and to prevent this from occurring the antioxidants dithioerythritol (1 mg) and diethylenetriaminopentaacetic acid (0.1 mg) must be present in the collection tube before addition of the sample. CSF is dripped directly into the collection tubes from the first drop. If the CSF is contaminated with blood, the tubes should be centrifuged and the clear CSF should be removed and placed into new, labeled tubes and then frozen as soon as possible and stored at −70 °C before shipping on dry ice. It is also critical that obtained values are compared to age-related reference ranges because concentrations of the pterins and the monoamine metabolites decrease with age.

The pterin and neurotransmitter metabolite profiles in CSF are characteristic for each of the disorders that affect BH$_4$ metabolism (Table 11-1). Each oxidation species of biopterin and neopterin can

Table 11-1   Neurotransmitter Metabolite Patterns Observed in CSF in the Inherited Disorders Affecting Catecholamine and Serotonin Metabolism

Disorder	HVA	5HIAA	3OMD	BH$_4$	BH$_2$	NEOP	SEP
GTPCH (recessive)	↓	↓	N	↓	↓	↓	N
GTPCH (dominant)	↓	↓/N	N	↓	↓	↓	N
PTS	↓	↓	N	↓	↓	↑	N
SR	↓	↓	N	↓	↑	N	↑
PCD	N	N	N	N	N	N	N
DHPR	↓	↓	N	↓/N	↑	N	N
TH	↓	N	N	N	N	N	N
TPH*	N	↓	N	N	N	N	N
AADC	↓	↓	↑	N	N	N	N
DβH*	↑	N	N	N	N	N	N
MAO	↓	↓	N	N	N	N	N
DAT	↑	N	N	N	N	N	N

AADC = aromatic L-amino acid decarboxylase, BH$_2$ = 7-8-dihydrobiopterin, BH$_4$ = tetrahydrobiopterin, DAT = dopamine transporter, DβH = dopamine β hydroxylase, DHPR = dihydropteridine reductase, GTPCH = GTP cyclohydrolase, 5-HIAA = 5-hydroxyindoloeacteic acid, HVA = homovanillic acid, MAO = monoamine oxidase, N = normal, NEOP = total neopterin, 3OMD = 3-O-methyldopa, PCD = pterin 4-α-carbinolamine dehydratase, PTS = 6-pyruvoyltetrahydropterin synthase, SEP = sepiapterin, SR = sepiapterin reductase, TH = tyrosine hydroxylase, TPH = tryptophan hydroxylase, ↓ = decreased, ↑ = elevated, * = predicted.

be measured directly using isocratic reversed-phase high-performance liquid chromatography (HPLC) with in-series electrochemical and then fluorescence detection *(8)* or they can be measured using isocratic reversed-phase HPLC with only fluorescence detection as total biopterin and total neopterin after all of the individual pterins have been converted to their fully oxidized forms *(9)*. This can be done using either manganese dioxide or iodine to perform the oxidation reaction. Figures 11-2 and 11-3 show example neurotransmitter metabolite and pterin chromatograms obtained from patients with each form of BH_4 deficiency. In GTPCH deficiency there are decreased concentrations of BH_4 and neopterin. In the central forms of PTS deficiency, BH_4 is low but there is an elevation of the neopterin precursor. In SR deficiency, BH_4 is low, neopterin is normal, and there is accumulation of BH_2 and sepiapterin. Sepiapterin analysis requires the use of a separate reversed-phase HPLC assay that is specific for yellow fluorescent pterins *(9)*. In DHPR deficiency, BH_4 and neopterin concentration are generally normal, but there is an elevation of BH_2. In all of the BH_4 defects that perturb the CNS there are also altered concentrations of neurotransmitter metabolites. These are measured using isocratic reversed-phase HPLC with electrochemical detection *(10)*. All lead to reduced concentrations of HVA and 5HIAA because of inhibited synthesis of dopamine and serotonin. In the dominant form of GTPCH deficiency, the major effect seen is on dopamine metabolism because of the reduction in TH protein concentration found in this condition.

Enzyme assays and mutation analysis are available for all of the defects of BH_4 metabolism. GTPCH can be measured in cytokine-stimulated fibroblasts; PTS in erythrocytes, fibroblasts, and amniocytes; SR in skin fibroblasts and amniocytes; and DHPR in erythrocytes, fibroblasts, amniocytes, and in dried filter paper blood spots *(9)*.

Oral phenylalanine loading can be used to help identify the presence of SR deficiency or dominantly inherited GTPCH deficiency. In these disorders there appears to be sufficient BH_4 in the liver to cope with a normal phenylalanine input, but if the system is stressed by administration of 100 mg/kg of oral phenylalanine, there is an inappropriate conversion of phenylalanine to tyrosine and monitoring the plasma phenylalanine:tyrosine ratio together with plasma biopterin can expose the defect. A caveat is that phenylketonuria (PKU) heterozygotes can have a similar abnormal profile *(11)*.

Treatment and Prognosis

Treatment of defects with associated hyperphenylalaninemia requires correction of the hyperphenylalaninemia and the CNS neurotransmitter deficit. BH_4 supplementation or a low-phenylalanine diet can reduce phenylalanine concentrations in autosomal-recessive GTPCH deficiency and PTS deficiency. BH_4 is generally ineffective in DHPR deficiency because the dose required is extremely large in the absence of the recycling mechanism. The interference with folate metabolism and the development of a CNS folate insufficiency in DHPR deficiency requires supplementation with folinic acid. The neurotransmitter deficit in all disorders is corrected by administration of the neurotransmitter precursors L-dopa and 5-hydroxytryptophan in conjunction with carbidopa. MAO inhibitors have also been given as adjunct therapy. In dominantly inherited GTPCH deficiency, low-dose L-dopa in combination with carbidopa generally produces an excellent clinical response. In all disorders anticholinergic agents have occasionally been supplemented to aid in dystonia control. Prognosis is good in all disorders if therapy is started early *(1)*.

PRIMARY DISORDERS OF CATECHOLAMINE AND SEROTONIN BIOSYNTHESIS

Primary defects in monoamine neurotransmitter synthesis include deficiencies of TH, AADC, and DBH. A defect with a defined pathogenic mutation(s) in the *TPH* gene has not yet been described.

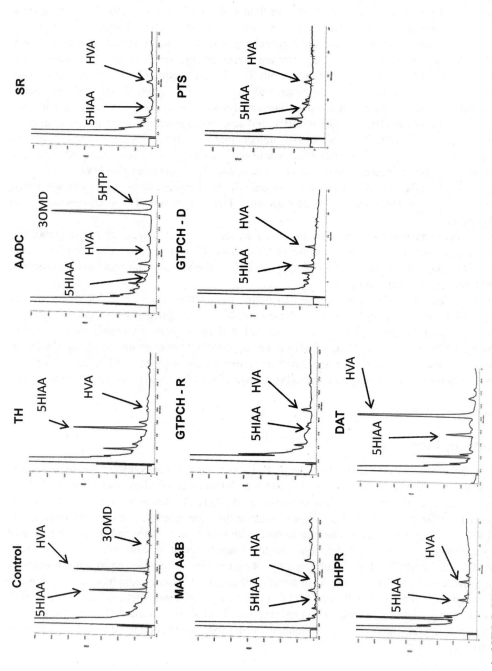

Figure 11-2 Typical HPLC CSF neurotransmitter metabolite chromatograms from patients with disorders of neurotransmitter metabolism. AADC = aromatic L-amino acid decarboxylase, DAT = dopamine transporter, DHPR = dihydropteridine reductase, GTPCH-D = autosomal-dominant GTP cyclohydrolase, GTPCH-R = autosomal-recessive GTP cyclohydrolase, 5HIAA = 5-hydroxyindoleacetic acid, 5HTP = 5-hydroxytryptophan, HVA = homovanillic acid, MAO A&B = combined monoamine oxidase A and B, 3OMD = 3-*O*-methyldopa, PTS = 6-pyruvoyltetrahydropterin synthase, SR = sepiapterin reductase, TH = tyrosine hydroxylase. Chromatograms were obtained using isocratic reversed-phase HPLC with electrochemical detection (*10*).

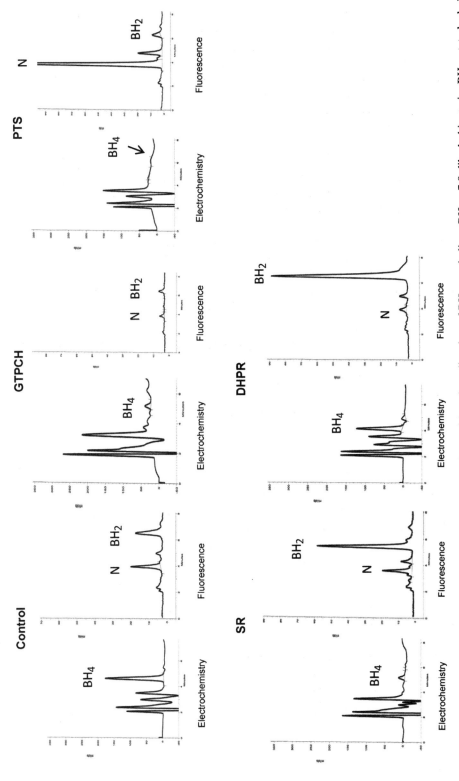

Figure 11-3 Typical HPLC CSF pterin chromatograms from patients with various disorders of BH₄ metabolism. BH₂ = 7,8-dihydrobiopterin, BH₄ = tetrahydrobiopterin, DHPR = dihydropteridine reductase, GTPCH = GTP cyclohydrolase, N = neopterin, PTS = 6-pyruvoyltetrahydropterin synthase, SR = sepiapterin reductase. Chromatograms were obtained using isocratic reversed-phase HPLC with in-series electrochemical and fluorescence detection (*10*).

Clinical Presentation

Clinical presentation is according to the disorder. On the basis of the presenting neurological features, TH deficiency can be divided in two phenotypes: an infantile-onset, progressive, hypokinetic-rigid syndrome with dystonia that presents anywhere between 2 months and 5 years of life (type A) and a complex encephalopathy with onset <3 years of age *(1)*. AADC deficiency generally presents in infancy, but later-onset cases have been reported. Presenting symptoms may include muscle hypotonia and oculogyric crises together with some type of movement disorder that can include athetosis, chorea, dystonia, or hypokinesia. There are also autonomic features that include excessive sweating and temperature instability *(1)*. DBH deficiency has mostly been diagnosed in adolescents or adults who have presented with severe orthostatic hypotension and noradrenergic failure. Retrospective case histories have demonstrated difficulties in the perinatal period, including delay in opening of eyes, ptosis of the eyelids, hypotension, hypothermia, and hypoglycemia. The symptoms of the disease become progressively worse with age. By early adulthood, individuals have profound orthostatic hypotension, greatly reduced exercise tolerance, ptosis of the eyelids, and nasal stuffiness. Apart from the autonomic abnormalities neurologic function is normal *(12)*.

Genetics and Pathogenesis

All of the primary defects affecting neurotransmitter synthesis are inherited in an autosomal-recessive manner.

TH Deficiency. TH deficiency is caused by mutations in the *TH* gene located at 11p15.5. The disorder leads to a lack of catecholamines because the enzyme is the first and rate-limiting enzyme required for dopamine and norepinephrine synthesis. Therefore, the clinical symptoms result from the central and peripheral catecholamine deficiency.

AADC Deficiency. AADC deficiency is caused by mutations in the *DDC* gene located at 7p12.3-p12.1. The disorder leads to a lack of serotonin and the catecholamines because the enzyme is required for the synthesis of both neurotransmitters. Deficiency also leads to an accumulation of the enzyme's substrates, L-dopa and 5HTP. L-dopa is methylated by a reaction catalyzed by COMT using *S*-adenosylmethionine as the methyl group donor. The continual drain on one-carbon metabolism can lead to homocystinemia and to 5MTHF deficiency within the periphery and CNS *(13)*. Lack of the PLP cofactor, as can be found in PNPO deficiency, can cause a secondary decrease in AADC activity *(1)*.

DBH Deficiency. DBH deficiency is caused by mutations in the *DBH* gene located at 9q34.2 *(12)*. The disorder leads to a lack of norepinephrine and epinephrine and to various peripheral autonomic symptoms.

Laboratory Diagnosis

Diagnosis of the primary disorders affecting neurotransmitter synthesis relies mostly on CSF neurotransmitter metabolite analysis for TH and AADC and on measurement of plasma catecholamine profiles in conjunction with physiological tests of autonomic function in DBH deficiency. The measurement of serum prolactin can be informative in all situations in which there is a CNS dopamine deficiency (including the defects of BH_4 metabolism) *(1)*. Pituitary prolactin secretion is regulated by neurosecretory dopamine neurons, which inhibit prolactin secretion. Elevations of blood prolactin may therefore be an indicator of CNS dopamine deficiency. It should be noted that normal prolactin does not exclude a CNS dopamine deficiency.

In TH deficiency there is a decrease in CSF HVA (Figure 11-2). A finding of a low HVA concentration in CSF does not guarantee the presence of TH deficiency. Confirmation of TH deficiency cannot be performed by enzyme analysis because TH is not present in any easily accessible peripheral tissue or cells. Absolute diagnosis therefore relies on a finding of pathogenic mutations in the *TH* gene.

In AADC deficiency there are decreases in HVA and 5HIAA and these are associated with an accumulation of the L-dopa and 5-hydroxytryptophan precursors. L-Dopa can be methylated to 3-*O*-methyldopa (3OMD) and accumulation of this metabolite in association with low HVA and 5HIAA is very characteristic for AADC deficiency. AADC deficiency is one of the few neurotransmitter disorders in which testing of peripheral fluids is useful. 3OMD can be further metabolized to vanillacetic acid. This compound can be detected on a urine organic acid screen. Confirmation of AADC deficiency can be accomplished by measurement of AADC activity in plasma *(14)* or by the finding of pathogenic mutations after gene sequencing.

CSF neurotransmitter metabolite concentrations in DBH deficiency have not been reported. It is presumed that MHPG concentrations would be decreased. The diagnosis of DBH deficiency is normally originally based on clinical findings, including poor cardiovascular regulation and other autonomic dysfunction with intact sweating. Definitive diagnosis may be made by analysis of plasma catecholamines using HPLC with electrochemical detection. The absence or presence of very low concentrations of norepinephrine and epinephrine and their metabolites with plasma dopamine concentrations elevated five- to tenfold above the reference range is likely pathognomonic of DBH deficiency. There may also be a two- to threefold increase in L-dopa. Confirmation of DBH deficiency relies on physiological autonomic testing and a finding of pathogenic mutations after gene sequencing. Plasma enzyme analysis may not be informative because there is a genetically determined interindividual variation in plasma DBH in normal adults, with 3–4% of the population having near-zero concentrations *(12)*.

Treatment and Prognosis

First-line treatment in TH deficiency relies on the use of L-dopa combined with carbidopa. These bypass the metabolic block and allow for catecholamine synthesis. Careful monitoring is required and initial dose should be low to avoid dyskinesis. Response to treatment is varied but in general is better in type A patients when compared with type B. In a large study, 67% of type A patients had normal cognitive capacities during follow-up, whereas 91% of type B patients were mentally retarded. Two type B patients died during follow-up because of infectious and respiratory complications.

Treatment of AADC deficiency is aimed at stimulating residual AADC activity, stimulating postsynaptic receptors, or preventing degradation of the limited neurotransmitters that are produced. AADC is a PLP-requiring enzyme and all patients should receive pyridoxine to test for pyridoxine responsiveness. MAO inhibitors are used to try and conserve the neurotransmitters and dopamine agonists have been used to try and stimulate dopaminergic neurotransmission. Response to treatment is generally limited. A mutation has been described in the *DDC* gene that affects the L-dopa binding site. In this particular case there was a significant clinical response to L-dopa administration *(15)*. Folate supplementation should be considered in all cases because of the disruption of one-carbon metabolism. Response to treatment varies, but in many cases the therapy shows little or no benefit.

DBH deficiency is treated with L-threo-3,4-dihydroxyphenylserine (droxidopa, DOPS). DOPS acts as a substrate for AADC in noradrenergic neurons where it is decarboxylated to norepinephrine. Correction of the norepinephrine defect alleviates the orthostatic hypotension and other symptoms. Long-term prognosis is excellent after initiation of DOPS therapy *(12)*.

DISORDERS OF NEUROTRANSMITTER CATABOLISM

The catabolism of serotonin and the catecholamines requires three enzymes: MAO, COMT, and aldehyde dehydrogenase (Figure 11-1). Of the three, only defects affecting MAO have been described. MAO exists in two distinct forms, MAOA and MAOB, and the genes for these are both located in close proximity to each other and to the Norrie disease (a syndrome characterized by congenital blindness, hearing loss, and variable mental retardation) gene (*NDP*) on the X chromosome. Deletions affecting *MAOA*, *MAOB*, and the *NDP* gene and just *MAOB* and the *NDP* gene have been described *(16, 17)*. In addition, microdeletions encompassing just *MAOA* and *MAOB* exist, as does an isolated defect affecting only *MAOA (18, 19)*. Isolated MAOB deficiency has never been documented.

Clinical Presentation

MAOA and MAOB play major roles in regulating the concentration of neurotransmitters in the brain. Patients missing these enzymes have distinct metabolic and neurologic abnormalities. An isolated defect affecting MAOA has been described in a single family *(19)*. Males showed cognitive impairment and impulsive aggressive behavior. The most prominent behavioral problem was excessive, sometimes violent aggression, often triggered by anger. No description is available concerning the early childhood behavioral characteristics associated with MAOA deficiency. Combined deficiencies of MAOA and MAOB are also known. These can occur in isolation or in association with Norrie disease. Clinical features in Norrie disease in which MAOA and MAOB are involved include severe mental retardation, autistic-like behavior, abnormal peripheral autonomic function, and atonic seizures *(16, 17)*. When there was involvement of the *NDP* gene and the *MAOB* gene, but an intact *MAOA* gene, there were no psychiatric symptoms or mental retardation *(17)*. This suggests that the adverse neurological symptoms mostly relate to the deficiency of MAOA and not to the lack of MAOB. Several patients have been described with a microdeletion affecting only *MAOA* and *MAOB*. These patients showed unique clinical features not seen in Norrie disease with associated deletion of *MAOA* and *MAOB*. These consisted of episodic hypotonia and stereotypic repetitive movements from early infancy *(18)*.

Genetics and Pathogenesis

MAOA and MAOB are encoded by separate genes that share approximately 70% overall homology in amino acid sequence. Both have been mapped to the X chromosome in the p11.23–11.4 region. MAOA deficiency is caused by mutations in the *MAOA* gene. Lack of the enzyme prevents the catabolism of serotonin and the catecholamines and leads to accumulation of these neurotransmitters and to decreased concentrations of their metabolites. MAOB deficiency has only been described in association with either Norrie disease or in association with MAOA deficiency. Comparison of the clinical features and biochemical changes seen in isolated MAOA deficiency, Norrie disease patients with combined MAOA and MAOB deficiency, and with a patient with Norrie disease with only MAOB deficiency has shown that MAOA is the most important enzyme required for monoamine catabolism. In contrast to the borderline mental retardation and abnormal behavioral phenotype seen in patients with selective MAOA deficiency and the severe mental retardation in patients with combined MAOA/ MAOB deficiency and Norrie disease, the MAOB-deficient patients do not exhibit abnormal behavior or mental retardation. In addition, significant changes are seen in monoamine and metabolite concentrations in which there is a MAOA defect but only minor alterations in the face of isolated MAOB deficiency. Several cases of a combined MAOA and MAOB deficiency (in the absence of Norrie disease) have been described *(18, 20)*. In these there were microdeletions on the X chromosome. All had low concentrations of serotonin and catecholamine metabolites in urine.

Laboratory Diagnosis

The laboratory diagnosis of MAOA and MAOB deficiency has relied mostly on neurotransmitter and metabolite analysis in peripheral fluids, although recently elevated serotonin and absent HVA and 5HIAA have been reported in a patient with combined MAOA and MAOB deficiency *(20)*. An example CSF chromatogram from this patient is seen in Figure 11-2. MAOB-deficient patients display normal plasma concentrations of catecholamines, O-methylated amine metabolites, and deaminated metabolites, with the only abnormality being a slight elevation in the urinary excretion of phenylethylamine. Confirmation of MAOB deficiency can be made by measurement of enzyme activity in platelets *(17)*.

MAOA-deficient patients have increased plasma concentrations of O-methylated amine metabolites and decreased plasma concentrations of deaminated metabolites, elevated urinary excretion of O-methylated metabolites and serotonin, decreased urinary excretion of deaminated metabolites, and increased concentrations of 5-HT in platelets. Patients with combined MAOA and MAOB deficiency have a similar biochemical profile to those with isolated MAOA deficiency. Confirmation of MAOA deficiency is made by measurement of the enzyme activity in dexamethasone-stimulated fibroblasts *(19)*.

Treatment and Prognosis

Tyramine and phenylethylamine, which are natural MAO substrates found in the diet, act as indirect sympathomimetics at sympathetic nerve terminals and in the adrenal glands. High concentrations of these compounds can cause dramatic elevations in systolic blood pressure, which can lead to cardiac arrhythmias, intracerebral hemorrhage, and cardiac failure. Treatment of MAOA deficiency is therefore aimed at initiating a diet low in naturally occurring biogenic amines to reduce the possibility of these events occurring. Of the few patients that have been described, a single case died unexpectedly at 5 years of age. The brain was mildly underweight and on microscopy showed small foci of perivascular calcification, occasional hemosiderin granules in the Virchow–Robin spaces, loss of Purkinje cells in the cerebellum, and some loss of neurons in the cortex *(18)*.

DISORDER OF MONOAMINE TRANSPORT

After the action of a neurotransmitter on pre- and postsynaptic receptors, there are several neurotransmitter-specific transporter proteins that remove them from the synaptic cleft, thereby terminating their action. These reuptake transporters exist for the catecholamines and serotonin. Thus far, only a defect affecting *DAT1* has been described.

Clinical Presentation

Patients present in early infancy with a complex movement disorder. This may consist of hyper- or hypokinesia or a mixture of the two. Parkinsonian features with axial hypotonia are often early features. Most develop a progressive generalized dystonia and pyramidal tract features during childhood. A recent review has been published *(2)*.

Genetics and Pathogenesis

DAT1 deficiency is inherited in an autosomal-recessive fashion and is caused by mutations in the *SLC6A3* gene located at 5p15.33. Deficiency of this protein leads to a reduced capacity to take dopamine back into the presynaptic nerve terminals from the synaptic cleft. The dopamine is metabolized to HVA, which accumulates to high concentrations in CSF. It is thought that the inability to reuptake dopamine leads to diminished presynaptic dopamine stores. The excess dopamine in the synaptic cleft also leads to feedback inhibition on dopamine synthesis, therefore exacerbating this effect. The resulting dopamine deficiency leads to the clinical symptoms.

Laboratory Diagnosis

The laboratory diagnosis of DAT1 deficiency relies on CSF analysis. In this disorder, HVA concentrations are highly elevated, whereas 5HIAA concentrations are normal (Figure 11-2). High concentrations of serum prolactin are seen in some patients. Confirmation of diagnosis is achieved by sequencing of the *SLC6A3* gene.

Treatment and Prognosis

Dopamine agonists have been tried as treatment, but with little clinical effect.

REFERENCES

1. Kurian M, Gissen P, Smith M, Heales SJ, Clayton PT. The monoamine neurotransmitter disorders: an expanding range of neurological syndromes. Lancet Neurol 2011;10:721–33.
2. Kurian MA, Li Y, Zhen J, Meyer E, Hai N, Christen HJ, et al. Clinical and molecular characterisation of hereditary dopamine transporter deficiency syndrome: an observational cohort and experimental study. Lancet Neurol 2011;10:54–62.
3. Werner ER, Blau N, Thony B. Tetrahydrobiopterin: biochemistry and pathophysiology. Biochem J 2011;438:397–414.
4. Blau N, Thony B, Cotton RG, Hyland K. Disorders of tetrahydrobiopterin and related biogenic amines. In: Scriver CR, Beaudet AL, Sly WS, Valle D, eds. The Metabolic and Molecular Bases of Inherited Disease. New York: McGraw-Hill, 2001:1725–76.
5. Thony B, Calvo AC, Scherer T, Svebak RM, Haavik J, Blau N, Martinez A. Tetrahydrobiopterin shows chaperone activity for tyrosine hydroxylase. J Neurochem 2008;106:672–81.
6. Kaufman S. Some metabolic relationships between biopterin and folate: implications for the "methyl trap hypothesis." Neurochem Res 1991;16:1031–6.
7. Hyland K. Clinical utility of monoamine neurotransmitter metabolite analysis in cerebrospinal fluid. Clin Chem 2008;54:633–41.
8. Howells DW, Hyland K. Direct analysis of tetrahydrobiopterin in cerebrospinal fluid by high performance liquid chromatography with redox electrochemistry: prevention of autoxidation during storage and analysis. Clin Chim Acta 1987;167:23–30.
9. Blau N, Thony B. Pterins and related enzymes. In: Blau N, Duran M, Gibson KM, eds. Laboratory Guide to the Methods in Biochemical Genetics. Berlin, Heidelberg: Springer-Verlag, 2008:665–701.
10. Hyland K, Surtees RA, Heales SJ, Bowron A, Howells DW, Smith I. Cerebrospinal fluid concentrations of pterins and metabolites of serotonin and dopamine in a pediatric reference population. Pediatr Res 1993;34:10–4.
11. Hyland K, Fryburg JS, Wilson WG, Bebin EM, Arnold LA, Gunasekera RS, et al. Oral phenylalanine loading in dopa-responsive dystonia: a possible diagnostic test. Neurology 1997;48:1290–7.
12. Robertson D, Garland EM. Dopamine beta-hydroxylase deficiency. In: Pagon RA, Bird TD, Dolan CR, Stephens K, eds. GeneReviews [Internet]. Seattle: University of Washington, 2010.
13. Brautigam C, Wevers RA, Hyland K, Sharma RK, Knust A, Hoffman GF. The influence of L-dopa on methylation capacity in aromatic L-amino acid decarboxylase deficiency: biochemical findings in two patients. J Inherit Metab Dis 2000;23:321–4.
14. Hyland K, Clayton PT. Aromatic L-amino acid decarboxylase deficiency: diagnostic methodology. Clin Chem 1992;38:2405–10.
15. Chang YT, Sharma R, Marsh JL, McPherson JD, Bedell JA, Knust A, et al. Levodopa-responsive aromatic L-amino acid decarboxylase deficiency. Ann Neurol 2004;55:435–8.
16. Collins FA, Murphy DL, Reiss AL, Sims KB, Lewis JG, Freund L, et al. Clinical, biochemical, and neuropsychiatric evaluation of a patient with a contiguous gene syndrome due to a microdeletion Xp11.3 including the Norrie disease locus and monoamine oxidase (MAOA and MAOB) genes. Am J Med Genet 1992;42:127–34.
17. Lenders JW, Eisenhofer G, Abeling NG, Berger W, Murphy DL, Konings CH, et al. Specific genetic deficiencies of the A and B isoenzymes of monoamine oxidase are characterized by distinct neurochemical and clinical phenotypes. J Clin Invest 1996;97:1010–9.
18. Whibley A, Urquhart J, Dore J, Willatt L, Parkin G, Gaunt L, et al. Deletion of MAOA and MAOB in a male patient causes severe developmental delay, intermittent hypotonia and stereotypical hand movements. Eur J Hum Genet 2010;18:1095–9.

19. Brunner HG, Nelen M, Breakefield XO, Ropers HH, van Oost BA. Abnormal behavior associated with a point mutation in the structural gene for monoamine oxidase A. Science 1993;262:578–80.
20. O'Leary R, Shih J, Hyland K, Kramer N, Tavyev Y, Graham J. De novo microdeletion of Xp11.3 targeting the monoamine oxidase A and B genes in a male infant with episodic hypotonia: a genomics approach to personalized medicine. Eur J Med Genetics 2012; In press.

Chapter 12

Creatine Deficiency Syndromes

V. Reid Sutton, William E. O'Brien, and Qin Sun

Creatine is critical for temporal and spatial regulation of the intracellular ATP energy pool *(1–3)*. The human endogenous biosynthesis pathway involves arginine:glycine amidinotransferase (AGAT) and guanidinoacetate methyltransferase (GAMT). In the first step, AGAT catalyzes the synthesis of ornithine and guanidinoacetate (GAA) from glycine and arginine. The subsequent conversion of GAA to creatine by GAMT requires *S*-adenosylmethionine (SAM) as a methyl donor and is the largest SAM-consuming reaction in humans. Figure 12-1 shows creatine synthesis and transport pathway. Most creatine synthesis occurs in the kidney, and the product is later taken up by creatine membrane transporters *(4)*.

Disorders have been described in creatine biosynthesis and its membrane transporter. Patients present in infancy and childhood with developmental delay, hypotonia, and, in some cases, seizures. Plasma determination of GAA by high-performance liquid chromatography (HPLC)/tandem mass spectrometry (MS/MS) is the preferred test for diagnosis of AGAT and GAMT deficiencies, whereas urinary creatine measurement is required for the diagnosis of creatine transporter deficiency. In AGAT-deficient patients, plasma GAA is extremely low. High plasma GAA concentrations are considered pathognomonic for GAMT deficiency. Magnetic resonance spectroscopy of the brain of these patients reveals creatine depletion and GAA phosphate accumulation *(5)*. X-linked creatine transporter (XCrT) deficiency is diagnosed based on an elevated urine creatine:creatinine ratio. It is worth noting that the plasma creatine concentration may be in the normal range because of diet or creatine supplementation in individuals with creatine deficiency syndromes.

CLINICAL PRESENTATION

Individuals with disorders of creatine biosynthesis and transport manifest a diverse spectrum of neurological phenotypes. The most common features include seizures, intellectual disability, autism, speech delay, and movement disorders. Although there is a significant amount of phenotypic overlap, the disorders are distinct in their presentation, pathogenesis, and treatment and therefore will be discussed individually.

AGAT Deficiency

AGAT deficiency seems to be the rarest of the three creatine deficiency disorders with only a handful of cases reported in the medical literature. The most prominent feature of AGAT deficiency is developmental delay/intellectual disability, with speech and language development being more impaired than gross- or fine-motor skills. Not all individuals with AGAT have seizures, and in those who do the reports are of occasional fever-induced seizures and not epilepsy *(6)*. IQ scores that are reported are in the mild-moderate intellectual disability range. Intellectual impairment seems to be static and developmental regression has not been reported. Failure to thrive has been identified in one sibling-pair, both of whom also had a reduction in the activity of mitochondrial respiratory chain complex function *(7)*.

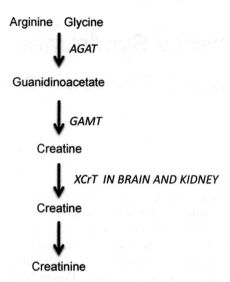

Arginine   Glycine

↓ *AGAT*

Guanidinoacetate

↓ *GAMT*

Creatine

↓ *XCrT IN BRAIN AND KIDNEY*

Creatine

↓

Creatinine

Figure 12-1   Pathway of creatine biosynthesis and transport. AGAT = arginine:glycine amidinotransferase, GAMT = guanidinoacetate methyltransferase, XCrT = X-linked creatine transporter.

"Autistic-like" behaviors have been mentioned but are not well described in case reports, so it is unclear whether this is referring to the severe language delay or whether other features of autism are seen *(8)*. Focal neurologic findings, such as pyramidal or extrapyramidal movement disorders, have not been reported in AGAT deficiency.

GAMT Deficiency

Severe intellectual disability, treatment-resistant epilepsy, and movement disorders are seen in most individuals with GAMT deficiency. Seizures typically present before 3 years of age and types of seizures include myoclonic, generalized tonic-clonic, partial complex seizures, and drop attacks. Autism, hyperactivity, and self-injurious behavior are common, and speech delay is severe with most children having fewer than ten single words *(9, 10)*. Developmental regression, mostly due to movement disorders, is reported. Characteristic findings on brain magnetic resonance imaging (MRI) include bilateral hyperintensities of the globi pallidi and delayed myelination. Creatine concentration on magnetic resonance spectroscopy of the brain is very low and GAA is elevated, although not invariably *(10)*.

XCrT Deficiency

Creatine transporter deficiency appears to be the most common of the creatine deficiency disorders with hundreds of cases described in the medical literature. This disorder appears to account for 1–2% of males with intellectual disability *(11, 12)* and over 4% of males with a family history indicating X-linked intellectual disability *(12)*. In males, intellectual disability can be in the mild to severe range and seizures can be present from early in life or may develop in childhood. Behavior problems, including hyperactivity, are reported and may be progressive. However, a study that sequenced the gene for creatine transporter in 100 males with autism in which "autistic features" are described did not detect any clearly pathogenic mutations *(13)*. Growth retardation, microcephaly, and decreased muscle bulk are seen in many males with creatine transporter deficiency. Half of carrier females have learning and behavior problems. Table 12-1 provides a summary of clinical symptoms in creatine disorders.

Table 12-1 Summary of Clinical Symptoms in Creatine Deficiency Syndromes

Disorder	Intellectual disability	Speech delay	Regression	Seizures	Epilepsy	Autistic features	Extra-pyramidal	Failure to thrive
AGAT	Mild-moderate	+	–	+/–	–	+/–	–	+
GAMT	Severe	++	+	+	+	+	+	
XCrT	Mild-severe	+	+/–	Rare	–	+	–	+/–

+ = present, – = absent.

GENETICS AND PATHOGENESIS

In humans, half of creatine comes from diet and half from endogenous biosynthesis. Creatine is synthesized by the enzymes AGAT and GAMT, principally in the liver and pancreas. Creatine is transported through the blood stream and is actively transported into muscle and brain, where it participates in the high-energy phosphate-buffering system. Creatine/creatine-phosphate regenerates and buffers ATP, which makes it critical in maintaining the high energy levels necessary for brain development and function (14). In addition, there is evidence from rat studies that creatine may serve as a brain neurotransmitter (15). In AGAT and creatine transporter deficiency, the phenotype is secondary to a deficiency of creatine in brain and muscle. In GAMT deficiency, the phenotype is due to creatine deficiency and elevated concentrations of GAA. GAA activates γ-aminobutyric acid (GABA)-A receptors and is thought to be the reason that seizures and movement disorders are more severe in GAMT deficiency as compared with other creatine deficiency syndromes (16).

AGAT and GAMT deficiencies are autosomal-recessive conditions. Creatine transporter is X linked with 50% of female carriers having some neurobehavioral symptoms.

LABORATORY DIAGNOSIS

Creatine and GAA concentration in both urine and plasma should be determined first in patients in whom a creatine deficiency syndrome is suspected. Plasma is preferred for the diagnosis of AGAT and GAMT deficiencies, whereas urine is required to rule out XCrT deficiency. Figure 12-2 shows elevated GAA values in a patient with GAMT deficiency. Because creatine intake from U.S. diet or supplementation increases the creatine:creatinine ratio in urine, it is suggested that an accompanying plasma specimen always be submitted. Simultaneous elevations of plasma and urine creatine imply dietary sources of creatine. In addition, repeat testing for confirmation is recommended before proceeding to DNA sequencing analysis.

Creatine and GAA, Plasma

Draw blood in a heparin-containing tube and separate plasma as soon as possible. Store the specimen frozen at –20 °C. Specimen may be stored frozen for up to 7 days. Ship frozen. It is interesting to note that plasma GAA is increased in combined methylmalonic aciduria and homocystinuria because of cobalamin deficiencies (17).

Creatine and GAA, Urine

Collect 2–4 mL of random urine. When possible, a first morning void or 24-h collection is preferred. Do not add preservatives. Store the specimen frozen at –20 °C and ship frozen. Creatinuria is also found after trauma, likely because of release from injured muscle (18). Such patients should be retested at a later date.

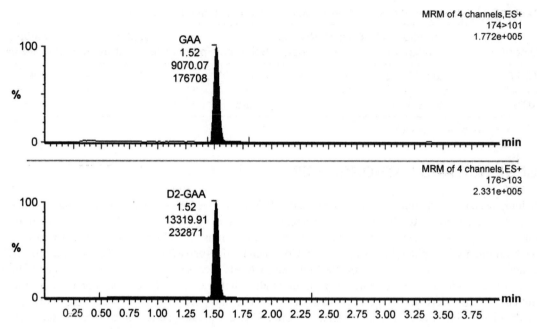

Figure 12-2 Chromatogram of a patient with GAMT deficiency. (Top) GAA at 10.8 μM (normal ranges 0.3–2.8 μM). (Bottom) D2-GAA used as internal standard.

DNA Sequence Analyses

Draw blood in an ethylenediaminetetraacetic acid-containing tube and ship the sample at room temperature.

TREATMENT AND PROGNOSIS

AGAT Deficiency

High-dose creatine has been shown to improve neurological symptoms and central nervous system development, but it does not produce normalization once symptoms have appeared. In one individual treated presymptomatically, development was normal at 18 months of age. Doses of creatine monohydrate of 300–400 mg/kg per day divided 3–6 times per day have been shown to be well tolerated and effective (8).

GAMT Deficiency

High-dose creatine has been shown to improve seizures, movement, and behavioral disorders, but it does not improve the intellectual disability or speech delay. Doses of creatine monohydrate of 300–400 mg/kg per day divided 3–6 times per day have been shown to be well tolerated and effective (8). In individuals who did not respond well to creatine alone, dietary restriction of arginine along with ornithine supplementation has been shown to improve seizures (19). Regimens that have been used restrict arginine to 15–25 mg/kg per day (which corresponds to 0.4–0.7 g/kg per day) and provide 100–800 mg ornithine/kg per day (19). Presymptomatic treatment has only been reported in one case of GAMT and may delay the onset of symptoms but does not prevent them entirely (20).

XCrT Deficiency

Creatine supplementation and arginine restriction have been used in males and females but have not been shown to be effective. Treatment is therefore only symptomatic.

REFERENCES

1. Monge C, Beraud N, Kuznetsov AV, Rostovtseva T, Sackett D, Schlattner U, et al. Regulation of respiration in brain mitochondria and synaptosomes: restrictions of ADP diffusion in situ, roles of tubulin, and mitochondrial creatine kinase. Mol Cell Biochem 2008;318:147–65.
2. Saks V, Kaambre T, Guzun R, Anmann T, Sikk P, Schlattner U, et al. The creatine kinase phosphotransfer network: thermodynamic and kinetic considerations, the impact of the mitochondrial outer membrane and modelling approaches. Subcell Biochem 2007;46:27–65.
3. Saks V, Kuznetsov A, Andrienko T, Usson Y, Appaix F, Guerrero K, et al. Heterogeneity of ADP diffusion and regulation of respiration in cardiac cells. Biophys J 2003;84:3436–56.
4. Braissant O, Bachmann C, Henry H. Expression and function of AGAT, GAMT and CT1 in the mammalian brain. Subcell Biochem 2007;46:67–81.
5. Schulze A, Hess T, Wevers R, Mayatepek E, Bachert P, Marescau B, et al. Creatine deficiency syndrome caused by guanidinoacetate methyltransferase deficiency: diagnostic tools for a new inborn error of metabolism. J Pediatr 1997;131:626–31.
6. Bianchi MC, Tosetti M, Fornai F, Alessandri MG, Cipriani P, De Vito G, et al. Reversible brain creatine deficiency in two sisters with normal blood creatine level. Ann Neurol 2000;47:511–3.
7. Edvardson S, Korman SH, Livne A, Shaag A, Saada A, Nalbandian R, et al. L-Arginine:glycine amidinotransferase (AGAT) deficiency: clinical presentation and response to treatment in two patients with a novel mutation. Mol Genet Metab;101:228–32.
8. Battini R, Leuzzi V, Carducci C, Tosetti M, Bianchi MC, Item CB, et al. Creatine depletion in a new case with AGAT deficiency: clinical and genetic study in a large pedigree. Mol Genet Metab 2002;77:326–31.
9. Mercimek-Mahmutoglu S, Stoeckler-Ipsiroglu S, Adami A, Appleton R, Araujo HC, Duran M, et al. GAMT deficiency: features, treatment, and outcome in an inborn error of creatine synthesis. Neurology 2006;67:480–4.
10. Dhar SU, Scaglia F, Li FY, Smith L, Barshop BA, Eng CM, et al. Expanded clinical and molecular spectrum of guanidinoacetate methyltransferase (GAMT) deficiency. Mol Genet Metab 2009;96:38–43.
11. Clark AJ, Rosenberg EH, Almeida LS, Wood TC, Jakobs C, Stevenson RE, et al. X-linked creatine transporter (SLC6A8) mutations in about 1% of males with mental retardation of unknown etiology. Hum Genet 2006;119:604–10.
12. Lion-Francois L, Cheillan D, Pitelet G, Acquaviva-Bourdain C, Bussy G, Cotton F, et al. High frequency of creatine deficiency syndromes in patients with unexplained mental retardation. Neurology 2006;67:1713–4.
13. Newmeyer A, deGrauw T, Clark J, Chuck G, Salomons G. Screening of male patients with autism spectrum disorder for creatine transporter deficiency. Neuropediatrics 2007;38:310–2.
14. Andres RH, Ducray AD, Schlattner U, Wallimann T, Widmer HR. Functions and effects of creatine in the central nervous system. Brain Res Bull 2008;76:329–43.
15. Almeida LS, Salomons GS, Hogenboom F, Jakobs C, Schoffelmeer AN. Exocytotic release of creatine in rat brain. Synapse 2006;60:118–23.
16. Neu A, Neuhoff H, Trube G, Fehr S, Ullrich K, Roeper J, et al. Activation of GABA(A) receptors by guanidinoacetate: a novel pathophysiological mechanism. Neurobiol Dis 2002;11:298–307.
17. Bodamer OA, Sahoo T, Beaudet AL, O'Brien WE, Bottiglieri T, Stockler-Ipsiroglu S, et al. Creatine metabolism in combined methylmalonic aciduria and homocystinuria. Ann Neurol 2005;57:557–60.
18. Threlfall CJ, Maxwell AR, Stoner HB. Post-traumatic creatinuria. J Trauma 1984;24:516–23.
19. Schulze A, Ebinger F, Rating D, Mayatepek E. Improving treatment of guanidinoacetate methyltransferase deficiency: reduction of guanidinoacetic acid in body fluids by arginine restriction and ornithine supplementation. Mol Genet Metab 2001;74:413–9.
20. Schulze A, Hoffmann GF, Bachert P, Kirsch S, Salomons GS, Verhoeven NM, et al. Presymptomatic treatment of neonatal guanidinoacetate methyltransferase deficiency. Neurology 2006;67:719–21.

Chapter 13

The Congenital Disorders of Glycosylation

Miao He, Dietrich Matern, Kimiyo M. Raymond, and Lynne Wolfe

The congenital disorders of glycosylation (CDG) are a rapidly expanding group of inborn errors of metabolism that result from defects in the synthesis of glycans. Since the first clinical description of a CDG in 1980 by Jaak Jaeken, over 50 disorders have been identified *(1–3, 4)*. (Table 13-1). Most of these are defects in protein glycosylation, although defects in lipid glycosylation and in dermatan and chondroitin chains on proteoglycans have been reported *(3)*. Glycosylation, the major posttranslational protein modification, is a complex process of addition and removal of branched linkages between various monosaccharides linked to mainly the amide group of asparagine (N-linked) or the hydroxyl group of serine or threonine (O-linked) *(4)*. It is believed that approximately 50% of all human proteins are glycosylated through N-linkage accounting for the wide phenotypic variability of CDG patients *(1)*. Many defects in this pathway are designated as CDGx because the underlying defect is still unknown and approximately 30% of patients in the United States with significant protein hypoglycosylation fall into the CDGx category. With an estimated 2% of the human genome encoding proteins for glycosylation and more than six different glycosylation pathways involving synthesis of different glycoconjugates, it can be expected that more CDG will be characterized in the future *(4)*.

Currently, 17 defects of N-glycosylation; 17 defects of O-glycosylation; several CDGs caused by either combined defects in N- and O-glycosylation, glycosphingolipid, and glycophosphatidylinositol (GPI)-anchor glycosylation; or defects in other glycosylation pathways are known (Table 13-1). These disorders were previously grouped as type I defects because they affect assembly and addition of glycans to proteins in the endoplasmic reticulum (ER) and as type II defects characterized by improper trimming and folding of glycoproteins. Because of the rapid changes in our understanding of these complex disorders and identification of new disorders, the original nomenclature was recently revised *(5)* so that the defective enzyme is identified by its gene name and conditions are grouped based on which kind of glycosylation site of a protein is affected. In this chapter, the new nomenclature is applied with the old CDG designation provided in parentheses.

The biosynthesis of N-glycans as well as O-glycans can be divided into three stages (Figure 13-1): (1) the biosynthesis and activation of monosaccharides, (2) the entry of nucleotide sugars bound to dolichol phosphate into the ER and of nucleotide sugars into the Golgi apparatus via specific antiporters, and (3) assembly and processing of the glycans in the ER and Golgi apparatus by specific glycosyltransferases and glycosidases *(4)*. Structure and function of N- and O-linked glycans in humans are highly variable and likely account for the phenotypic variation seen in these disorders.

N-linked glycosylation plays important roles in protein folding and stability, protein-protein complex formation, imparting protease resistance, inter- and intracellular transporting, and cell-cell recognition and signaling. O-linked glycosylation plays roles in antibacterial immune defense, lymphocyte targeting as part of inflammatory responses, and ABO blood type determination. N- and O-linked glycosylation are also important for early human development (including embryogenesis), and many functions of glycosylation are yet to be discovered *(6)*.

Table 13-1   Known Genetic Defects in CDG

Enzyme deficiency	CDG designation (#OMIM)
Disorders of dolichol biosynthesis or recycling	
Dehydrodolichyl diphosphate synthase; *cis-prenyl chain elongation*	DHDDS-CDG (#608172) (autosomal-recessive retinitis pigmentosa type 59)
Steroid 5-α-reductase 3; *probable polyprenol reductase*	SRD5A3-CDG (CDG-Iq) (#612379) (CHIME syndrome)
Dolichol kinase	DOLK-CDG (CDG-Im) (#610768)
Dolichol-phosphate mannosyltransferase polypeptide 1, catalytic subunit; *synthesize Dol-P-Man from GDP-mannose and* *dolichol phosphate*	DPM1-CDG (CDG-Ie) (#608799)
Dolichol-phosphate mannosyltransferase polypeptide 3	DPM3-CDG (CDG-Io) (#612937)
Mannose-phosphate dolichol utilization defect 1	MPDU1-CDG (CDG-If) (#609180)
Disorders of mannose metabolism in cytoplasm	
Mannosephosphate isomerase	MPI-CDG (CDG-Ib) (#602579)
Phosphomannomutase-2	PMM2-CDG (CDG-Ia) (#601785)
Disorders of asparagine-linked glycosylation (ALG, N-linked)	
Asparagine-linked glycosylation 1, β-1,4- mannosyltransferase homolog (*S. cerevisiae*); *GDP-Man:GlcNAc(2)-PP-Dol β-1,4-* *mannosyltransferase*	ALG1-CDG (CDG-Ik) (#608540)
Asparagine-linked glycosylation 2, α-1,3- mannosyltransferase homolog (*S. cerevisiae*); *GDP-Man:Man(1)GlcNAc(2)-PP-Dol α-1,3-* *mannosyltransferase*	ALG2-CDG (CDG-Ii) (#607906)
Asparagine-linked glycosylation 11, α-1,2- mannosyltransferase homolog (*S. cerevisiae*); *GDP-Man:Man(3)GlcNAc(2)-PP-Dol α-1,2-* *mannosyltransferase*	ALG11-CDG (CDG-Ip) (#613661)
Asparagine-linked glycosylation 3, α-1,3- mannosyltransferase homolog (*S. cerevisiae*); *Dol-P-Man:Man(5)GlcNAc(2)-PP-Dol α-1,3-* *mannosyltransferase*	ALG3-CDG (CDG-Id) (#601110)
Asparagine-linked glycosylation 9, α-1,2- mannosyltransferase homolog (*S. cerevisiae*); *Dol-P-Man:Man(6)GlcNAc(2)-PP-Dol α-1,2-* *mannosyltransferase*	ALG9-CDG (CDG-Il) (#608776)
Asparagine-linked glycosylation 12, α-1,6- mannosyltransferase homolog (*S. cerevisiae*); *Dol-P-Man:Man(7)GlcNAc(2)-PP-Dol α-1,6-* *mannosyltransferase*	ALG12-CDG (CDG-Ig) (#607143)
Asparagine-linked glycosylation 6, α-1,3- glucosyltransferase homolog (*S. cerevisiae*); *Dol-P-Glc:Man(9)GlcNAc(2)-PP-Dol α-1,3-* *glucosyltransferase*	ALG6-CDG (CDG-Ic) (#603147)
Asparagine-linked glycosylation 8, α-1,3- glucosyltransferase homolog (*S. cerevisiae*); *Dol-P-Glc:Glc(1)Man(9)GlcNAc(2)-PP-Dol* *α-1,3-glucosyltransferase*	ALG8-CDG (CDG-Ih) (#608104)
Dolichyl-phosphate (UDP-N-acetylglucosamine) N-acetylglucosaminephosphotransferase 1; *GlcNAc-1-phosphate transferase, add GlcNAc* *to dolichol phosphate*	DPAGT1-CDG (CDG-Ij) (#608093)

Table 13-1   Known Genetic Defects in CDG *(Continued)*

Enzyme deficiency	CDG designation (#OMIM)
Disorders of asparagine-linked glycosylation (ALG, N-linked) *(continued)*	
Flippase of Man5GlcNAc2-PP-Dol; *translocate Man5GlcNAc2-PP-Dol from cytoplasmic to luminal side of ER membrane*	RFT1-CDG (CDG-In) (#612015)
Tumor suppressor candidate 3; *oligosaccharyltransferase subunit 3A*	TUSC3-CDG (#611093) (autosomal-recessive nonsyndromic intellectual disability)
Magnesium transporter 1; *oligosaccharyltransferase subunit 3B*	MAGT1-CDG (#160995) (X-linked nonsyndromic intellectual disability)
Mannosidase, α, class 1B, member 1; *ER mannosidase 1, trimming Man9GlcNAc to Man5-6GlcNAc*	MAN1B1-CDG (#604346) (autosomal recessive nonsyndromic intellectual disability)
Mannosyl-oligosaccharide glucosidase; *α-1,2 glucosidase 1, the first step of glucose trimming in ER*	MOGS-CDG (CDG-IIb) (#606056)
Mannosyl(α-1,6-)-glycoprotein β-1,2-*N*-acetylglucosaminyltransferase; *Golgi N-acetylglucosaminyltransferase 2*	MGAT2-CDG (CDG-IIa) (#602616)
O-Linked glycosylation defects	
Exostosin 1; *glucuronosyl-N-acetylglucosaminyl-proteoglycan 4-α-N-acetylglucosaminyltransferase for chain elongation in heparan sulfate biosynthesis in Golgi*	EXT1-CDG (#608177) (AD multiple cartilaginous exotoses)
Exostosin 2; *N-acetylglucosaminyl-proteoglycan 4-β-N-acetylglucosaminyltransferase for chain elongation in heparin sulfate biosynthesis in Golgi*	EXT2-CDG (#608210) (AD multiple cartilaginous exotoses)
Chondroitin synthase 1; *UDP-GlcUA: chondroitin β-1,3-GlcUA transferase, and UDP-GalNAc: chondroitin β-1,4-GalNAc transferase*	CHSY1-CDG (#605282) (Temtamy preaxial brachydactyly syndrome [TPBS])
β-1,3-Glucuronyltransferase 3; *glucuronosyltransferase, synthesis of dermatan sulfate, chondroitin sulfate, and heparin sulfate proteoglycans*	B3GAT3-CDG (#245600) (multiple joint dislocations, short stature, craniofacial dysmorphism, and congenital heart defects)
Carbohydrate sulfotransferase 14; *dermatan-4-O-sulfotransferase 1, catalyzes the 4-O-sulfation of GalNAc residues in dermatan sulfate*	CHST14-CDG (#601776) (Ehlers-Danlos syndrome, musculo-contractural type, adducted thumbs, clubfeet, and progressive joint and skin laxity)
Carbohydrate (chondroitin 6) sulfotransferase 3; *chondroitin-6-O-sulfotransferase 3, catalyzes the 6-O-sulfation of GalNAc residue in chondroitin sulfate*	CHST3-CDG (#143095) (spondyloepiphyseal dysplasia with congenital joint dislocations)
Carbohydrate sulfotransferase 6; *corneal GlcNAc-6-O-sulfotransferase, catalyzes the 6-O-sulfation of GlcNAc or galactose residue in keratan sulfate*	CHST6-CDG (#217800) (macular corneal dystrophy)
Xylosylprotein β-1,4-galactosyltransferase, polypeptide 7; *use UDP-galactose as exclusive substrate, attach the first galactose to O-xylosylproteoglycan*	B4GALT7-CDG (#130070) (EDS progeroid form)

Table 13-1   Known Genetic Defects in CDG *(Continued)*

Enzyme deficiency	CDG designation (#OMIM)
O-Linked glycosylation defects *(continued)*	
UDP-*N*-acetyl-α-D-galactosamine:polypeptide *N*-acetylgalactosaminyltransferase 3; *GalNAc-transferase 3, transfer first GalNAc to OH group of serine or threonine*	GALNT3-CDG (#211900) (tumoral calcinosis)
Solute carrier family 35 (UDP-glucuronic acid/ UDP-N-acetylgalactosamine dual transporter), member D1; *participate in glucuronidation and/or chondroitin sulfate biosynthesis*	SLC35D1-CDG (#269250) (Schneckenbecken dysplasia)
Protein-*O*-mannosyltransferase 1 or 2; *POMT1 requires POMT2 for enzyme function (ER enzyme)*	POMT1/POMT2-CDG (#613156) (congenital muscular dystrophy spectrum)
Protein O-linked mannose β-1,2-*N*-acetylglucosaminyl-transferase; *Golgi O-linked GlcNAc transferase*	POMGNT1-CDG (#613151) (congenital muscular dystrophy spectrum)
Fukutin; *may be a glycosyltransferase*	FKTN-CDG (#613152) (congenital muscular dystrophy spectrum)
Fukutin-related protein	FKRP-CDG (#613153) (congenital muscular dystrophy spectrum)
Like-glycosyltransferase; *N-acetylglucosaminyltransferase-like protein*	LARGE-CDG (#613154) (congenital muscular dystrophy spectrum)
O-Fucosylpeptide β-1,3-*N*-acetylglucosaminyl-transferase; *elongation of O-fucose on NOTCH*	LFNG-CDG (#609813) (spondylocostal dysostosis type 3)
β-1,3-Galactosyltransferase-like; *β-1,3-glucosyltransferase that transfers glucose to O-linked fucosylglycans*	B3GALTL-CDG (#261540) (Peters plus syndrome)
Glycosphingolipid and glycosylphosphatidylinositol (GPI) anchor disorders	
ST3 β-Galactoside α-2,3-sialyltransferase 5; *ganglioside GM3 synthase using lactosylce-ramide as the substrate*	ST3GAL5-CDG (#609056) (Amish infantile epilepsy)
Phosphatidylinositol glycan anchor biosynthesis, class M; *encodes a mannosyltransferase GPI-MT-1, transfer the first mannose to GPI at ER*	PIGM-CDG (#610293) (glycosylphosphatidylinositol deficiency)
Phosphatidylinositol glycan anchor biosynthesis, class V; *encodes a mannosyltransferast GPI-MT-II, transfer the second mannose to GPI back-bone at ER*	PIGV-CDG (#239303) (hyperphosphatasia with MR: Mabry syndrome)
Multiple glycosylation defects	
UDP-Gal:β-GlcNAc β-1,4-galactosyltransferase, polypeptide 1; *Golgi galactose transferase*	B4GALT1-CDG (CDG-IId) (#607091) (clinical presentation uncertain)
Glucosamine (UDP-*N*-acetyl)-2-epimerase/ *N*-acetyl-mannosamine kinase; *bifunctional enzyme in CMP-sialic acid synthesis pathway*	GNE-CDG (HIBM) (#600737) (autosomal recessive, hereditary inclusion body myopathy, Nonaka myopathy)
Glucosamine (UDP-N-acetyl)-2-epimerase/ *N*-acetyl-mannosamine kinase; *feedback effects produce excessive sialic acid in carrier of certain mutations*	GNE-CDG (sialuria) (autosomal dominant, sialuria)

Table 13-1   Known Genetic Defects in CDG (Continued)

Enzyme deficiency	CDG designation (#OMIM)
Multiple glycosylation defects (continued)	
Solute carrier family 35 (CMP-sialic acid transporter), member A1	SLC35A1-CDG (CDG-IIf) (#603585)
Solute carrier family 35, member C1; *GDP-fucose transporter deficiency*	SLC35C1-CDG (CDG-IIc) (#605881) (leukocyte adhesion deficiency type II, LAD II)
ATPase, H+ transporting, lysosomal V0 subunit a2; *one of the five subunits of V0 domain of vacuolar ATPase (v-ATPase), essential for the acidification of diverse cellular components*	ATP6V0A2-CDG (#219200) (cutis laxa type II)
Sec23 homolog B; *component of COPII, coat protein complex for vesicle budding from the ER*	SEC23B-CDG (#224100) (congenital dyserythropoietic anemia type II)
Conserved oligomer Golgi (COG) defects	
Component of oligomeric Golgi complex 1; *conserved oligomer Golgi (COG) subunit 1*	COG1-CDG (CDG-IIg) (#611209)
Component of oligomeric Golgi complex 4; *COG subunit 4*	COG4-CDG (CDG-IIj) (#613489)
Component of oligomeric Golgi complex 5; *COG subunit 5*	COG5-CDG (CDG-IIi) (#613612)
Component of oligomeric Golgi complex 6; *COG subunit 6*	COG6-CDG (CDG-III) (#606977)
Component of oligomeric Golgi complex 7; *COG subunit 7*	COG7-CDG (CDG-IIe) (#608779)
Component of oligomeric Golgi complex 8; *COG subunit 8*	COG8-CDG (CDG-IIh) (#611182)

ER = endoplasmic reticulum.

CLINICAL PRESENTATION

Defects of Protein N-linked Glycosylation

To our knowledge, the most common initial presentation of diagnosed patients with N-linked CDG is developmental delay, followed by failure to thrive, microcephaly, coagulopathy, abnormal brain magnetic resonance imaging (MRI) including cerebral and/or cerebellar atrophy, cell migration abnormalities, and immune dysfunction. Patients with N-linked CDGs present with highly variable multisystem involvement throughout life (1). Given the extreme phenotypic variation, a clinical suspicion for CDG should arise in all clinical settings, in particular once testing for more common causes of the patient's presentation have been excluded (3). Fortunately, most N-linked CDGs can be detected biochemically by serum transferrin analysis and, if negative, N-glycan structural analysis of total plasma or serum glycoproteins. Most N-linked CDG types present with a phosphomannomutase deficiency, PMM2-CDG (CDG-Ia)-like multisystem disorder with a few exceptions as described below. Particularly MPI-CDG (CDG-Ib) is different from other subtypes because most of these patients have minimal neurological deficits.

PMM2-CDG (CDG-Ia) is by far the most prevalent protein N-glycosylation disorder (2). Approximately 60% of patients with congenital hypoglycosylation of transferrin have PMM2-CDG (CDG-Ia). The clinical spectrum of PMM2-CDG (CDG-Ia) is highly variable, but the nervous system is always affected. Three phenotypes of this disorder have been described: an infantile multisystem disease, a late-infantile/childhood ataxia-intellectual disability variant, and an adult stable disability (2). The infantile multisystem variant is characterized by increased mortality in the first two years of life because

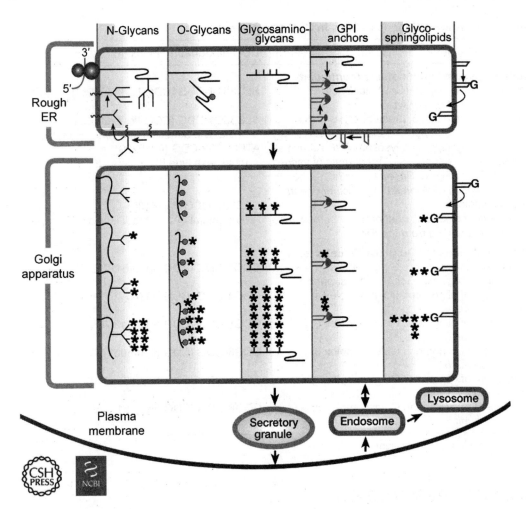

Figure 13-1   Initiation and maturation of the major types of eukaryotic glycoconjugates in relation to subcellular trafficking in the ER-Golgi–plasma membrane pathway. This illustration outlines the different mechanisms and topology for initiation, trimming, and elongation of the major glycan classes in animal cells. Asterisks represent the addition of outer sugars to glycans in the Golgi apparatus. N-Glycans and GPI-anchors are initiated by the en bloc transfer of a large preformed precursor glycan to a newly synthesized glycoprotein. O-Glycans and sulfated glycosaminoglycans are initiated by the addition of a single monosaccharide, followed by extension. The most common glycosphingolipids are initiated by the addition of glucose to ceramide on the outer face of the ER-Golgi compartments, and the glycan is then flipped into the lumen to be extended. Reprinted with permission from *(6)*.

of vital organ involvement or severe infection *(2)*. The neurological symptoms include strabismus, abnormal eye movements, axial hypotonia, psychomotor retardation, ataxia, hyporeflexia, seizures, and olivopontocerebellar hypoplasia. During infancy, feeding problems are common and often require gastrostomy tube placement. Symptoms such as anorexia, vomiting, and diarrhea can contribute to severe failure to thrive. Other variably present features include excessive subcutaneous fat over the buttocks and suprapubic region, microcephaly, and inverted nipples. Hepatomegaly, skeletal abnormalities, pericardial effusion, or cardiomyopathy may also be present. After infancy, symptoms include stroke-like episodes, peripheral neuropathy, retinitis pigmentosa, joint contractures, and skeletal deformities, and most patients are bound to a wheelchair *(2)*. During adulthood, most patients have stable intellectual disability, whereas thoracic and spinal deformities progress. Females lack secondary sexual development with primary ovarian failure, and males may exhibit decreased testicular volume. Other features can include peripheral neuropathy, hyperprolactinemia, insulin resistance, coagulopathy, renal cysts, and proximal tubulopathy *(2)*.

MPI-CDG (CDG-Ib) is mainly a hepatic-intestinal disorder. More than 20 patients have been reported. Symptoms start between one and 11 months of age and consist of variable combinations of recurrent vomiting, abdominal pain, protein-losing enteropathy, recurrent thromboses, gastrointestinal bleeding, liver disease, and hypoglycemia. This is the only CDG that is currently treatable (D-mannose supplementation) *(2)*.

ALG6-CDG (CDG-Ic) is the second most common disorder in protein N-glycosylation with at least 30 patients identified. The clinical feature of CDG-Ic is similar to PMM2-CDG (CDG-Ia), including axial hypotonia, strabismus, seizures, areflexia, ataxia, moderate to severe psychomotor retardation, feeding difficulties, and coagulopathy, particularly deficiencies of clotting factor XI. Inverted nipples and cardiomyopathy may also be present *(2)*.

The second most common CDG after PMM2-CDG (CDG-Ia) in France *(7)* is ALG1-CDG (CDG-Ik), with overall at least 20 patents identified *(7)*. Severe neurological complications are constant features, particularly seizures. Acquired microcephaly is also relatively common, but dysmorphic features are rare and highly variable if present. Optic atrophy has also been reported.

ALG12-CDG (CDG-Ig) has been identified in seven patients with a phenotype similar to PMM2-CDG (CDG-Ia), including psychomotor retardation, hypotonia, seizures, facial dysmorphism, inverted nipples, and subcutaneous fat pads. Immune deficiency and skeletal dysplasia have been described and may be prominent in the severely affected patients *(3)*.

RFT1-CDG (CDG-In) was first described in 2008, and seven patients have been reported. The rapid identification of these patients is likely related to its striking feature of sensorineuronal deafness associated with intellectual disability, hypotonia, seizures, optic atrophy, and feeding problems. Some of them also have inverted nipples, microcephaly, coagulopathy, and kyphoscoliosis *(3)*.

ALG3-CDG (CDG-Id) has been reported in six patients. Neurological impairment was reported in all six patients including dysmorphic facial features, hypotonia, seizures, visual impairment, cerebellar hypoplasia, and psychomotor retardation *(3)*. Some had liver and intestinal involvement. Hyperinsulinemic hypoglycemia and coloboma were reported in one ALG3-CDG (CDG-Id) patient.

ALG8-CDG (CDG-Ih) has been reported in five patients who presented with multiorgan involvement including neurological features as well as hepatomegaly and protein-losing enteropathy similar to PMM2-CDG (CDG-Ia) *(3)*. ALG9-CDG (CDG-Il) and ALG11-CDG (CDG-Ip) have been reported in very few patients who suffered severe multiorgan involvement in infancy in a way similar to PMM2-CDG (CDG-Ia). Inverted nipples and lipodystrophy were reported in one of the affected infants with ALG9-CDG (CDG-Il) *(8)* and deafness was reported in ALG11-CDG (CDG-Ip) patients *(9)*.

DPAGT1-CDG (CDG-Ij) has been reported in one patient with a severe clinical presentation including microcephaly, severe hypotonia, intractable seizures, developmental delay, exotropia, and micrognathia *(10)*. She developed infantile spasms at 4 months of age, within 72 h after DPT (diphtheria, tetanus, pertussin) immunization. A few more patients have been recently identified (unpublished data).

One patient has been reported with ALG2-CDG (CDG-Ii). The child was normal at birth except for bilateral colobomas of the iris, which were discovered along with a unilateral cataract at 2 months old. In the first year of life, she developed a multisystem disorder with mental retardation, seizures, hypomyelination, hepatomegaly, and coagulation abnormalities *(11)*.

TUSC3(OST3A)-CDG and MAGT1(OST3B)-CDG, the only known X-linked recessive CDGs, are caused by defects in subunits of the oligosaccharyltransferase (OST) complex. Both disorders present with nonsyndromic mental retardation *(3)*. Of note, the transferrin isoform profile is normal in these CDGs. Nine genes encode the subunits of two different human OST complexes. Each OST complex consists of seven different subunits and differs by the presence of the TUSC3(OST3A) or MAGT1(OST3B) subunit. It has been proposed that the relative mild clinical and biochemical findings observed in TUSC3(OST3A)-CDG and MAGT1(OST3B)-CDG may be related to functional compensation between these two subunits. A novel DDOST(OST)-CDG has recently been detected and the affected patient had an abnormal transferrin profile, but normal N-glycan and lipid-linked oligosaccharide profiles (12). Additional, yet undiscovered CDGs are likely caused by defects in the other OST subunits.

MAN1B1-CDG was newly described in 12 patients from five families with autosomal-recessive nonsyndromic intellectual disability (13). MAN1B1 encodes an ER α-1,2 mannosidase I, an enzyme involved in trimming of N-linked Man9GlcNAc2 in the ER-associated degradation (ERAD) of glycoproteins. The characterization of MAN1B1-CDG suggests that the ERAD pathway may play a role in the pathogenesis of CDGs.

MGAT2 –CDG (CDG-IIa) was the first identified N-glycan processing defect (CDG type II), but only four patients have been reported. Their presentation included generalized hypotonia, severe intellectual disability, seizures, stereotypic behavior (hand-washing movement, head-banging), macrocephaly, large dysplastic ears, and gum hypertrophy (3). Some were also affected by coagulopathy, skeletal abnormalities, gastrointestinal disturbance, and growth failure.

MOGS-CDG (CDG-IIb) was first reported in a female newborn of consanguineous parents who was delivered at 36 weeks gestation after an uncomplicated pregnancy. Subsequently, multiple congenital anomalies, severe hypotonia with hypermobile joints, hepatomegaly, and low immunoglobulin A were noted. Her hospital course was complicated by seizures, poor feeding, growth failure, polyneuropathy, hearing loss, visual impairment, and respiratory failure, leading to her death at 74 days of age (14). A decade later, the Undiagnosed Disease Program (UDP) at the National Institutes of Health (NIH) identified a second and third patient at the ages of 6 and 11 years and born to nonconsanguineous parents (15). The 6-year-old presented with neonatal seizures and had secondary cerebral folate deficiency that was treated with folinic acid at 1 mg/kg per day leading to resolution of her seizures and improvement of hypotonia. Both siblings identified through the UDP also presented with congenital hypotonia, profound global developmental delay, progressive generalized cerebral atrophy, optic atrophy, sensorineural hearing loss, and hypo/agammopathy without frequent viral infections.

Defects of O-Linked Glycosylation

Defects have been identified in the synthesis of O-xylosylglycans (EXT1/EXT2-CDG, CHST14-CDG, CHSY1-CDG, B3GAT3-CDG, CHST6-CDG, and B4GALT7-CDG), O-N-acetylgalactosaminylglycans (GALNT3-CDG), O-xylosyl/N-acetylgalactosaminylglycans (SLC35D1-CDG), O-mannosylglycans (POMT1/POMT2-CDG, POMGNT1-CDG, LARGE-CDG), and O-fucosylglycans (LFNG-CDG and B3GALTL-CDG). Different O-linked glycans often have different linkage, composition, and tissue distribution (4); thus, there is not a single blood-based biochemical test that will detect all O-linked disorders. Particularly, transferrin isoform analysis will not detect isolated O-glycosylation disorders because there is no O-linked glycosylation on transferrin.

Skeletal and skin findings appear profound in the group of CDGs that affect the synthesis of glycosaminoglycans on the O-xylosylproteoglycans including EXT1/EXT2-CDG, CHST14-CDG, CHSY1-CDG, B3GAT3-CDG, CHST3-CDG, B4GALT7-CDG, SLC35D1-CDG, and GALNT3-CDG with the exception of CHST4-CDG, which is a deficiency in an enzyme mainly expressed in the cornea. These deficiencies in proteoglycan biosynthesis are often detected by reduced immunostaining by specific antibodies toward different glycosaminoglycan chains in cells or tissues and confirmed by molecular genetic analysis (16).

EXT1/EXT2-CDG represents over 70% of cases with hereditary multiple exostoses with autosomal-dominant inheritance. It is characterized by osteochondromas at the end of the long bones. Patients have a higher risk of developing chondrosarcomas and osteosarcomas (3). The exostosin (EXT) gene family encodes glycosyltransferases involved in heparan sulfate biosynthesis and five human members have been cloned to date. EXT1 and EXT2 are believed to form a hetero-oligomeric complex located in the Golgi apparatus and to catalyze the chain elongation step in heparan sulfate biosynthesis.

CHST14-CDG is the cause of the musculocontractural type of Ehlers-Danlos (EDS VIB) also known as adducted thumb-clubfoot syndrome (ATCS). CHST14 encodes a dermatan-4-O-sulfotransferase in dermatan sulfate biosynthesis. Thus far, about 24 cases have been reported who presented with distinct craniofacial features (large fontanels, hypertelorism, and short and downslanting palpebral fissure), multiple congenital contractures, progressive joint and skin laxity, and multisystem fragility similar to the kyphoscoliosis type of EDS *(17)*.

CHST3-CDG causes spondyloepiphyseal dysplasia with congenital joint dislocation. It is also known as chondrodysplasia with multiple dislocations or humerospinal dysostosis *(18)*. More than 18 patients have been reported. The disorder is usually evident at birth with short stature and multiple joint dislocations or subluxations, in a way similar to autosomal-recessive Larsen syndrome. The dislocations often improve over time, and features of spondyloepiphyseal dysplasia (SED) become apparent, leading to arthritis of the hips and spine with intervertebral disc degeneration, rigid kyphoscoliosis, and trunk shortening by late childhood. Congenital heart defects, clubfeet, abnormal hands, deafness, dysmorphic facial features, microdontia, and delayed dentition were observed in some patients. All patients have normal intelligence.

CHSY1-CDG has been identified to be the cause of autosomal-recessive Temtamy preaxial brachydactyly syndrome (TPBS), which is characterized by limb malformations, short stature, and hearing loss. Affected patients have bilateral symmetrical digital anomalies mainly in the form of preaxial brachydactyly and hyperphalangism of digits I-III. CHSY1 encodes a chondroitin sulfate synthase 1 and the deficiency disrupts NOTCH and bone morphogenetic protein (BMP) signaling *(19, 20)*. CHSY1-CDG was reported in at least six consanguineous families.

B3GAT3 encodes a glucuronyltransferase, which is involved in the synthesis of dermatan sulfate, chondroitin sulfate, and heparan sulfate *O*-xylosylproteoglycans. Five siblings from one consanguineous family were reported with B3GAT3-CDG *(21)*. The clinical presentation includes multiple joint dislocations, short stature, craniofacial dysmorphism, and congenital heart defect including bicuspid aortic valve (BAV) and aortic root dilatation. The affected children described have normal skin and no contractures.

SLC35D1-CDG causes Schneckenbecken dysplasia, a rare, severe, lethal skeletal dysplasia comprising platyspondyly, extremely short long bones, and small ilia with snail-like appearance *(3)*. SLC35D1 encodes a UDP-glucuronic acid and UDP-*N*-acetylgalactosamine dual transporter. Thus, glucuronidation and/or chondroitin sulfate biosynthesis of proteoglycans are affected, which may explain the severe phenotype of the affected patients.

Three patients with B4GALT7-CDG presented with EDS progeroid form, with premature aging; macrocephaly; loose, elastic skin; thin, atrophic scars; joint hyperlaxity; hypotonia; and psychomotor retardation *(3)*. B4GALT7 encodes a galactose transferase, adding the first galactose on the *O*-xylosylproteoglycans.

GALNT3-CDG is one of the major causes for hyperphosphatemic familial tumoral calcinosis (HFTC). Patients present with recurrent painful calcified subcutaneous masses of up to 1 kg, often resulting in secondary infection and incapacitating self-mutilation, and some of them developed deep periarticular tumors. All of them have hyperphosphatemia due to increased renal phosphate retention with normal calcium, parathyroid hormone, and 1,25-hydroxyvitamin D3 *(3)*.

LFNG-CDG is a form of autosomal-recessive spondylocostal dysotosis type 3 with extensive vertebral anomalies and camptodactyly of fingers. This disorder is due to defective O-linked fucose O-glycosylation of the epidermal growth factor (EGF)-like repeats of NOTCH and alters NOTCH binding to its ligand Delta *(22)*.

Another *O*-fucose defect is B3GALTL-CDG, responsible for Peters plus syndrome. This disorder is characterized by eye malformations including corneal opacities and irido-corneal adhesions in addition to mental retardation, seizures, mild facial dysmorphism, occasionally cleft lip and/or palate, and multiple other organ involvement *(3)*.

Thus far, there are six O-mannosylation genetic defects associated with the congenital muscular dystrophy (CMD) spectrum: POMT1-CDG, POMT2-CDG, POMGNT1-CDG, FKRP-CDG, FKTN-CDG, and LARGE-CDG. Of these six CDGs, the most commonly seen in the Caucasian population is FKRP-CDG. FKRP-CDG is associated with an extremely wide spectrum of clinical severity, and more recent data suggest this may be a common theme for the other ones *(23)*. A characteristic and diagnostic feature of all six of these CDGs is the abnormal O-mannosylated glycans of α-dystroglycan.

The defects in O-mannosylglycans caused by mutations in POMT1/POMT2-CDG cause Walker-Warburg syndrome (WWS), a rare neuronal migration disorder characterized by brain and eye involvement associated with CMD. These patients have multiple brain anomalies including "cobblestone" lissencephaly, agenesis of the corpus callosum, cerebellar hypoplasia, hydrocephaly, and sometimes encephalocele. This condition is usually fatal during the first year of life (24).

FKTN-CDG, another O-mannosylglycan defect, formerly designated as Fukuyama congenital muscular dystrophy (FCMD) (24), presents with clinical features varying from severe muscle, eye, and brain anomalies (WWS) to a milder limb-girdle myopathy without mental retardation. Some of the FKTN-CDG patients have developed a severe dilated cardiomyopathy before the symptoms of proximal muscle weakness were noted. FKRP-CDG is relatively common and has a similar phenotype to FKTN-CDG. POMGNT1-CDG is also known as muscle-eye-brain disease (MEB), which is similar to WWS but less severe (25). The clinical features of LARGE-CDG are similar to FKTN or FKRP-CDG with a wide spectrum of severity.

Defects of Multiple Glycosylation and Other Pathways

This group comprises three dolichol (SRD5A3-CDGIq, DOLK-CDGIm, DHDDS-CDG) and three dolichol sugar synthesis (DPM1-CDGIe, DPM3-CDGIo, MPDU1-CDGIf) defects, two Golgi nucleotide sugar transport defects (SLC35A1-CDG-IIf, SLC35C1-CDG-IIc), two defects in sialic acid synthesis (GNE-CDG(IBM2) and GNE-CDG [sialuria]), six defects in conserved oligomer Golgi (COG) complex, one defect in a vacuolar-type proton pump-ATPase (ATP6V0A2-CDG), and one defect in the COPII component (SEC23B-CDG) (1).

Among the dolichol synthesis defects, SRD5A3-CDG (CDG-Iq) has been reported in more than 11 patients. Mutations in SRD5A3 have been found in patients with CHIME syndrome (ocular colobomas, congenital heart disease, early-onset ichthyosiform dermatosis, mental retardation, and ear anomalies), a distinct neuroectodermal disease. Patients presented with psychomotor retardation, cerebellar atrophy, hypotonia, nystagmus, elevated liver enzymes, and coagulopathy. In addition, visual loss and/or coloboma and hypoplasia of the optic disc or cataracts in combination with ichthyosiform erythroderma were common. One patient had cardiac hypertrophy. Transferrin analysis may be normal. Accordingly, molecular genetic analysis of SRD5A3 should be considered in patients presenting with coloboma or cataracts in combination with intellectual impairment (3, 25).

Four DOLK-CDG (CDG-Im) patients were reported in 2007 with a severe clinical phenotype causing death in early infancy. All of them presented with ichthyosis and sparse hair at birth or progressive hair loss during the neonatal period. Hypotonia was a common finding. Two patients presented with dilated cardiomyopathy, one with recurrent ketotic hypoglycemia, and one with seizures and acquired microcephaly (3).

Six children have been reported with DPM1-CDG (CDG-Ie). They all showed severe neurological involvement (3). One DPM3-CDG (CDG-Io) patient presented with mild muscle weakness and cardiomyopathy (26).

Four patients have been diagnosed with MPDU1-CDG (CDGIf) due to a mannose-phosphate-dolichol (MPD) utilization defect. All of these patients presented with severe psychomotor retardation, seizures, failure to thrive, dry and scaling skin with erythroderma, and vision impairment (3).

SLC35C1-CDG (CDG-IIc) is caused by GDP-fucose Golgi transporter deficiency. It is better known as leukocyte adhesion deficiency type II syndrome (LAD II), a rare condition characterized by microcephaly, short stature, severe intellectual disability, cortical atrophy, seizures, hypotonia, and failure to thrive. In addition, affected patients suffer from immune deficiency with marked neutrophilia, absence of pus formation, and recurrent bacterial infections (otitis media, periodontitis, and pneumonia). All patients had the rare Bombay (hh) blood phenotype in which erythrocytes lack H-antigen and markedly reduced neutrophil motility (3).

SLC35A1-CDG (CDG-IIf) is due to CMP-sialic acid transporter deficiency. Only one patient has been described. This patient presented with spontaneous and recurrent episodes of bleeding, recurrent bacterial infections, thrombocytopenia, and neutropenia (27).

GNE-CDG comprises different phenotypes. Inclusion body myopathy 2 (IBM2) is an autosomal-recessive defect of a bifunctional protein UDP-GlcNAc 2-epimerase/N-acetylmannosamine kinase, which is part of the CMP-sialic acid synthesis pathway. More than 200 patients with IBM2 have been described. The condition is characterized by a slowly progressive distal and proximal muscle weakness that begins in the late teens to early adulthood with gait disturbance and foot drop secondary to anterior tibialis muscle weakness but sparing of the quadriceps muscles. Muscle histology shows rimmed vacuoles and characteristic filamentous inclusions. The other phenotype associated with mutations in GNE is autosomal-dominant *sialuria (28)*. In this disorder, the mutations affect the epimerase, resulting in overproduction of sialic acid. Fewer than ten patients have been reported who presented with different degrees of developmental delay, coarse facial features, and hepatomegaly *(29)*.

ATP6V0A2-CDG is autosomal-recessive cutis laxa type 2A. It is caused by a defect in the A2 subunit of the V0 domain of the vesicular ATPase H^+-pump *(3)*. Affected patients have furrowing of the skin during infancy that improves with time and may not be notable by the age of 2 years. An enlarged anterior fontanel, congenital hip dislocation, myopia, inguinal hernias, and an abnormal distribution of subcutaneous fat have also been described. Most patients had seizures, and MRI of the brain revealed cortical and cerebellar malformations such as partial pachygyria and Dandy-Walker malformation as well as seizures that developed at any point over the lifespan. Dysmorphic facial features included mid-face hypoplasia, a long philtrum, flat face, low set ears, down slanting palpebral fissures, strabismus, short and anteverted nares, a small mouth, and a high-arched palate with submucosal clefting. Some of the facial features overlap with Noonan syndrome. Of note, cutis laxa has also been observed in some COG7-CDG (CDG-IIe) patients *(30)*.

SEC23B-CDG is also known as congenital dyserythropoietic anemia type II (CDAII). SEC23B encodes a component of coat protein complex II (COPII)-coated vesicles, which facilitate the transport of proteins from the ER to the Golgi apparatus *(3)*. SEC23B-CDG is the most frequent CDA with autosomal-recessive inheritance. More than 300 patients have been reported. CDAII is characterized by ineffective erythropoiesis, hemolysis, morphological erythroblast abnormalities, and hypoglycosylation of band 3 protein (anion exchange protein, a major erythrocyte membrane protein). This disorder appears to be limited to the erythroblast lineage, and a SEC23A isoform in other tissues might compensate for SEC23B deficiency.

COG-CDGs are due to defects in one of the eight subunits of the COG complex. COG complex comprises lobes A (COG 2-4) and B (COG 5-7), with COG1 and COG8 bridging these lobes *(4)*. The following CDGs caused by defects in COG have been identified: COG1-CDG (CDG-IIg), COG4-CDG (CDG-IIj), COG5-CDG (CDG-IIi), COG6-CDG (CDG-III), COG7-CDG (CDG-IIe), and COG8-CDG (CDG-IIh). Patients with COG1-CDG, COG6-CDG, COG7-CDG, and COG8-CDG appear to suffer more severe phenotypes than those with COG4-CDG and COG5-CDG. Common features include global developmental delay, microcephaly, cerebral or cerebellar atrophy, dysmorphic facial features, hypotonia, and feeding problems *(3)*. COG1-CDG (CDG-IIg) may present with skeletal abnormalities that appear as a cerebro-costo-mandibular-like syndrome. Eight patients have been reported with COG7-CDG (CDG-IIe), all with fevers of unknown origin. Some also had wrinkled skin (cutis laxa) and adducted thumbs *(30)*. Only three patients have been identified with COG8-CDG (CDG-IIh). Neuromuscular features in COG8-CDG (CDG-IIh) may resemble mitochondrial disorders *(31)*.

Defects of Glycosphingolipid and GPI-Anchor Glycosylation

Four disorders have been reported as GPI-anchor glycosylation disorder: ST3GAL5-CDG (Amish infantile epilepsy), PIGM-CDG (GPI deficiency), PIGV-CDG (Mabry syndrome), and PIGA deficiency (paroxysmal nocturnal hemoglobinuria [PNH]). Deficiencies in GPI-anchor glycosylation are often diagnosed by flow cytometry after reduction of GPI-anchor proteins, such as CD24 and CD59. This flow cytometry test is often known as a screening test for PNH, an acquired clonal disorder associated with somatic mutations of the X-linked PIGA gene in hematopoietic cells. PIGA encodes GPI *N*-acetylglucosamine (GlcNAc) transferase, which transfers GlcNAc from UDP-GlcNAc to phosphatidylinositol (PI). Note that PNH is not a CDG, but a PNH test is useful for the diagnosis of CDGs that are associated with GPI-anchor glycosylation defects. Any glycoprotein-based CDG testing will not detect this group of disorder.

ST3GAL5-CDG (Amish infantile epilepsy) is an infantile-onset epilepsy syndrome associated with developmental delay and blindness. ST3GAL5 encodes GM3 synthase, a lactosylceramide α-2,3 sialytransferase. Eight patients within one Amish pedigree have been reported *(3)*.

PIGM-CDG is the first CDG identified in the GPI-anchor biosynthesis pathway and caused by diminished expression of the mannnosyltranferase that transfers the first mannose from dolichol-phosphate-mannose to PI. This is an autosomal-recessive condition, characterized by a propensity for venous thrombosis and seizures. Three affected patients from two families were reported with positive Ham tests, indicating absence of the GPI-linked complement inhibitor CD59 from the erythrocyte surface. However, none of the patients showed clinical evidence of hemolysis or bone marrow failure. The acetylation status of the PIGM locus promotes PIGM expression. Butyrate, a histone deacetylase inhibitor, markedly increases PIGM expression, thus allowing for at least partial treatment *(3)*.

PIGV-CDG is better known as Mabry syndrome characterized by hyperphosphatasia and mental retardation. PIGV encodes the second mannosyltransferase in the GPI-synthesis pathway. Mutations have been described in a subgroup of patients with Mabry syndrome who had facial dysmorphism (hyperterlorism, long palpebral fissures, a broad nasal bridge and tip, thin upper lip) and variable neurological features. The hyperphosphatasia is due to defective alkaline phosphatase, a GPI-anchored protein *(3)*.

GENETICS AND PATHOGENESIS

Most CDGs are inherited as autosomal-recessive disorders except MAGT1-CDG, which is X-linked recessive, and EXT1/EXT2-CDG and GNE-CDG (sialuria), which are autosomal dominant.

Although the specific enzyme defects were identified for most CDGs, the pathophysiology of a specific defect remains obscure. This comes as no surprise given the abundant roles that glycosylation plays and the potential effect of defects on various pathways. First, many cellular transport proteins (such as glucose, calcium transporters), clotting factors, immunoglobulins, signaling proteins (such as sonic hedgehog), hormones (such as growth hormone, thyroid hormone, gonadal steroids) and their receptors, and lysosomal hydrolases are glycosylated proteins. Decreased glycosylation of these proteins will affect their function and lead to the variable clinical manifestations. Furthermore, the degree of protein glycosylation often changes during development, which may have consequences on any treatment options over time. Second, glycosylation of proteins also plays a major role in cellular protein folding quality control. About half of the newly synthesized proteins are faulty and defective protein quality control leads to activation of the unfolded protein response (UPR) pathway and disrupts the regulation of ERAD *(32)*. The poorly folded glycoproteins may also be dysfunctional or unstable. Third, accumulation of potentially toxic intermediates such as glycoproteins or glycolipids with abnormal glycan structures or free oligosaccharides (as in the case of MOGS-CDG (CDG-IIb)) may occur because of disrupted pathways.

DIAGNOSTIC TESTING AND EVALUATION

CDGs should be included in the differential diagnosis of any unexplained multisystem syndrome or single tissue disorder. Of note, the initial clinical presentation varies not only between patients with the same CDG, but also within families. New phenotypes are likely to be identified and described over time in most of the rare CDGs. Global developmental delay/intellectual disability in childhood are the most common feature in CDGs. Failure to thrive because of chronic vomiting, diarrhea, and/or amino-aciduria also are relatively common initial symptoms and further support the need to consider CDGs in patients with a wide range of nonspecific symptoms *(33)*.

The classic biochemical diagnosis of CDGs is based on isoelectric focusing (IEF) of serum transferrin. This method relies on a cathodic shift of serum transferrin isoforms being indicative of a CDG. Because this method cannot differentiate between the change of molecular weight and change of surface charge of the protein, it can lead to an underdiagnosis of CDGs, in particular MOGS-CDG (CDG-IIb), SLC35C1-CDG (CDG-IIc), and SLC35A1-CDG (CDG-IIf). In addition, a mixed CDG type I/type II was discovered *(34)* that could not be differentiated from other CDGs by the IEF method. Conversely, false-positive transferrin IEF results can occur because of (benign) amino acid variants of the transferrin protein itself. To overcome these limitations, mass spectrometric (MS) techniques have been applied to transferrin isoform analysis (Figure 13-2, A and B); these techniques provide better resolution and specificity than IEF *(35)*. Analysis of other serum proteins, such as apolipoprotein C, by IEF or MS has proven useful to detect hyposialylation of the mucin-type core 1 O-glycan *(36)* because 75% of patients with uncharacterized CDG type II have an abnormal O-glycan profile.

Although MS-based serum transferrin analysis has overcome some limitations of IEF, screening and diagnosis of CDG type II and COG deficiencies still remain a challenge with protein-based tests because of limited resolution and quantification of glycans with different structure and components. Therefore, new strategies have recently been developed to profile both N- and O-linked glycan chain structures from whole serum or plasma glycoproteins as shown in Figure 13-2, C and D *(37)*. By detecting the glycan structural abnormalities, diagnosis of the CDG type II and COG defects or the combined CDG type II and I can be better achieved. The major advantage of N- and O-glycan profiles of the total glycoproteins in plasma or serum are their abilities to detect the glycans that are not present on transferrin or apolipoprotein C, including high-mannose, glucosylated, fucosylated, and hybrid glycans or mucin core 2 O-glycans *(38)*. For example, SLC35C1-CDG (CDG-IIc) and MOGS-CDG (CDG-IIb) are difficult to diagnose by transferrin analysis but can be detected by N-glycan profiling *(39)*. Some CDG type I subtypes can be detected by N-glycan profiling in plasma or serum through their unique glycan signature, including PMM2-CDG (CDG-Ia), MPI-CDG (CDG-Ib), ALGI-CDG (CDG-Ik), ALG8-CDG (CDG-Ih) (unpublished data). Usually only a small amount of blood is needed for any of the biochemical testing approaches. One to two milliliters of heparin or EDTA blood is often sufficient for transferrin, N-glycan, and O-glycan profile analyses.

The analysis of GPI-anchor proteins on cell surfaces by flow cytometry is being used to diagnose GPI-anchor protein deficiencies *(40)* in which protectin (CD59) is reduced on leukocytes and erythrocytes and CD24 is reduced on granulocytes as well as B cells. However, the reduction of CD59 may only be seen in a small fraction of leukocytes and erythrocytes, making necessary further testing in fibroblast cultures.

Immunostaining of glycosaminoglycans on proteoglycans on the cell surface could also serve as a screening method for proteoglycan biosynthesis defects *(18, 21)*. However, this analysis is currently not clinically available.

Altered glycosylation also occurs in other pathologies. For example, some malignant cells synthesize large N-glycans (known as the Warren-Glick phenomenon) *(41)*. Inflammatory diseases (e.g., rheumatoid arthritis) and some genetic (e.g., classic galactosemia, hereditary fructose intolerance, peroxisomal biogenesis defects) and nongenetic conditions (e.g. hepatitis, chronic alcohol abuse) that cause liver dysfunction can lead to at least intermittent undergalactosylation, undersialylation, and overfucosylation of N-glycan chains. Hemolytic uremic syndrome (HUS) because of infection with neuraminidase-secreting bacteria can also cause abnormal glycosylation patterns.

Urine free oligosaccharide and glycoamino acid analysis by matrix-assisted laser desorption ionization–time of flight (MALDI-TOF) or other MS methods can identify additional CDGs, such as MOGS-CDG (CDG-IIb) and should be considered as additional diagnostic tools to diagnose CDGs. The defect in O-fucosylated glycosylation, such as in B3GALTL-CDG (Peters plus syndrome), has a deficiency in glycosylated amino acids, such as Glc-fuc-threonine, a fucosylated amino acid that can be detected in urine.

Despite the advances in biochemical technologies that allow for the analysis of glycosylation at much higher resolution, molecular genetic analysis of disease-causing genes in CDGs remains the

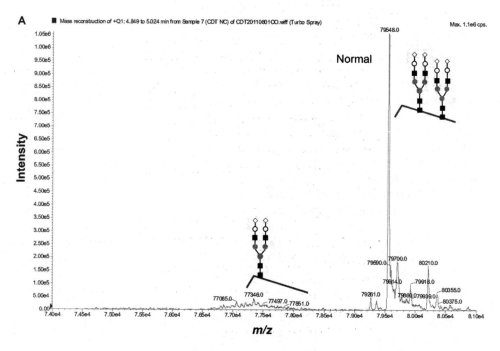

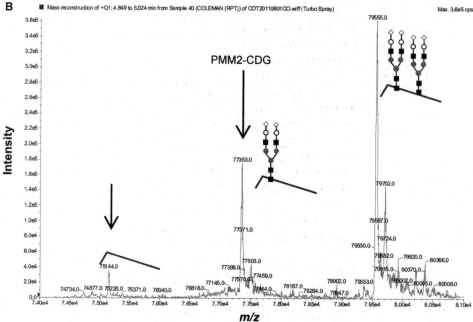

Figure 13-2   Electrospray ionization MS and MALDI profiles of CDG assays. Panels A and B show samples of the normal transferrin profile and the profile of a PMM2-CDG (CDG-Ia), respectively. The arrows point to the transferrin with no glycan (aglycosylated) and the transferrin with only one glycan (monoglycosylated), which are elevated in patients with CDG type I. Panel C shows an overlay of a normal N-glycan profile (black) and a typical abnormal N-glycan profile of a known patient with COG7-CDG (gray). High-mannose glycans and truncated undergalactosylated and undersialylated glycans are increased in most of the patients with genetic defects in COG subunits, whereas normal multiantennary glycans are reduced in these patients. Dashed arrows point to one of the high-mannose glycans, one of the undergalactosylated glycans, and one of the triannentary glycans. Panel D shows a MALDI profile of O-glycans from normal. Arrows point to different O-glycan species identified. ● = mannose, O = galactose, ◇ = sialic acid, □ = N-acetylgalactosamine, ■ = N-acetylglucosamine, ◀ = fucose.

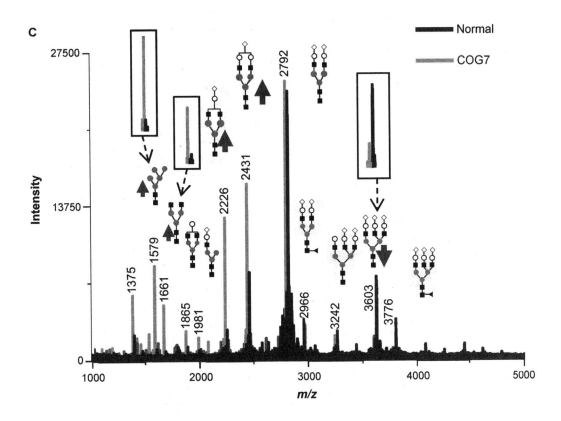

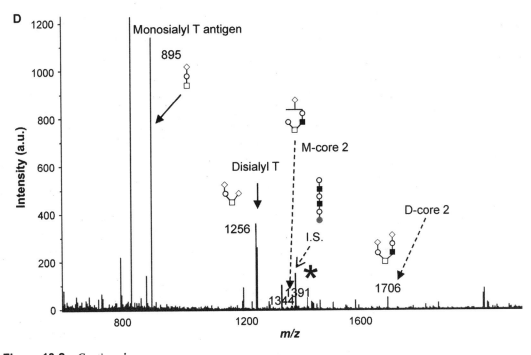

Figure 13-2 *Continued*

only blood-based diagnostic tool to differentiate certain CDG subtypes. In addition, many glycocon-jugates are tissue specific and not present in blood. For example, *O*-mannosylglycans are only present in muscle and brain. The blood-based biochemical assays, such as O-glycan analysis, are only useful when a substantial amount of muscle proteins break down into the blood stream. With the advance of next-generation sequencing, now almost all known CDG-causing genes can be sequenced using only a small amount of DNA. However, in the absence of reliable genotype/phenotype correlations and the currently still high cost of molecular genetic testing, biochemical analysis at functional and metabolic levels will remain the first step in the laboratory diagnosis of CDGs as outlined in Figure 13-3.

Some of the more routine clinical assays are also important in providing additional evidence for the diagnosis and monitoring of at least some CDGs. A complete blood cell count and peripheral smear may identify an unusual anemia (as observed in SEC23B-CDG), thrombocytopenia or a coagulopathy. Interestingly, prothrombin time and partial prothomboplastin time are often normal despite decreased plasma clotting factors II, V, IX, XI, antithrombin III, protein C, and protein S *(2)*. On the other hand, some clotting factors may be quantitatively normal while being dysfunctional. The clotting abnormali-ties are most common in N-linked and mixed glycosylation disorders with the exception of MOGS-CDG (CDG-IIb) *(15)*. This agrees with the fact that sialylated N-glycan production is only mildly reduced in MOGS-CDG (CDG-IIb) because of an alternative pathway from glucosidase I through endomannosidase. Recurrent venous thrombosis has been reported in MPI-CDG (CDG-Ib), RFT1-CDG (CDG-In), and the GPI-anchor disorder (PIGM-CDG). Thrombocytopenia has been identified in ALG8-CDG (CDG-Ih) and SLC35A1-CDG (CDG-IIf) without the apparent clinical implications noted to date.

A leukocyte differential can reveal leukocystosis, leukopenia, neutropenia, or elevated neutrophils, and these abnormalities have been identified in MOGS-CDG (CDG-IIb), SLC35A1-CDG (CDG-IIc) (LAD II), and SLC35A1-CDG (CDG-IIf) *(2)*. Quantitative immunoglobulin analysis is often performed as part of a failure-to-thrive evaluation and may reveal hypo- or agammopathy that may reveal B-cell or plasma cell abnormalities associated with recurrent bacterial infections. SLC35A1-CDG (CDG-IIc) (LAD II) is likely the most severe in this regard; however, MOGS-CDG (CDG-IIb) and some others, such as ALG8-CDG (CDG-Ih), can exhibit similar although milder recurrent infections with hypo- or agammopathy and leukocyte count abnormalities *(1)*.

Chemistry panels for electrolytes, glucose, liver and kidney function, creatine phosphate kinase (CPK), and a lipid panel may reveal organ-specific abnormalities that require further evaluation. Mark-edly abnormal liver function tests have been observed in infants with DPM1-CDG (CDG-Ie), ALG1-CDG (CDG-Ik), MOGS-CDG (CDG-IIb), and B4GALT1-CDG (CDG-IId). Often these abnormalities improve or normalize by 5 years old *(2)*. Low albumin and/or total cholesterol may also be found in some CDGs.

Two dolichol disorders, DPM1-CDG (CDG-Ie) and DPM3-CDG (CDG-Io), as well as MOGS-CDG (CDG-IIb) and B4GALT1-CDG (CDG-IId), have been associated with persistently elevated CPK concentrations. Elevated CPK concentrations and hyperthermia suggestive of malignant hyperther-mia was observed in COG7-CDG (CDG-IIe) *(2)*. In one of the MOGS-CDG (CDG-IIb) siblings, an elevated CPK concentration was found during intermittent illness even without any fever, seizures, and in the face of profound hypotonia *(15)*.

An endocrinology evaluation should be considered in most patients with CDG because hormones and hormone receptors are also subjected to glycosylation and treatable symptoms may be uncov-ered. In CDG-Ia, many females have absent secondary sexual characteristics whereas males appear to undergo normal puberty but may have low testosterone concentrations, micropenis, and small testes *(1, 42)*. In other CDGs, males had elevated testosterone concentrations. Hypothyroidism, growth hor-mone deficiency, and hyperinsulinemia have also been observed in CDG patients.

Skeletal surveys can provide helpful diagnostic clues because skeletal dysplasias, dyostosis, rhi-zomelia, and/or clubfeet have been documented in most CDGs *(43)*. Long bone tumors can occur in GALNT3-CDG as well as EXT1/EXT2-CDGs. Multiple skeletal abnormalities associated with low truncal tone including pectus excavatum, scoliosis, and kypho-scoliosis are common in PMM2-CDG

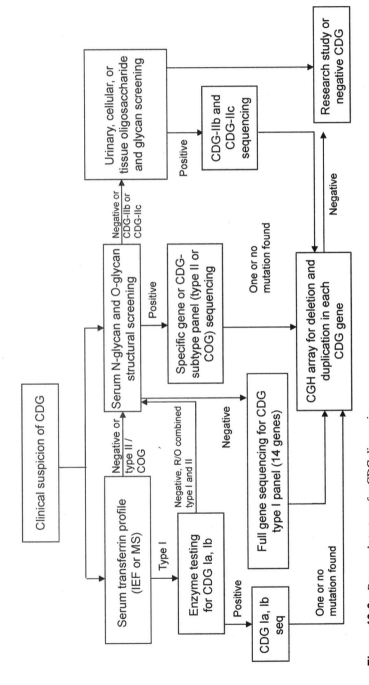

Figure 13-3 Proposed strategy for CDG diagnosis.

(CDG-Ia) and others. Osteopenia is common to most CDGs. For example, the older MOGS-CDG (CDG-IIb) sibling had severe osteopenia and a history of atraumatic long bone fractures but his lateral femur dual-energy X-ray absorptiometry scan was normal as were bone histomorphometric studies. He was subsequently diagnosed with severe vitamin D deficiency and hyperparathyroidism, which resolved after 3 months of vitamin D and calcium supplementation *(15)*. It may therefore be prudent to monitor vitamin D status in CDG patients and treat as needed to prevent bone loss.

Cardiomyopathy has been reported at all ages in patients with PMM2-CDG (CDG-Ia), ALG12-CDG (CDG-Ig), ALG8-CDG (CDG-Ih), ALG1-CDG (CDG-Ik), DOLK-CDG (CDG-Im), DPM3-CDG (CDG-Io), COG1-CDG (CDG-IIg), COG7-CDG (CDG-IIe), and SRD5A3-CDG (CDG-Iq). Accordingly, cardiac evaluation by electro- and echocardiograms can provide diagnostic clues and be indicated for long-term follow-up *(44)*.

Neurological evaluation including electroencephalogram and neuroimaging (e.g., MRI and MRS) can help identify generalized atrophy, cerebellar atrophy, migrational defects, thin or absent corpus callosum, leukoencephopathy, hydrocephalus, and/or stroke, all of which have been reported in CDGs. However, although seizures are common, no specific EEG pattern has been reported *(1)*.

Ophthalmology evaluations may reveal diagnostic hints. For example, nystagmus, optic atrophy, retinitis pigmentosa, and cataract/corneal opacities were observed in CDG patients. Eye abnormalities characteristic of DHDDS-CDG, CHST6-CDG, and B3GALTL-CDG (Peters plus syndrome) and CDGs in protein O-mannosylation are particularly important to identify because neither of these are associated with abnormal transferrin isoforms. Targeted mutation analysis should be considered to diagnose DHDDS-CDG, whereas urine glycoamino acids or platelet glycopeptides may be useful in B3GALTL-CDG (Peters plus syndrome). Microphthalmia, retinal detachment, or pigmentation change and glaucoma are most commonly identified in the O-linked glycosylation defects and are often associated with migrational defects. Colobomas have been reported in PMM2-CDG (CDG-Ia), ALG3-CDG (CDG-Id), ALG2-CDG (CDG-Ii), and SRD5A3-CDG (CDG-1q). Cortical blindness is also frequently observed in other CDGs.

TREATMENT

Treatment for most CDGs remains symptomatic and palliative given the fact that many CDGs cause irreversible damage already in utero. Only four CDGs are at least partially treatable. MPI-CDG (CDG-Ib) is the only known CDG that is effectively treated by oral D-mannose supplementation (1 g/kg body weight per day, divided in 4–6 doses) *(2)*.

Some patients with SLC35C1-CDG (CDG-IIc) respond to fucose supplementation, at least with respect to the problem of recurrent infections *(1, 45)*. Butyrate, a histone deacetylase inhibitor, was used in a PIGM-CDG patient with promoter mutations because butyrate increases PIGM expression leading to seizure control *(46)*. Sialic acid and its precursor ManNAc were shown to be beneficial in the animal model of IBM2-CDG due to GNE deficiency and clinical trials are now underway *(47)*.

As our understanding of the pathophysiology of CDGs advances, more treatment options will undoubtedly become available. Treatment strategies will need to be developed at the metabolic and genetic levels. For patients with missense mutations and a small amount of residual activity of the defective enzyme, strategies that lead to increasing the amount of available substrate or enzyme cofactors could be considered. For example, D-mannose supplementation could be predicted to increase the GDP-mannose concentration, a substrate of several mannosyltransferases. Therefore, provision of D-mannose might be effective in treating some of the eight known mannosyltransferase deficiencies. ManNAc and sialic acid may be potentially used for certain sialic acid transporter or sialyltransferase defects. With discovery of more metabolic pathways that are associated with protein glycosylation *(38)*, treatment that takes advantage of alternative metabolic pathways will emerge. For the patients with nonsense mutations, pharmaceutical compounds that allow ribosomes to read through the premature stop codon may be used as part of treatment for CDG in the near future.

PROGNOSIS

The prognosis of CDG varies among different subtypes and is not well known given the few patients identified for most CDGs. Only for PMM2-CDG (CDG-Ia) have natural history studies been conducted as described earlier in this chapter *(2)*.

REFERENCES

1. Jaeken J. Congenital disorders of glycosylation (CDG): it's (nearly) all in it! J Inherit Metab Dis 2011;34:853–8.
2. Sparks S, Krasnewich D. Congenital disorders of glycosylation overview. GeneReviews 2011.
3. Jaeken J. Congenital disorders of glycosylation. Ann N Y Acad Sci 2010;1214:190–8.
4. Freeze HH. Genetic defects in the human glycome. Nat Rev Gen 2006;7:537–51.
5. Jaeken J, Hennet T, Freeze HH, Matthijs G. On the nomenclature of congenital disorders of glycosylation (CDG). J Inherit Metab Dis 2008;31:669–72.
6. Varki A, Cummings RD, Esko JD, Freeze HH, Stanley P, Bertozzi CR, et al., eds. Essentials of Glycobiology, 2nd ed. New York: Cold Spring Harbor Laboratory Press, 2009.
7. Dupre T, Vuillaumier-Barrot S, Chantret I, Yaye HS, Le Bizec C, Afenjar A, et al. Guanosine diphosphate-mannose:GlcNAc2-PP-dolichol mannosyltransferase deficiency (congenital disorders of glycosylation type Ik): five new patients and seven novel mutations. J Med Genet 2010;47:729–35.
8. Frank CG, Grubenmann CE, Eyaid W, Berger EG, Aebi M, Hennet T. Identification and functional analysis of a defect in the human ALG9 gene: definition of congenital disorder of glycosylation type IL. Am J Hum Genet 2004;75:146–50.
9. Rind N, Schmeiser V, Thiel C, Absmanner B, Lubbehusen J, Hocks J, et al. A severe human metabolic disease caused by deficiency of the endoplasmatic mannosyltransferase hALG11 leads to congenital disorder of glycosylation-Ip. Hum Mol Genet 2010;19:1413–24.
10. Wu X, Rush JS, Karaoglu D, Krasnewich D, Lubinsky MS, Waechter CJ, et al. Deficiency of UDP-GlcNAc:dolichol phosphate N-acetylglucosamine-1 phosphate transferase (DPAGT1) causes a novel congenital disorder of glycosylation type Ij. Hum Mutat 2003;22:144–50.
11. Thiel C, Schwarz M, Peng J, Grzmil M, Hasilik M, Braulke T, et al. A new type of congenital disorders of glycosylation (CDG-Ii) provides new insights into the early steps of dolichol-linked oligosaccharide biosynthesis. J Biol Chem 2003;278:22498–505.
12. Jones MA, Ng BG, Bhide S, Chin E, Rhodenizer D, He P, et al. DDOST mutations identified by whole-exome sequencing are implicated in congenital disorders of glycosylation. Am J Hum Genet 2012;90:363–8.
13. Rafiq MA, Kuss AW, Puettmann L, Noor A, Ramiah A, Ali G, et al. Mutations in the alpha 1,2-mannosidase gene, MAN1B1, cause autosomal-recessive intellectual disability. Am J Hum Genet 2011;89:176–82.
14. Volker C, De Praeter CM, Hardt B, Breuer W, Kalz-Fuller B, Van Coster RN, Bause E. Processing of N-linked carbohydrate chains in a patient with glucosidase I deficiency (CDG type IIb). Glycobiology 2002;12:473–83.
15. Golas GA, He M, Xia B, Song X, Cummings R, Adams DR, et al. Further characterization of Congenital Disorder of Glycosylation IIb in siblings [Abstract]. Society for Inherited Metabolic Disorders Annual Meeting, Pacific Grove, CA, 2011.
16. Zhang L, Muller T, Baenziger JU, Janecke AR. Congenital disorders of glycosylation with emphasis on loss of dermatan-4-sulfotransferase. Prog Mol Biol Transl Sci 2010;93:289–307.
17. Kosho T, Miyake N, Hatamochi A, Takahashi J, Kato H, Miyahara T, et al. A new Ehlers-Danlos syndrome with craniofacial characteristics, multiple congenital contractures, progressive joint and skin laxity, and multisystem fragility-related manifestations. Am J Med Genet A 2010;152A:1333–46.
18. Thiele H, Sakano M, Kitagawa H, Sugahara K, Rajab A, Hohne W, et al. Loss of chondroitin 6-O-sulfotransferase-1 function results in severe human chondrodysplasia with progressive spinal involvement. Proc Natl Acad Sci U S A 2004;101:10155–60.
19. Li Y, Laue K, Temtamy S, Aglan M, Kotan LD, Yigit G, et al. Temtamy preaxial brachydactyly syndrome is caused by loss-of-function mutations in chondroitin synthase 1, a potential target of BMP signaling. Am J Hum Genet 2010;87:757–67.
20. Tian J, Ling L, Shboul M, Lee H, O'Connor B, Merriman B, et al. Loss of CHSY1, a secreted FRINGE enzyme, causes syndromic brachydactyly in humans via increased NOTCH signaling. Am J Hum Genet 2010;87:768–78.

21. Baasanjav S, Al-Gazali L, Hashiguchi T, Mizumoto S, Fischer B, Horn D, et al. Faulty initiation of proteogly-can synthesis causes cardiac and joint defects. Am J Hum Genet 2011;89:15–27.

22. Sparrow DB, Chapman G, Wouters MA, Whittock NV, Ellard S, Fatkin D, et al. Mutation of the LUNATIC FRINGE gene in humans causes spondylocostal dysostosis with a severe vertebral phenotype. Am J Hum Genet 2006;78:28–37.

23. Muntoni F, Torelli S, Brockington M. Muscular dystrophies due to glycosylation defects. Neurotherapeutics 2008;5:627–32.

24. Mercuri E, Messina S, Bruno C, Mora M, Pegoraro E, Comi GP, et al. Congenital muscular dystrophies with defective glycosylation of dystroglycan: a population study. Neurology 2009;72:1802–9.

25. Mohamed M, Cantagrel V, Al-Gazali L, Wevers RA, Lefeber DJ, Morava E. Normal glycosylation screening does not rule out SRD5A3-CDG. Eur J Hum Genet 2011;19:1019.

26. Lefeber DJ, Schonberger J, Morava E, Guillard M, Huyben KM, Verrijp K, et al. Deficiency of Dol-P-Man synthase subunit DPM3 bridges the congenital disorders of glycosylation with the dystroglycanopathies. Am J Hum Genet 2009;85:76–86.

27. Martinez-Duncker I, Dupre T, Piller V, Piller F, Candelier JJ, Trichet C, et al. Genetic complementation reveals a novel human congenital disorder of glycosylation of type II, due to inactivation of the Golgi CMP-sialic acid transporter. Blood 2005;105:2671–6.

28. Seppala R, Lehto VP, Gahl WA. Mutations in the human UDP-N-acetylglucosamine 2-epimerase gene define the disease sialuria and the allosteric site of the enzyme. Am J Hum Genet 1999;64:1563–9.

29. Eisenberg I, Grabov-Nardini G, Hochner H, Korner M, Sadeh M, Bertorini T, et al. Mutations spectrum of GNE in hereditary inclusion body myopathy sparing the quadriceps. Hum Mutat 2003;21:99.

30. Wu X, Steet RA, Bohorov O, Bakker J, Newell J, Krieger M, et al. Mutation of the COG complex subunit gene COG7 causes a lethal congenital disorder. Nat Med 2004;10:518–23.

31. Kranz C, Ng BG, Sun L, Sharma V, Eklund EA, Miura Y, et al. COG8 deficiency causes new congenital disor-der of glycosylation type IIh. Hum Mol Genet 2007;16:731–41.

32. Cantagrel V, Lefeber DJ, Ng BG, Guan Z, Silhavy JL, Bielas SL, et al. SRD5A3 is required for converting polyprenol to dolichol and is mutated in a congenital glycosylation disorder. Cell 2010;142:203–17.

33. Ficicioglu C, An Haack K. Failure to thrive: when to suspect inborn errors of metabolism. Pediatrics 2009;124:972–9.

34. Mandato C, Brive L, Miura Y, Davis JA, Di Cosmo N, Lucariello S, et al. Cryptogenic liver disease in four children: a novel congenital disorder of glycosylation. Pediatr Res 2006;59:293–8.

35. Lacey JM, Bergen HR, Magera MJ, Naylor S, O'Brien JF. Rapid determination of transferrin isoforms by immunoaffinity liquid chromatography and electrospray mass spectrometry. Clin Chem 2001;47:513–8.

36. Wopereis S, Grunewald S, Huijben KM, Morava E, Mollicone R, van Engelen BG, et al. Transferrin and apoli-poprotein C-III isofocusing are complementary in the diagnosis of N- and O-glycan biosynthesis defects. Clin Chem 2007;53:180–7.

37. Faid V, Chirat F, Seta N, Foulquier F, Morelle W. A rapid mass spectrometric strategy for the characterization of N- and O-glycan chains in the diagnosis of defects in glycan biosynthesis. Proteomics 2007;7:1800–13.

38. Hayee B, Antonopoulos A, Murphy EJ, Rahman FZ, Sewell G, Smith BN, et al. G6PC3 mutations are as-sociated with a major defect of glycosylation: a novel mechanism for neutrophil dysfunction. Glycobiology 2011;21:914–24.

39. Guillard M, Morava E, van Delft FL, Hague R, Korner C, Adamowicz M, et al. Plasma N-glycan profiling by mass spectrometry for congenital disorders of glycosylation type II. Clin Chem 2011;57:593–602.

40. Almeida AM, Murakami Y, Layton DM, Hillmen P, Sellick GS, Maeda Y, et al. Hypomorphic promoter muta-tion in PIGM causes inherited glycosylphosphatidylinositol deficiency. Nat Med 2006;12:846–51.

41. Kobata A. Structural alterations of the N-linked sugar chains of glycoproteins produced by tumor cells and their clinical application. Yakugaku Zasshi 1992;112:375–92.

42. Miller BS, Freeze HH. New disorders in carbohydrate metabolism: congenital disorders of glycosylation and their impact on the endocrine system. Rev Endocr Metab Disord 2003;4:103–13.

43. Coman D, Irving M, Kannu P, Jaeken J, Savarirayan R. The skeletal manifestations of the congenital disorders of glycosylation. Clin Genet 2008;73:507–15.

44. Footitt EJ, Karimova A, Burch M, Yayeh T, Dupré T, Vuillaumier-Barrot S, et al. Cardiomyopathy in the con-genital disorders of glycosylation (CDG): a case of late presentation and literature review. J Inherit Metab Dis 2009 Sep 7 [Epub ahead of print].

45. Lubke T, Marquardt T, Etzioni A, Hartmann E, von Figura K., Korner C. Complementation cloning identifies CDG-IIc, a new type of congenital disorders of glycosylation, as a GDP-fucose transporter deficiency. Nat Genet 2001;28:73–6.
46. Almeida AM, Murakami Y, Baker A, Maeda Y, Roberts IA, Kinoshita T, et al. Targeted therapy for inherited GPI deficiency. N Engl J Med 2007;356:1641–7.
47. Noguchi S, Malicdan MC, Nishino I. Animal model of distal myopathy with rimmed vacuoles/hereditary inclusion body myopathy and preclinical trial with sugar compounds. Brain Nerve 2010;62:601–7.

Chapter 14

Lactic Acidemia and Mitochondrial Disorders

Devin Oglesbee and Bryce A. Heese

Mitochondria are multimembrane organelles that are responsible for most cellular oxygen consumption and they house key components of important metabolic processes such as heme biosynthesis, amino acid metabolism, fatty acid oxidation, and nitrogen clearance. Mitochondria are distinctive in the fact that they contain their own 16,569-bp genome, called mtDNA, which encodes for 13 protein products and its own translational machinery with a unique set of DNA codons. Although mtDNA is maternally inherited, it is presumptuous to assume that all defects in mitochondrial metabolism are inherited via the maternal lineage. Indeed, there are hundreds, if not thousands, of protein products that are imported into the mitochondrion by transmembrane apparati and that are required for mitochondrial homeostasis. As the main source of oxygen consumption, mitochondrial disorders have been classically defined as disorders of enzyme or enzyme complexes that are important for oxidative phosphorylation. This includes enzymes involved in pyruvate utilization, the citric acid cycle, the respiratory chain, and the maintenance of the mitochondrial genome (Figures 14-1 and 14-2). Defects in mitochondrial enzymes typically lead to a loss in energy production and accumulation of toxic metabolic intermediates. The decline of mitochondrial activity results in a failure of ATP production to keep up with cellular energy requirements, leading to progressive organ dysfunction, especially in tissues with high energetic demand, such as brain, heart, skeletal muscle, retina, and liver. There is considerable phenotypic overlap between individual mitochondrial disorders, which can be attributed to the accumulation of detrimental metabolites that may have an inhibitory effect on numerous enzymes, the utilization of common redox cofactors, such as NAD^+ and FAD, and the inheritance of genetic mutations in translational machinery, such as tRNAs, which are needed for expression of mtDNA-encoded proteins. In addition to maternal inheritance, mitochondrial disorders can also be inherited recessively, dominantly, or X-linked with variable expression or penetrance. This chapter will touch on the clinical and laboratory diagnosis of a subset of well-defined mitochondrial disorders.

As a clinical entity, mitochondrial disease should be considered for patients presenting at any age with a variation of symptoms including neuromuscular and others involving independent organ systems. The disease progression is often variable, but it is frequently progressive and may be punctuated by periods of stability or even clinical improvement.

In children, mitochondrial disorders frequently present with severe manifestations, including intrauterine growth restriction, encephalomyopathic disease, dysmorphic features, and cerebral malformations. In adults, clinical features tend to express as progressive myopathic disease. In both circumstances, laboratory tests can support a clinical diagnosis. However, there are some situations when a clinical presentation, and concurrent laboratory testing, are insufficient to conclusively diagnose an individual with a mitochondrial disease. Current practice has unfortunately adopted less-than-ideal clinical criteria that include labels such as "definite, probable, possible, and unlikely" to describe levels of certainty regarding the presence of a mitochondrial disease *(1)*.

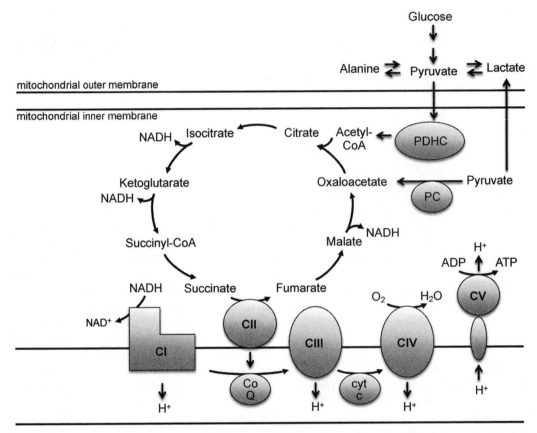

Figure 14-1 Mitochondrial energy metabolism. CI = complex I or NADH:ubiquinone oxidoreductase, CII = complex II or succinate dehydrogenase. CIII = complex III or ubiquinone:cytochrome c oxidoreductase, CIV = complex IV or cytochrome c oxidase, CoQ = coenzyme Q, CV = complex V or ATP synthase, Cyt c = cytochrome c, PC = pyruvate carboxylase, PDHC = pyruvate dehydrogenase complex.

PYRUVATE CARBOXYLASE DEFICIENCY

Clinical Presentation

Pyruvate carboxylase (PC) is a biotin-containing, nuclear-encoded, mitochondrial-localized enzyme that is critical for the conversion of pyruvate to oxaloacetate, which is an important component of the citric acid cycle as well as gluconeogenesis and neurotransmitter synthesis. PC deficiency is a rare mitochondrial disorder that is characterized into three clinical subphenotypes according to the severity of clinical and biochemical findings (2, 3). There is an infantile-onset form (type A or North American form) that presents as relatively moderate infantile lactic acidemia with neurological abnormalities, including developmental delay, hypotonia, ataxia, and early death (4). There is also a rigorous neonatal form (type B or French form) that presents with severe lactic acidemia, respiratory distress, hyperammonemia, tremor, and seizures and is often fatal within months. Lastly, there is a relative mild form (type C) that presents with variable severity, including intermittent attacks of ketolactic acidosis, mild developmental delays, or even normal neurological outcomes (4).

Genetics and Pathogenesis

PC deficiency is an autosomal-recessive genetic disorder caused by mutations in the PC gene on chromosome 11q13.2, which encodes for a biotin-containing tetrameric enzyme important for gluconeogenesis,

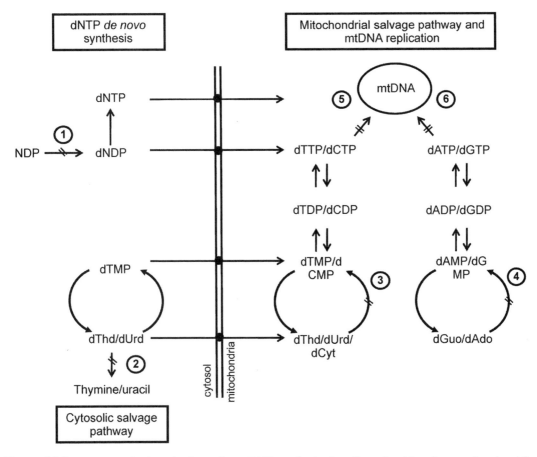

Figure 14-2 dNTP synthesis and salvage for mtDNA synthesis. 1 = ribonucleotide reductase, 2 = thymidine phosphorylase, 3 = thymidine kinase, 4 = mitochondrial deoxyguanosine kinase, 5 = mtDNA helicase, twinkle, 6 = mtDNA polymerase g. dAdo = deoxyadenosine, dADP = deoxyadenosine diphosphate, dAMP = deoxyadenosine monophosphate, dATP = deoxyadenosine triphosphate, dCDP = deoxycytidine diphosphate, dCMP = deoxycytidine monophosphate, dCTP = deoxycytidine triphosphate, dCyt = deoxycytidine, dGDP = deoxyguanosine diphosphate, dGMP = deoxyguanosine monophosphate, dGTP = deoxyguanosine triphosphate, dGuo = deoxyguanosine, dNDP = deoxyribonucleoside diphosphate, dNTP = deoxyribonucleoside triphosphate, dTDP = thymidine diphosphate, dThd = thymidine, dTMP = thymidine monophosphate, dTTP = thymidine triphosphate, dUrd = deoxyuridine, NDP = nucleoside diphosphate.

lipogenesis, and neurotransmitter synthesis. The incidence of PC deficiency is very low (1:250,000), but there are regional variations in the prevalence of this condition, such as an increased incidence among some native North Americans and Europeans of Arab descent *(5)*. The lack of sufficient PC activity leads to the accumulation of pyruvate and a concomitant reduction in oxaloacetate. Excess pyruvate is subsequently converted to lactate by lactate dehydrogenase, which causes an increase in the concentration of plasma lactate. As expected, blood pyruvate elevations are also found in PC deficiency, leading to a normal lactate:pyruvate ratio for some PC deficiencies, especially for types A and C. In addition, the loss of oxaloacetate production impedes the citric acid cycle, which has the downstream effect of reducing the production of NADH from NAD^+ and limiting the oxidation of acetyl-CoA in several organs, such as liver. Outcomes of these metabolic imbalances include elevated lactate and pyruvate in blood and cerebrospinal fluid (CSF), elevated ketone bodies (3-hydroxybutyrate acid and acetoacetate) in blood, hyperammonemia, and alterations in plasma and urine amino acid profiles, such as elevated alanine and proline from the shunting of pyruvate and increased citrulline and lysine concentrations from secondary urea cycle inhibition and hyperammonemia, respectfully. There is not a strong genotype-phenotype correlation for PC deficiency, and an attempt to explain this finding has included theories about somatic mosaicism. Most PC-deficient individuals have missense mutations in the PC gene, but splice-site, single-nucleotide duplications and small deletions also occur. Indeed, it is generally accepted that molecular alterations that lead to absent or low amounts of PC mRNA or protein will cause a more severe phenotype.

Laboratory Diagnosis

A diagnosis of PC deficiency relies heavily on the identification of abnormal analyte values from proper laboratory testing. When PC deficiency is suspected, consider plasma lactate and pyruvate, amino acid profiles from serum and urine, blood ammonia, and ketone body measurements. PC activity in skin fibroblasts, leukocytes, and other tissue, such as muscle, is commonly found to be ≤10% than that observed in normal controls.

For type A PC deficiency, plasma concentrations of lactate are typically <10 mmol/L but may vary depending on metabolic status. The lactate:pyruvate (L/P) ratio is commonly normal (<20). Amino acid profiles from plasma and urine usually have significantly elevated concentrations of alanine and proline, whereas the elevation of other amino acids may fluctuate depending on illness and diet. PC activity in skin fibroblasts is consistently low, and molecular analysis of the PC gene can confirm the presence of two DNA sequence alterations.

For type B PC deficiency, plasma lactate concentrations are generally >10 mmol/L and may be as high as >20 mmol/L (6). The plasma L/P ratio is consistently >20. Amino acid elevations include moderate to markedly increased concentrations of alanine, proline, lysine, and citrulline. Blood ammonia concentrations are elevated, as are total ketone bodies. Hypoglycemia may also be commonplace (6). PC activity in skin fibroblasts is typically very low (<5%), but there have been cases with residual PC activity in the 10% of normal control range (6).

For type C PC deficiency, plasma lactate and blood pyruvate concentrations are elevated during an episode of ketoacidosis, but lactate will not reach >10 mmol/L and the L/P will remain <20. Total ketone bodies will be moderately elevated and plasma amino acids may be normal. PC activity in skin fibroblasts will show a reduction in PC activity to 10% of normal control values.

Molecular genetic testing for PC deficiency is clinically available to help confirm the diagnosis.

Treatment

Current treatments focus on providing alternative energy sources, inducing residual PC activity with additional cofactor supplementation, hydration, and correction of the metabolic acidosis during an acute crisis. There is evidence that citrate supplementation will assist with reducing the metabolic acidosis and that aspartate supplementation will bypass secondary urea cycle inhibition (7). Biotin supplementation is commonly provided with limited recorded success, but triheptanoin, an odd-chain triglyceride, may correct the biochemical abnormalities in individuals with type B PC deficiency, as will liver transplantation.

Prognosis

The prognosis for type A and B PC deficiencies is generally poor because of the severity of the metabolic derangement on liver and brain function. Indeed, the median lifespan for type B PC deficiency has been reported to be 60 days from a French cohort (6). In contrast, the prognosis for individuals with type C PC deficiency is considerably superior, especially if ketoacidotic episodes are properly treated and controlled.

PYRUVATE DEHYDROGENASE COMPLEX (PDHC) DEFICIENCY

Clinical Presentation

Pyruvate dehydrogenase complex (PDHC) is a large mitochondrial enzyme that is integral for glucose metabolism because of its ability to metabolize pyruvate to acetyl-coA, which is required for the citric acid cycle. An inherited deficiency in at least one of the three different PDHC activities impairs the oxidation of pyruvate in the mitochondria and promotes its cytoplasmic reduction to lactate. PDHC deficiency is a frequent cause of congenital lactic acidosis and is also found with progressive neurological and neuromuscular degeneration that often ends in death in childhood (8). Clinical symptoms frequently occur by 1 year of age; however, it should also be recognized that a portion (approximately one third) of PDHC deficiency cases present between 1 year and adolescence. The clinical presentation of PDHC deficiency varies with age of onset and gender. Neonatal PDHC deficiency typically manifests with encephalopathy and brain malformations of the cortex and/or corpus callosum with lactic acidosis; added attributes may include microcephaly, facial dysmorphism, and seizures, which are seemingly more common in female neonates. Another infantile presentation comprises acute brainstem dysfunction with/ or without basal ganglia abnormalities typical for Leigh syndrome. Childhood presentations include psychomotor retardation combined with neuropathy and ataxia or chronic neuropathy with recurrent ataxia and motor deficiency without mental retardation (9). Blood lactate concentrations are consistently elevated but typically do not reach concentrations seen for PC type B deficiency, nor do lactate/pyruvate ratios typically surpass 20 unless clinical manifestations are compounded by respiratory distress.

Genetics and Pathogenesis

PDHC is composed of three enzymatic subunits—pyruvate dehydrogenase (E1), dihydrolipoamide transacylase (E2), dihydrolipoamine dehydrogenase (E3)—as well as an E3 binding protein (E3BP). Its activity is regulated by pyruvate dehydrogenase phosphatases (PDP) and pyruvate dehydrogenase kinases (PDK). PDHC also requires thiamine and lipoic acid as cofactors. The E1 enzyme component is composed of two E1α and two E1β protein subunits, of which the E1α protein is encoded on the X chromosome whereas the additional PDHC-related peptides are encoded in the nucleus. Therefore, the inheritance of PDHC deficiency is either autosomal recessive for deficiencies of E2 (*DLAT*), E3 (*DLD*), E3BP (*PDHX*), E1β (*PDHB*), and pyruvate dehydrogenase phosphatase (*PDP1*) but X-linked recessive for E1α (*PDHA1* gene) deficiency. Loss of PDHC function and the concomitant reduction of energy production, alongside increases in pyruvate and lactate concentrations, comprise the biochemical alterations leading to this heterogeneous neurological disorder. A surprising observation about PDHC deficiency is the fact that a large proportion of cases are due to E1α deficiency, which is in turn caused by a high frequency of de novo, germ-line mutations affecting male and female individuals in equal portion (9). Although hemizygotic males are generally symptomatic, heterozygous females will have a random pattern of X-chromosome inactivation with variable expression of mutant and normal gene products in different tissues. This can significantly complicate tissue-specific, enzyme-based laboratory testing. Indeed, among other X-linked recessive disorders, females with PDHC deficiency due to a *PDHA1* mutation often demonstrate unexpectedly severe disease that begins earlier than males (on average at 1 month of age vs 4 months of age for males) but with disproportionate residual PDHC activity levels (8).

Laboratory Diagnosis

Unfortunately, there are no clinical, neuroimaging, or classic biochemical signs that help to unequivocally categorize individuals with PDHC deficiency into representative phenotypes with possible E1α, E1β, E2, PDP1, or E3BP defects. An exception to this rule of thumb is E3 deficiency. These individuals can have biochemical findings that overlap with maple syrup urine disease (branched-chain α-ketoacid dehydrogenase complex deficiency) and α-ketoglutarate dehydrogenase deficiency as the E3 protein is a component of these three complexes. Thus, patients with E3 deficiency can also have lactic acidosis with elevated plasma branched-chain amino acids and allo-isoleucine concentrations and increased excretion of ketoacids with prominent α-ketoglutarate by urinary organic acid analysis.

For all possible PDHC defects, once a mitochondrial disorder is suspected through clinical findings, elevated lactate in blood and/or CSF, urinary organic acids, plasma amino acids, and/or abnormal magnetic resonance imaging (MRI), PDHC deficiency should be excluded by assessing its three functions in tissue lysates (lymphoblasts, muscle, or cultured skin fibroblasts). It is noteworthy that a correlation between residual PDHC activity and symptoms has been observed with more mildly affected individuals having higher residual PDHC activity (as high as 80% of normal co-run controls). Because of this biochemical graduation, it may be necessary to consider additional testing of PDHC activity in more than one tissue.

The gold standard for PDHC activity is the assessment of radiolabeled pyruvate catabolism with and without pretreatment with dichloroacetic acid (DCA). Approximately 25–30% of PDHC from normal cultured skin fibroblasts is found to be inactive. Pretreatment with DCA permits the assessment of total PDHC activity, which can be helpful to determine whether lactic acidosis is from the deficiency of a core PDHC subunit or the loss of PDH phosphatase (PDP1) activity. PDHC core subunit defects will have low native PDHC activity that cannot be activated to normal levels whereas PDP1 deficiency will have low native PDHC activity that can be induced to normal levels through DCA incubation.

Additional laboratory tests using immunochemical methods to detect the presence of PDHC subunits have shown to be helpful in some specific circumstances. In particular, females with *PDHA1* mutations may have ambiguous PDHC enzyme results in different tissues because of randomized X-chromosome inactivation. Immunohistochemical staining for PDHC E1α protein in cultured skin fibroblasts can help elucidate mosaicism for E1α deficiency *(9, 10)*. Western blotting tissue lysates for PDHC subunits have also shown to be helpful for identifying some cases of E1β and E3BP deficiency from other subunit defects, but a normal immunochemical analysis does not exclude an enzymatic deficiency *(11, 12)*.

Molecular genetic testing is clinically available for all subunits of PDHC.

Treatment

No specific treatment of PDHC deficiency exists. Acute clinical management of PDHC deficiency includes the administration of sodium bicarbonate as a temporary treatment of acid-base decompensation. Thiamine supplementation is often commonplace, especially if molecular analysis suggests a disruption of thiamine pyrophosphate binding to the E1α subunit. Some patients are prescribed a ketogenic diet to increase the production of energy through the mitochondrial fatty acid oxidation. DCA is often prescribed for the acute treatment of lactic acidemia. However, the efficacy of chronic oral treatment with DCA has been questioned by the observation that DCA causes a toxic neuropathy in mitochondrial myopathy, encephalopathy, lactic acidosis, and stroke-like episodes (MELAS) *(13)*. Nevertheless, interventions for PDHC deficiency have yet to be evaluated in a randomized controlled trial.

Prognosis

The prognosis of PDHC deficiency seems to be closely correlative to age of diagnosis, blood lactic acid concentration, and residual PDHC activity level. Individuals with a younger age of presentation (≤ 3 months), higher blood lactate concentrations (≥ 11 mmol/L), and lower residual PDHC activity ($\leq 40\%$ of normal) have a shorter time of survival than individuals with less severe clinical and biochemical phenotypes *(8)*.

MITOCHONDRIAL ENCEPHALOMYELOPATHY, LACTIC ACIDOSIS, AND STROKE-LIKE EPISODES (MELAS)

Clinical Presentation

MELAS is a severe multisystem disorder that typically presents in childhood with symptoms of generalized tonic-clonic seizures, recurrent headaches, and vomiting. Proximal limb weakness can also be an initial symptom. Symptoms commonly initiate between 2 and 15 years of age with 90%

of patients presenting before the age of 30 *(14)*. Seizures are associated with stroke-like episodes of transient hemiparesis and cortical blindness. These episodes are often recurrent and lead to cumulative effects that gradually impair motor abilities, cognition, and vision, leading to eventual death. Hearing loss and gastrointestinal pseudo-obstruction can also occur during disease progression. Early psychomotor development is typically normal but there is recognition of frequent growth failure and a history of motor and speech delays in some cases. The prevalence of MELAS, as indicated by the carrier rate of the m.3243A>G mutation, has been determined to range from 1:6,135 in a northern Finish population to as high as 1:434 found in an Australian study *(15, 16)*. An additional study on the frequency of mtDNA mutations in the general population of England has suggested that the prevalence of carrier status for m.3243A>G could approach 1:704, but clinically presenting MELAS is much rarer *(17)*.

Genetics and Pathogenesis

MELAS is a diagnosis that is based on a combination of clinical, biochemical, and molecular genetic findings. Most genetic mutations that lead to MELAS are maternally transmitted by inheritance of mtDNA. As with all mtDNA mutations, the clinical expression of MELAS is dependent on three factors: the level of heteroplasmy or mutational load (the amount of mutant vs normal mtDNA), the tissue distribution of mutant mtDNA, and the susceptibility of specific tissues to mutational load (also called threshold effect). The individual variability of mutation load and tissue distribution may account for the differences in clinical presentation because most mothers of MELAS patients are obligate carriers, yet many do not express disease. There is no contribution to mutational load by fathers of MELAS patients. The most common mutation in MELAS is the m.3243A>G mutation in *MT-TL1*, which encodes for mitochondrial tRNA leucine *(18)*. The m.3243A>G mutation, and additional mutations in *MT-TL1*, such as m.3271T>C and m.3252A>G, account for almost 80% of MELAS cases. Mutations causing MELAS have been found other mtDNA genes, including *MT-ND5* (m.13513G>A), *MT-ND1*, and *MT-ND6*, which encode for subunits of the NADH:ubiquinone oxidoreductase complex (CI), other tRNA genes (*MT-TC*, *MT-TK*, *MT-TV*, *MT-TQ*, *MT-TF*, *MT-TS1*, *MT-TS2*, and *MT-TW*), and other protein-encoding genes (*MT-CO1*, *MT-CO2*, *MT-CO3*, and *MT-CYB*).

The pathogenesis of MELAS is not fully understood, and there are two different theories to explain clinical symptoms: one hypothesis claims that the disease occurs from ischemic vascular events that are caused by "mitochondrial angiopathy" and the other hypothesis focuses on the toxic outcome of generalized cytopathy, which is caused by "mitochondrial cytopathy." A combination of angiopathy and cytopathy due to mitochondrial dysfunction is likely a driver of MELAS progression. The molecular mechanism of mitochondrial dysfunction is relatively less opaque. Most mtDNA mutations are found in tRNA genes, and these mutations decrease the lifespan of the affected tRNA molecules, increase the amount of uncharged tRNAs, lead to the accumulation of RNA intermediates, impede protein translation, and cause general mitochondrial function. However, it is uncertain how mutations in mitochondrial-encoded oxidative phosphorylation complexes (complex I, III, and IV) lead to a MELAS phenotype beyond their ability to diminish mitochondrial oxidative phosphorylation.

Laboratory Diagnosis

In individuals with MELAS, lactate concentrations are commonly elevated in blood and persistently elevated in CSF. These concentrations can be induced after exercise, seizure, or a stroke-like event. Evidence of a mitochondrial myopathy can be detected in a muscle biopsy by the appearance of ragged red fibers (RRFs) that are also positive for increased cytochrome c oxidase (complex IV or CIV) activity as detected by a modified Gomori trichrome stain *(19)*. In addition, intramuscular blood vessels will show strong succinate dehydrogenase (SDH) reactivity by an SDH stain. These muscle-staining patterns are in juxtaposition to other mtDNA-related disorders, such as Kearns-Sayre syndrome (KSS) and myoclonic epilepsy ragged red fibers (MERRF).

The biochemical analysis of mitochondrial oxidative phosphorylation enzymes in muscle extracts or skin fibroblasts will frequently demonstrate partial deficiencies of CI and or complex IV (CIV). It is not infrequent that enzyme results are uninformative because the tissue distribution of mtDNA mutations may not correlate with severity of symptoms. Nevertheless, partial or severe mitochondrial oxidative phosphorylation enzyme deficiencies should be seriously considered as supportive of a mitochondrial disease, especially when correlative with blood lactate concentrations and a multisystem presentation.

Sequencing of the mitochondrial genome and/or targeted mutation analysis for common mutations associated with MELAS are available to help make a diagnosis. However, disorders of mtDNA such as MELAS are confounded by heteroplasmy, which can lead to varying proportions of mutated DNA in different tissues.

Treatment

There is no specific treatment for MELAS. A cocktail of mitochondrial-related vitamins and supplements has been advocated by many. The components of a "mitochondrial cocktail" vary widely in clinical practice, and its use is based largely on theoretical benefit and anecdotal reports of clinical improvement. Some reports do suggest that the administration of coenzyme Q_{10} (CoQ_{10}) and L-carnitine may modestly reduce resting lactate concentrations in MELAS. There are additional experimental therapies that are under investigation, including a clinical trial of idebenone. L-Arginine administration, which was shown to ameliorate the stroke-like symptoms when given during an acute event, may also be beneficial. Lastly, oral succinate for slowing MELAS progression is also under investigation.

Prognosis

There is substantial clinical variability in the manifestation and progression of MELAS. It is very difficult, if not impossible, to provide a prediction of disease progression on the presence of a specific mutation. Additional factors such as mutational load and tissue distribution potentially have a profound effect on MELAS expressivity. It is important to keep this in mind when counseling asymptomatic carriers of MELAS mutations. For symptomatic patients, there is evidence that the survival time from onset of neurological disease, such as seizures and stroke, may average 16.9 years *(14)*.

MYOCLONIC EPILEPSY AND RAGGED RED FIBERS (MERRF) SYNDROME

Clinical Presentation

MERRF is a mitochondrial disease that presents with myoclonic seizures as the first symptom, but it is often followed by generalized epilepsy, ataxia, muscle weakness, hearing loss, lactic acidemia, and dementia. Onset is frequently in childhood subsequent to normal early development. Short stature, optic atrophy, and cardiomyopathy are a few additional clinical findings. The clinical diagnosis is classically based on the identification of RRFs in a muscle biopsy alongside myoclonus, ataxia, and generalized epilepsy. Nevertheless, normal muscle histochemical studies cannot completely exclude MERRF.

Genetics and Pathogenesis

MERRF syndrome is caused by mutations in mtDNA and is maternally inherited. Four mutations (m.8344A>G, m.8356T>C, m.8363G>A, and m.8361G>A) in *MT-TK*, which encodes for mitochondrial tRNA lysine, account for almost 90% of all mutations in individuals with MERRF *(20)*. Other genes with mutations associated with MERRF include *MT-TL1*, *MT-TH*, *MT-TS1*, *MT-TS2*, and *MT-TF*.

A MERRF/MELAS overlap syndrome has occurred with mutations in *MT-ND5 (21)*. Although muscle and brain tissues are predominantly affected in individuals with MERRF, causative mtDNA mutations can be found in just about every tissue tested. Therefore, mutation analysis of a blood sample is frequently sufficient to identify the MERRF-related mtDNA mutation and its mutational load. In MERRF syndrome, there is often uniform distribution of mutational load, and MERRF individuals generally have a high percentage of mutant mtDNA, reaching as high as >99% in some cases. The incidence of MERRF is rare, but there is a calculated prevalence of 0.25:100,000 individuals in a northeast England population on the basis of the identification of m.8344A>G *(22)*.

The pathogenesis of MERRF-related mtDNA mutations is uncertain. It has been found that a high mutational load of m.8344A>G is associated with decreased protein synthesis and reduced cytochrome c oxidase (CIV) function in isolated cells. It is thought that the protein synthesis impairment may be a direct result of reduced mutant tRNA lysine affinity, thereby preferentially impeding the synthesis of peptides with a higher proportion of lysine residues. Indeed, mtDNA-encoded subunits of CIV contain a significant proportion of lysine residues than other mtDNA genes, and this protein complex's activity is preferentially reduced in MERRF patient tissues. However, this molecular mechanism does not explain why there is such a profound effect on brain and muscle but other tissues are left relatively unscathed even with a high level of mutation load.

Laboratory Diagnosis

In individuals with MERRF, blood and CSF concentrations of lactate and pyruvate are elevated at rest, and lactate concentrations can substantially increase after exercise or a seizure. A histochemical analysis of muscle tissue typically shows RRFs that fail to stain for CIV activity but have fibers that are hyperactive for SDH staining. However, patients without RRFs have been described *(23)*. The analysis of mitochondrial oxidative phosphorylation enzymes in muscle or skin fibroblast extracts usually shows a deficiency of CIV; however, diminished activities of other mitochondrial enzymes with mtDNA-encoded subunits may also be observed. It is also not too infrequent that enzymatic studies are inconclusive or normal. Therefore, it is pertinent to consider molecular genetic testing for the four mtDNA mutations (m.8344A>G, m.8356T>C, m.8363G>A, and m.8361G>A) frequently found in MERRF patients from a blood sample. In rare circumstances, a pathogenic mutation might not be detected, and it would be worthwhile to consider other tissues, such as muscle or skin fibroblasts, or to consider sequencing for mutations in other mtDNA genes associated with MERRF.

Treatment

Although there are no specific treatments for MERRF, conventional antiepileptic therapy can help control seizure manifestations. In particular, there is greater acceptance of levetiracetam (Keppra) for suppressing myoclonus in MERRF, and an increasing avoidance of valproic acid, which can cause secondary carnitine deficiency, thereby resulting in additional mitochondrial toxicity, and should not be considered, if at all possible, for individuals with MERRF. In addition, it is not uncommon to find a cocktail of mitochondrial-related vitamins and supplements used by MERRF individuals in the hopes of stimulating mitochondrial function. CoQ_{10} and L-carnitine are common components of this mitochondrial vitamin cocktail. Indeed, supplementation with L-carnitine is needed if valproic acid is prescribed to control drug-resistant status epilepticus.

Prognosis

MERRF syndrome is a progressive condition, and unfortunately there is not a clear correlation between mutation and clinical phenotype for affected individuals. The severity of this condition varies greatly, and individuals with reduced cerebral symptoms may have prolonged survival. All patients with

MERRF should be regularly evaluated at proper intervals for possible cardiac, ophthalmologic, or audiologic manifestations.

NEUROPATHY, ATAXIA, AND RETINITIS PIGMENTOSA (NARP) SYNDROME

Clinical Presentation

NARP is a clinically heterogeneous condition that frequently presents with a combination of developmental delay, retinitis pigmentosa, ataxia, muscle weakness, and sensory neuropathy from childhood into adulthood (24). Seizures may also accompany severe, early-onset forms of NARP, but they are rare in cases with adult-aged presentations. It has a slowly progressive clinical course with developmental delay and hypotonia often being the initial findings, followed by blindness due to optic atrophy or retinitis pigmentosa and finally neuropathy. However, severe infantile- and neonatal-onset cases of NARP have been described, and its clinical manifestations are part of a phenotypic continuum of subacute necrotizing encephalomyelopathy, or Leigh syndrome, with a maternally inherited pattern called maternally inherited Leigh syndrome (MILS) (25).

Genetics and Pathogenesis

NARP is maternally inherited and associated with mutations (more often m.8993T>G and less frequent m.8993T>C, m.9176T>G, or m.9176T>C) in *MT-ATP6*, which encodes for subunit 6 of the ATP synthase on the mitochondrial genome. The phenotypic spectrum of NARP is related to the level of mutation load, with severe presentations having a higher level of heteroplasmy. Clinical symptoms are thought to arise from diminished mitochondrial ATP synthesis activity because of the conversion of a conserved leucine 156 residue to arginine (for m.8993T>G). However, the leucine 156 to proline (for m.8993T>C) mutation does not seem to affect ATP synthesis in vitro, and the molecular mechanism for the m.9176T>C/G alterations have yet to be unequivocally elucidated. Nevertheless, it is apparent that NARP arises from only a few *MT-ATP6* mutations because the severe presentation of MILS is more often observed in families carrying the less-common alterations, m.8993T>C and m.9176T>C. The prevalence of NARP is not completely known. Recent population studies of the m.8993T>G mutation failed to find it among the normal English population (22).

Laboratory Diagnosis

A laboratory diagnosis of NARP is made by correlating clinical findings with focused laboratory analyses. In NARP, presenting individuals may have indications of lactic acidemia by moderately elevated lactate concentrations in blood and CSF. In addition, plasma amino acids may demonstrate relative hypocitrullinemia with normal concentrations of other urea-cycle-related amino acids (ornithine and arginine) (Table 14-1). In cases of MILS, hyperammonemia is a compounding factor. Oxidative phosphorylation enzyme activities in muscle and skin fibroblasts from NARP patients are frequently diminished; in particular, deficiencies of CIV and/or CI are observed. If available, oligomycin-sensitive ATPase activity in muscle or skin fibroblast mitochondria isolates or homogenates should be considered because it is often reduced, but clinically available testing of this activity is almost impossible to find. In contrast to MERRF and MELAS, NARP does not typically have evidence of a mitochondrial myopathy in a muscle biopsy. Indeed, histochemical analyses of muscle samples may often be normal. Thus, confirmation of a suspected diagnosis is often dependent on molecular genetic analysis for the frequent *MT-ATP6* mutation, m.8993T>G. If the common NARP mutation is not identified, complete *MT-ATP6* gene sequencing may be warranted. There is not evidence of substantial tissue variation for NARP mutations; therefore, it is possible to use whole blood for mutation analysis.

Table 14-1 Selective Laboratory Results for Different Mitochondrial Disorders

Disorder	Lactate	L/P	Citrulline (P)	Alanine (P)	Glutamine (P)	Skin fibroblast enzyme	Muscle enzyme
PC	↑-↑↑	↑-N	↓-N	↑	↑	↓↓	↓↓
PDHC	↑-↑↑	N	N	↑	N	↓	↓
MELAS	↑	↑-N	↓-N	↑-N	N	↓-N (CI and/or CIV)	↓-N (CI and/or CIV)
MERRF	↑	↑-N	N	↑-N	N	↓-N (CIV)	↓-N (CIV)
NARP	↑	↑-N	↓-N	↑-N	↑-N	↓-N (CI, CIV, and/or CV)	↓-N (CI, CIV, and/or CV)
Kearns-Sayre syndrome	↑	↑-N	N	↑-N	N	N	↓-N (CI, CIII, and/or CIV)
Pearson syndrome	↑	↑	N	↑	N	N	↓-N (CI, CIII, and/or CIV)
Mitochondrial DNA depletion syndrome	↑-↑↑	↑	↑-N	↑	↑-N	N	↓-N (CI, CIII, CIV and/or CV)

CI = OXPHOS complex I, CIII = OXPHOS complex III, CIV = OXPHOS complex IV, CV = OXPHOS complex V, L/P = lactate/pyruvate ratio, N = normal, P = plasma.

Treatment

There is no specific treatment for NARP, and current interventions are supportive and specific to the symptoms. Previous studies have hinted that it may be theoretically possible to increase some NARP cell survival with α-ketoglutarate/aspartate-supplemented media, suggesting that progression of the condition could be slowed with similar supplementations in patients. α-Ketoglutarate and aspartate provide increased flux through the citric acid cycle, thereby stimulating ATP production in a non-ATP synthase manner.

Prognosis

There is remarkable clinical variability of NARP manifestations, which complicates the ability to reliably provide a prognosis. It is a progressive condition with a deterioration of clinical symptoms over time, but there is some evidence that a higher mutational load might be predictive of a more severe clinical phenotype. It is also noteworthy that the clinical presentation of NARP may worsen in subsequent generations, often precipitating as MILS.

KEARNS-SAYRE SYNDROME (KSS)

Clinical Presentation

KSS is a multisystem condition that was first recognized in 1958 as a collection of ocular symptoms (e.g., ophthalmoplegia, pigmentary retinitis, and ptosis) in early adulthood with heart conduction defects (26). Since that time, individuals with KSS have been found to present before the age of 20 years with ocular findings and progressive manifestations of one or more of the following: heart conduction block or cardiomyopathy, hearing loss, ataxia, myopathy, endocrine dysfunction (diabetes), and renal dysfunction (27). There is substantial variability of symptoms because the progression of disease to new organ systems is sporadic, but it can also be sudden, leading to severe handicap and reduced life expectancy. The prevalence of KSS is rare, with approximately 200 cases reported in the literature.

Genetics and Pathogenesis

Most KSS cases are due to the sporadic occurrence of tissue-specific mtDNA rearrangements (deletions or duplications), which can be different sizes, but they have been classically described as a "common" heteroplasmic, 4,977-bp mtDNA deletion in muscle *(28)*. Indeed, most patients with KSS have mtDNA deletions around this size, which encompass approximately 10 mtDNA-encoded genes, including tRNAs and subunits of CI, CIV, and CV. Although the inheritance of this condition is rare, rearranged mtDNA is detectable in human oocytes and increases the risk of transmitting mtDNA deletions *(29)*. However, it is presumed that inherited forms of KSS could be due to autosomal-recessive mutations in nuclear genes needed for mtDNA maintenance, such as *RRM2B*, which encodes for a ribonucleotide reductase subunit that is important for mtDNA synthesis. Although the extent of mtDNA rearrangements varies, there have been identical mtDNA deletions found in KSS and two other mitochondrial diseases—Pearson syndrome and chronic progressive external ophthalmoplegia (CPEO)—suggesting that these conditions may constitute a continuum of clinically related entities *(30)*. Nevertheless, additional understanding about the natural history of KSS would assist with its clinical classification, which is an area of debate *(30)*. Traditionally, the variation in tissue-specific mutational load, with KSS having a high level of muscle- and central nervous system (CNS)-localized mutant mtDNA, has been thought to account for the differences in clinical presentation between these conditions.

The pathogenesis of KSS seems to be related to the failure of sufficient ATP production in specific tissues because of a high percentage of mtDNA with a rearrangement. Because KSS deletions often include one of three common breakpoints where there are 10- to 13-bp direct repeats in the mitochondrial genome, it is often observed that genes encoding for subunits of ATP synthase, CI, and CIV are deleted, leading to reduced respiratory capacity in affected tissues. In KSS, the affected tissues include muscle and CNS, which have a high energetic demand. Blood samples from KSS patients do not have an appreciatively elevated amount of mutant mtDNA. Although it is uncertain how the deletions observed in KSS arise and remain maintained, it is likely that they occur somatically, leading to the tissue-specificity and clinical phenotype.

Laboratory Diagnosis

A laboratory diagnosis of KSS is based on the correlation of clinical findings with other indications of possible mitochondrial disease, including elevated lactic and pyruvate concentrations in blood and CSF (Table 14-1). In CSF studies, increased protein concentrations (>100 mg/dL) alongside diminished 5-methyltetrahydrofolate concentrations are also found in KSS individuals, but they are not entirely specific for this condition. Muscle histology and morphology of KSS patients typically contain ragged-red and CIV-deficient fibers, but a normal muscle result does not exclude KSS. The confirmation of a suspected diagnosis is made by the detection of an mtDNA rearrangement of appreciable mutational load (>40 %) in a tissue sample. Most mtDNA rearrangements can be detected by Southern blot analysis from total DNA isolated from a nondividing cell line, such as muscle. Probing for mtDNA-specific bands using radio-labeled, purified whole mtDNA permits the detection of an abnormal banding pattern that indicates an mtDNA rearrangement. However, there are considerable pitfalls to using Southern blot for rearrangement analysis. In particular, it is difficult to characterize mtDNA molecules that contain a partial deletion and partial duplication because the resulting rearranged DNA size may be essentially indistinguishable from the parent molecule. In addition, the tissue specificity of KSS is such that a DNA analysis with an inconclusive result in one tissue type does not exclude KSS and it may be necessary to sample a second tissue.

Treatment

There is no specific treatment for KSS, and current therapies are supportive on the basis of the organ systems involved. A cardiac conduction block may be treated with a pacemaker and is often necessary because of the risk for a sudden cardiac event in some KSS patients. Oral CoQ_{10} supplementation has been reported to modestly reduce the L/P ratio and to significantly reduce the protein concentration in CSF with an improvement in cardiac conductivity for a few patients *(31)*. There are ongoing clinical studies on the efficacy of CoQ_{10} derivatives for KSS and other mitochondrial disorders. Lastly, cell studies have shown that KSS-related biochemical abnormalities can be reversed with RNA-mediated gene therapy for missing mtDNA genes, but human gene therapy studies await future work.

Prognosis

KSS is a slowly progressive condition for which prognosis is difficult to assess for affected patients. However, there is increasing evidence that the age of symptom onset, the length of the mtDNA deletion, and the percentage of mutational load in affected tissues may have some strength in predicting progression. In particular, an earlier age of onset, larger deletion size, and a higher percentage of mutant mtDNA may be indicative of a more severe prognosis and shorter lifespan.

PEARSON SYNDROME

Clinical Presentation

Pearson syndrome is a rare, sporadic mitochondrial disease with clinical variability, but it typically presents in the neonatal period with a small birth weight and the clinical features of hyporegenerative anemia with pancytopenia and exocrine pancreatic dysfunction *(32, 33)*. Additional features include neuromuscular manifestations, such as hypo/hypertonia, tremor, or lethargy; metabolic findings, such as hypoglycemia and persistent lactic acidemia; or additional multiple organ involvement, such as cardiac dysfunction, renal cysts, or hydrops fetalis *(34)*. This condition often results in death during infancy or early childhood. If survival is beyond early infancy, normalization of hematological findings can occur, but there is an increased risk of developing KSS, including diabetes and a cardiac conduction block. The incidence of Pearson syndrome is unknown, and approximately 80 cases have been reported in the literature *(34)*

Genetics and Pathogenesis

Pearson syndrome is caused by the sporadic occurrence of distinct, heteroplasmic mtDNA deletions, with the common 4,977-bp mtDNA deletion accounting for up to 25% of all described cases *(34)*. Other Pearson-related mtDNA rearrangements include mtDNA deletions from 3 kb to as large as 9 kb that overlap with regions missing in the common mtDNA deletion *(34)*. In addition, complex mixtures of mtDNA rearrangements have been observed (e.g., an mtDNA duplication in the presence of an mtDNA deletion) in tissue samples from a few Pearson syndrome cases.

The pathogenesis of Pearson syndrome is uncertain. It appears that the mutant mtDNA load varies from tissue to tissue because it is commonly observed that blood contains the highest amount (up to ~80% mutant) of mutant mtDNA, but other tissues have detectable amounts of mtDNA deletions. It is thought that the mtDNA deletions will lead to decreased mitochondrial energy production. However, its distinctly variable phenotype may be the result of differences in mutant load, tissue distribution of abnormal mtDNA, and the evolution of this tissue distribution over time.

Laboratory Diagnosis

A laboratory diagnosis of Pearson syndrome is made through the correlation of clinical symptoms with laboratory findings, such as a complete blood count indicating anemia with or without leukocytopenia or thrombopenia *(34)*. Bone marrow aspiration will frequently show hypocellularity with vacuolization of bone marrow precursors. Hypoglycemia and an acid/base imbalance are also very common findings. In fact, Pearson syndrome should be excluded in cases of neonatal metabolic acidosis and lactic acidemia despite the absence of anemia *(34)*. It is not surprising that an elevated blood lactate concentration (>2 mmol/L) and a L/P ratio >20 is frequently observed and may be the main sign of a potential mitochondrial disorder. Plasma amino acids will demonstrate an elevated alanine concentration (>500 nmol/mL), and urine amino acids may have nonspecific aminoaciduria. Urinary organic acids from Pearson syndrome patients have been described to contain elevated concentrations of lactate with citric acid cycle intermediates, but quantitative data to support this observation have not been fully corroborated.

The laboratory finding most consistent with Pearson syndrome is the identification of a large mtDNA deletion in total blood DNA through the genetic analysis of the mitochondrial genome by Southern blotting or polymerase chain reaction (PCR). Complex mtDNA rearrangements, as seen for KSS, are less frequently observed in Pearson syndrome, and the presence of large mtDNA deletions covering the common mtDNA deletion region is sufficient to confirm a diagnosis. Enzyme analysis of skin or muscle may not be informative or demonstrate nonspecific deficiencies of several respiratory chain enzymes because the primary tissue affected is the bone marrow.

Treatment

There is no specific treatment for Pearson syndrome. Because of the pancreatic dysfunction, pancreatic enzyme replacement is often used to manage manifestations alongside common therapies to normalize glucose concentrations and acid/base concentrations. A cocktail of oral CoQ_{10}, L-carnitine, and other mitochondrial-related cofactor supplementation is commonplace, but there is little information about the efficacy of these supplements for this condition.

Prognosis

Pearson syndrome often results in death during infancy or early childhood. However, there have been several cases described with survival beyond early infancy and in which normalization of hematological abnormalities occurred. In this circumstance, there is an increased risk of developing KSS, including diabetes and a cardiac conduction block, in individuals with long-term survival.

MITOCHONDRIAL DNA DEPLETION SYNDROME

Clinical Presentation

mtDNA depletion syndrome (MDS) is a group of heterogeneous, progressive disorders that are unified by the fact that they associated with a severe reduction of mtDNA copy number in affected tissues *(35)*. Their clinical manifestations often occur during infancy or childhood, but their phenotypes may overlap and change as a condition progresses with age. In addition, adult presentations of MDS have recently been recognized *(36)*. As a group, the prevalence of MDS is rare, and the overall incidence is not known. There are four distinct varieties of MDS, including myopathic, encephelomyopathic, hepatocerebral, and cardiomyopathic types *(37, 38)*. There are a growing number of genetic causes of MDS that involve enzymes important for mtDNA replication, maintenance of mitochondrial nucleotide pools and nucleotide membrane transport (Figure 14-2), and a mitochondrial protein of presently undetermined function.

The myopathic form was traditionally recognized as severe infantile myopathy with motor regression, lactic acidemia, and early death because of respiratory insufficiency *(39)*. However, the clinical spectrum currently also includes infantile mitochondrial myopathy, proximal muscular atrophy, and a milder myopathic phenotype without motor regression and with long-term survival. In addition, adult individuals with slowly progressive myopathy, with or without ptosis or facial weakness, have been described and suggest that this phenotype is likely underappreciated *(36)*.

The hepatocerebral form of MDS is in its own right a clinically diverse entity and likely one of the most common variants of MDS. As indicated by its name, it presents as severe liver impairment with or without neurological disease. Although neonatal liver impairment is a common finding, some forms of hepatocerebral MDS may also present by childhood with lactic acidemia, liver failure, developmental delay, and hypotonia (40). Other forms may present within the first year of life with hypoglycemia, liver failure, neuropathy, and leukodystrophy (41). Lastly, clinical manifestations of Alpers-Huttenlocher syndrome are part of the hepatocerebral form of MDS. Alpers-Huttenlocher syndrome is a childhood-onset, progressive encephalopathy with seizures and liver failure, including an infantile myocerebrohepatopathy spectrum that presents between the first few months of life and up to 3 years of age. Presentation of Alpers-Huttenlocher syndrome includes developmental delay, lactic acidemia, liver disease, myopathy, and failure to thrive (42, 43).

Encephelomyopathic MDS is noteworthy for the symptomatology that spares hepatic function but may fatally impair other organ systems, such as brain, kidney, and the digestive system. The clinical manifestations include fatal neonatal lactic acidemia, moderate methylmalonic aciduria, hypotonia, deafness, and Leigh-like syndrome findings (44). There is an infantile form with progressive neurological deterioration, infantile onset of hypotonia, deafness, hyperkinesia, lactic acidemia, moderate methylmalonic aciduria, and brain MRI showing basal ganglion lesions suggestive of Leigh syndrome (45). The predicted frequency of this infantile form of MDS has been found to be has high as 1:2,500 in the Faroese population, but it is considerably rarer in other populations (45). There are additional neonatal and infantile forms of encephalomyopathic MDS that do not excrete methylmalonic acid but do present with a renal tubulopathy or gastrointestinal dysmotility in the context of hypotonia, lactic acidemia, seizures, and progressive muscle weakness (46). Lastly, there is a late-onset (by age 13–20 years) MDS that is recognized by peripheral neuropathy, gastrointestinal dysmotility with other symptoms (nausea, vomiting, or diarrhea), ptosis and/or ophthalmoparesis, leukoencephalopathy, and moderate lactic acidemia (47). Called mitochondrial neurogastrointestinal encephalopathy syndrome (MNGIE), this is a progressive condition with survival that does not exceed 40 years of age.

Recently, a fourth variety of MDS has been recognized as a possible cardiomyopathic form because of the constellation of symptoms that includes lactic acidemia, cardiomyopathy, congenital cataracts, skeletal myopathy, and normal mental development (38). Individuals with this collection of manifestations were first described in 1975 by Sengers et al. and were since labeled as having Sengers syndrome (48). The clinical course of Sengers syndrome varies from a severe infantile form with bilateral cataracts and progressive hypertrophic cardiomyopathy to less rigorous forms that permit survival into the fourth decade. In either circumstance, heart failure because of progressive hypertrophic cardiomyopathy is often the cause of death.

Genetics and Pathogenesis

MDS are autosomal-recessive disorders that are associated with various mutations in at least ten different genes. The identification of causative mutations within MDS-related genes has helped elucidate the pathogenesis of these heterogeneous conditions, enhanced the ability to confirm a putative diagnosis, and pinpointed specific biological processes that are targets for additional mutation discovery. As a group, the gene products related to MDS are involved in either the maintenance or replication of mtDNA, thereby reducing the amount of intact mtDNA required for energy metabolism and healthy tissue function. One way in which mtDNA maintenance can be disrupted is through reducing the amount of available substrates needed for mtDNA replication, or by the disruption of enzymes required for mtDNA replication. In the case of MDS, most gene products limit the level of deoxyribonucleotide (dNTP) pools within mitochondria, thereby inhibiting mtDNA replication by diminishing substrate concentrations required for appropriate mtDNA maintenance.

In general, myopathic MDS is caused by the disruption of a single gene, *TK2*, which encodes for a mitochondrial thymidine kinase that is found in certain tissues to be reduced to <50% of normal function (39). This protein phosphorylates thymidine, deoxycytidine, and deoxyuridine and is important for salvaging dNTPs *(39)*. Encoded on chromosome 16q21, defects in *TK2* are frequently point mutations or small insertions and deletions; however, there is a single case report of a 5.8-kb deletion in siblings with MDS that leads to myopathic MDS with hepatic failure, but this is a rare finding for *TK2*-related MDS *(49)*.

Hepatocerebral forms of MDS are frequently caused by mutations in several different genes. In particular, mutations are found in the mitochondrial deoxyguanosine kinase gene, *DGUOK*, which is important for ensuring normal dNTP levels *(50)*; in the mitochondrial helicase, Twinkle, which is encoded by *PEO1* and is important for mtDNA replication *(51)*; and in *MPV17*, which encodes for an inner mitochondrial membrane protein of unknown function *(52)*. Alpers-Huttenlocher syndrome is due to mutations in *POLG1*, the mtDNA polymerase γ-protein that is critical for mtDNA replication *(42)*. However, *POLG1* mutations are not specific for MDS alone, and other mutations in this gene can cause different mitochondrial ataxia syndromes as well as autosomal recessive and dominant forms of external ophthalmoplegia *(40)*. Mutations in *POLG* are frequently claimed to be a common cause of mitochondrial disease and should be considered when attempting to investigate a patient with a putative mitochondrial disorder.

The encephalomyopathic forms of MDS are caused by distinct pathogenic entities. One entity interrupts the function of mitochondrial succinyl-CoA synthetase, an enzyme important for succinyl-CoA synthesis, through the loss of function of α or β subunits because of mutations in *SUCLG1* and *SUCLA2*, respectfully *(44, 53)*. These forms of MDS are noteworthy for their moderately elevated excretion of methylmalonic acid, which is not seen in other MDS varieties, and their severe lactic acidosis and Leigh-like encephalopathy. The encephalopathic form of MDS with renal tubulopathy is due to mutations in *RRM2B*, a gene that encodes for p53-induced ribonucleotide reductase small subunit (p53R2) that is likely needed for generating dNTPs for DNA synthesis *(46)*. The loss of p53R2 function may inhibit mtDNA synthesis by limiting the amount of specific of nucleotide pools. Why there is specifically kidney damage in this form of MDS is unknown because *RRM2B* is ubiquitously expressed in all tissues *(46)*. The clinical manifestations of the last variety of encephalomyopathic MDS, called MNGIE, are frequently due to mutations in *TYMP*, a gene encoding for a thymidine phosphorylase (TP), which leads to loss of TP function and aberrant thymidine metabolism, skeletal muscle mtDNA depletion, and multiple mtDNA deletions *(54)*. The pathogenesis of MNGIE due to loss of TP function is presumed to be caused by impediment of the mitochondrial deoxynucleotide salvage pathway; however, the mechanism that leads to the tissue selectivity of this disorder is not completely understood.

Cardiomyopathic MDS, otherwise known as Sengers syndrome, is caused by mutations in the *AGK* gene on chromosome 7q34, which encodes for an acylglycerol kinase (AGK) *(55)*. The pathogenesis of Sengers syndrome is unresolved. AGK is a lipid kinase that catalyzes phosphorylation of diacylglycerol (DAG) and monoacylglycerol generating phospholipid precursors, phosphatidic and lysophosphatidic acid. Sengers syndrome is also associated with a deficiency of adenine nucleotide translocator 1 (ANT), but the connection between a potential loss of lipid kinase function and ANT protein stability is unclear. It may be related to a posttranslational defect in ANT inner mitochondrial membrane assembly. It is also uncertain how a loss of AGK function directly leads to mtDNA depletion in only specific tissues but other organ systems are left relatively unscathed.

Laboratory Diagnosis

A laboratory diagnosis of MDS is difficult and relies on specific biochemical clues along with, in some circumstances, a molecular analysis as a first-tier approach. Plasma and CSF lactate and pyruvate, urine organic acids, plasma and urine amino acid profile, plasma acylcarnitine profile, plasma and urine purines and pyrimidines, serum creatine phosphokinase, and liver enzymes (alanine aminotransferase and aspartate aminotransferase) are a handful of biochemical laboratory analyses that must be considered for every possible case of MDS.

A muscle biopsy is also very informative in suspected MDS. First, analysis of mitochondrial respiratory chain activities will frequently demonstrate a combined deficiency of OXPHOS CI, CIII, CIV, and/or CV with normal, or elevated, activity levels of CII. Second, DNA isolation from muscle is useful for determining the relative amount of mtDNA levels by Southern blotting or real-time PCR. MDS will consistently display a depletion of relative mtDNA levels that are <15–20 % of normal control muscle. Sequencing analysis of specific genes associated with a certain variety of MDS that is based on clinical findings, biochemical laboratory results, and muscle biopsy results is clinically available for almost all MDS. However, a false-negative result because of possible exonic deletions cannot be excluded without additional analyses for deletions and duplications *(49)*. Therefore, a negative DNA sequencing result must be interpreted with caution.

There is a subset of biochemical laboratory results that can aid in narrowing the field of putative MDS. These diagnostic clues are sensitive and specific when placed in the context of clinical findings. For instance, an elevated serum creatine phosphokinase (>2 times normal) is suggestive of thymine kinase 2 deficiency, the myopathic form of MDS, and this elevation is not observed for other MDS types *(56)*. The isolated elevation of the plasma acylcarnitines propionylcarnitine and methymalonyl-carnitine (C3 and C4DC) alongside urinary excretion of moderate amounts of methylmalonic acid (20- to 50-times normal) without methylcitric acid but with marked lactic aciduria is sensitive for encephalomyopathic MDS because of *SUCLA2* or *SUCLG1* mutations *(44, 53)*. MNGIE syndrome is noteworthy because patients with this condition excrete large amounts of thymidine and deoxyuridine and have increased amounts of these compounds in plasma; these are present at undetectable concentrations in controls or carriers. In addition, MNGIE patients will have TP activity levels in leukocytes that are <10% of the mean activity of normal controls.

A handful of MDS varieties rely on DNA sequencing assays to obtain a diagnosis. In particular, the hepatocerebral forms of MDS are difficult to discern by basic biochemical laboratory testing alone. Therefore, DNA sequencing for *DGUOK*, *MPV17*, *PEO1*, and *POLG1* is essential for confirming a potential diagnosis. Likewise, the ability to obtain a diagnosis of MDS associated with renal tubulopathy and cardiomyopathy would be enhanced by the availability of DNA analyses of *RRM2B* and *AGK*, respectfully. However, clinical testing may not be easily available for all of these genes.

Treatment

Clinical management of MDS is largely supportive and centered on conventional therapy, such as antiepileptic drugs for seizures, physical therapy, mechanical assistance for mobility, dietary support to ensure sufficient caloric intake, and cochlear implants for hearing loss. Valproic acid and its derivatives, such as sodium divalproate, should be specifically avoided because they have been shown to induce liver damage in some cases of MDS. For children with hepatomyopathic MDS, liver transplantation does not provide additional survival benefit but may be desirable for cases with isolated liver involvement and *DGUOK* mutations. In MNGIE, experimental therapies under investigation include stem cell transplantation.

Prognosis

The prognosis for MDS is poor. These are progressive conditions with varying rates of clinical digression and decompensation. Lifespan is shortened by reoccurring complications of disease or by infection.

REFERENCES

1. Bernier FP, Boneh A, Dennett X, Chow CW, Cleary MA, Thorburn DR. Diagnostic criteria for respiratory chain disorders in adults and children. Neurology 2002;59:1406–11.
2. Robinson BH, Oei J, Sherwood WG, Applegarth D, Wong L, Haworth J, et al. The molecular basis for the two different clinical presentations of classical pyruvate carboxylase deficiency. Am J Hum Genet 1984;36:283–94.

3. Arnold GL, Griebel ML, Porterfield M, Brewster M. Pyruvate carboxylase deficiency. Report of a case and additional evidence for the "mild" phenotype. Clin Pediatr (Phila) 2001;40:519–21.
4. Hamilton J, Rae MD, Logan RW, Robinson PH. A case of benign pyruvate carboxylase deficiency with normal development. J Inherit Metab Dis 1997;20:401–3.
5. Carbone MA, MacKay N, Ling M, Cole DE, Douglas C, Rigat B, et al. Amerindian pyruvate carboxylase deficiency is associated with two distinct missense mutations. Am J Hum Genet 1998;62:1312–9.
6. García-Cazorla A, Rabier D, Touati G, Chadefaux-Vekemans B, Marsac C, de Lonlay P, Saudubray JM. Pyruvate carboxylase deficiency: Metabolic characteristics and new neurological aspects. Ann Neurol 2006;59:121–7.
7. Ahmad A, Kahler SG, Kishnani PS, Artigas-Lopez M, Pappu AS, Steiner R, et al. Treatment of pyruvate carboxylase deficiency with high doses of citrate and aspartate. Am J Med Genet 1999;87:331–8.
8. Patel KP, O'Brien TW, Subramony SH, Shuster J, Stacpoole PW. The spectrum of pyruvate dehydrogenase complex deficiency: clinical, biochemical and genetic features in 371 patients. Mol Genet Metab 2012; 105:34–43.
9. Imbard A, Boutron A, Vequaud C, Zater M, de Lonlay P, Ogier de Baulny H, et al. Molecular characterization of 82 patients with pyruvate dehydrogenase complex deficiency. Structural implications of novel amino acid substitutions in E1 protein. Mol Genet Metab 2011;104:507–16.
10. Lib MY, Brown RM, Brown GK, Marusich MF, Capaldi RA. Detection of pyruvate dehydrogenase E1 alpha-subunit deficiencies in females by immunohistochemical demonstration of mosaicism in cultured fibroblasts. J Histochem Cytochem 2002;50:877–84.
11. Brown RM, Head RA, Boubriak II, Leonard JV, Thomas NH, Brown GK. Mutations in the gene for the E1beta subunit: a novel cause of pyruvate dehydrogenase deficiency. Hum Genet 2004;115:123–7.
12. Geoffroy V, Fouque F, Benelli C, Poggi F, Saudubray JM, Lissens W, et al. Defect in the x-lipoyl-containing component of the pyruvate dehydrogenase complex in a patient with neonatal lactic acidemia. Pediatrics 1996;97:267–72.
13. Kaufmann P, Engelstad K, Wei Y, Jhung S, Sano MC, Shungu DC, et al. Dichloroacetate causes toxic neuropathy in MELAS: A randomized, controlled clinical trial. Neurology 2006;66:324–30.
14. Kaufmann P, Engelstad K, Wei Y, Kulikova R, Oskoui M, Sproule DM, et al. Natural history of MELAS associated with mitochondrial DNA M.3243A>G genotype. Neurology 2011;77:1965–71.
15. Majamaa K, Moilanen JS, Uimonen S, Remes AM, Salmela PI, Kärppä M, et al. Epidemiology of A3243G, the mutation for mitochondrial encephalomyopathy, lactic acidosis, and strokelike episodes: prevalence of the mutation in an adult population. Am J Hum Genet 1998;63:447–54.
16. Manwaring N, Jones MM, Wang JJ, Rochtchina E, Howard C, Mitchell P, Sue CM. Population prevalence of the MELAS A3243G mutation. Mitochondrion 2007;7:230–3.
17. Elliott HR, Samuels DC, Eden JA, Relton CL, Chinnery PF. Pathogenic mitochondrial DNA mutations are common in the general population. Am J Hum Genet 2008;83:254–60.
18. Goto Y, Nonaka I, Horai S. A mutation in the TRNA(Leu)(UUR) gene associated with the MELAS subgroup of mitochondrial encephalomyopathies. Nature 1990;348:651–3.
19. Sproule DM, Kaufmann P. Mitochondrial encephalopathy, lactic acidosis, and strokelike episodes: basic concepts, clinical phenotype, and therapeutic management of MELAS syndrome. Ann N Y Acad Sci 2008;1142:133–58.
20. Shoffner JM, Lott MT, Lezza AM, Seibel P, Ballinger SW, Wallace DC. Myoclonic epilepsy and ragged-red fiber disease (MERRF) is associated with a mitochondrial DNA TRNA(Lys) mutation. Cell 1990;61:931–7.
21. Naini AB, Lu J, Kaufmann P, Bernstein RA, Mancuso M, Bonilla E, et al. Novel mitochondrial DNA ND5 mutation in a patient with clinical features of MELAS and MERRF. Arch Neurol 2005;62:473–6.
22. Chinnery PF, Johnson MA, Wardell TM, Singh-Kler R, Hayes C, Brown DT, et al. The epidemiology of pathogenic mitochondrial DNA mutations. Ann Neurol 2000;48:188–93.
23. Mancuso M, Petrozzi L, Filosto M, Nesti C, Rocchi A, Choub A, et al. MERRF syndrome without ragged-red fibers: The need for molecular diagnosis. Biochem Biophys Res Commun 2007;354:1058–60.
24. Holt IJ, Harding AE, Petty RK, Morgan-Hughes JA. A new mitochondrial disease associated with mitochondrial DNA heteroplasmy. Am J Hum Genet 1990;46:428–33.
25. Tatuch Y, Christodoulou J, Feigenbaum A, Clarke JT, Wherret J, Smith C, et al. Heteroplasmic mtDNA mutation (T–G) at 8993 can cause Leigh disease when the percentage of abnormal mtDNA is high. Am J Hum Genet 1992;50:852–8.
26. Kearns TP, Sayre GP. Retinitis pigmentosa, external ophthalmophegia, and complete heart block: unusual syndrome with histologic study in one of two cases. AMA Arch Ophthalmol 1958;60:280–9.

27. Maceluch JA, Niedziela M. The clinical diagnosis and molecular genetics of Kearns-Sayre syndrome: a complex mitochondrial encephalomyopathy. Pediatr Endocrinol Rev 2006;4:117–37.
28. Lestienne P, Ponsot G. Kearns-Sayre syndrome with muscle mitochondrial DNA deletion. Lancet 1988;1:885.
29. Chen X, Prosser R, Simonetti S, Sadlock J, Jagiello G, Schon EA. Rearranged mitochondrial genomes are present in human oocytes. Am J Hum Genet 1995;57:239–47.
30. Berenberg RA, Pellock JM, DiMauro S, Schotland DL, Bonilla E, Eastwood A, et al. Lumping or splitting? "Ophthalmoplegia-plus" or Kearns-Sayre syndrome? Ann Neurol 1977;1:37–54.
31. Ogasahara S, Nishikawa Y, Yorifuji S, Soga F, Nakamura Y, Takahashi M, et al. Treatment of Kearns-Sayre syndrome with coenzyme q10. Neurology 1986;36:45–53.
32. Rötig A, Cormier V, Blanche S, Bonnefont JP, Ledeist F, Romero N, et al. Pearson's marrow-pancreas syndrome. A multisystem mitochondrial disorder in infancy. J Clin Invest 1990;86:1601–8.
33. Pearson HA, Lobel JS, Kocoshis SA, Naiman JL, Windmiller J, Lammi AT, et al. A new syndrome of refractory sideroblastic anemia with vacuolization of marrow precursors and exocrine pancreatic dysfunction. J Pediatr 1979;95:976–84.
34. Manea EM, Leverger G, Bellmann F, Stanescu PA, Mircea A, Lèbre AS, et al. Pearson syndrome in the neonatal period: two case reports and review of the literature. J Pediatr Hematol Oncol 2009;31:947–51.
35. Moraes CT, Shanske S, Tritschler HJ, Aprille JR, Andreetta F, Bonilla E, et al. mtDNA depletion with variable tissue expression: a novel genetic abnormality in mitochondrial diseases. Am J Hum Genet 1991;48:492–501.
36. Béhin A, Jardel C, Claeys KG, Fagart J, Louha M, Romero NB, et al. Adult cases of mitochondrial DNA depletion due to TK2 defect: an expanding spectrum. Neurology 2012;78:644–8.
37. Suomalainen A, Isohanni P. Mitochondrial DNA depletion syndromes—many genes, common mechanisms. Neuromuscul Disord 2010;20:429–37.
38. Calvo SE, Compton AG, Hershman SG, Lim SC, Lieber DS, Tucker EJ, et al. Molecular diagnosis of infantile mitochondrial disease with targeted next-generation sequencing. Sci Transl Med 2012;4:118ra10.
39. Saada A, Shaag A, Mandel H, Nevo Y, Eriksson S, Elpeleg O. Mutant mitochondrial thymidine kinase in mitochondrial DNA depletion myopathy. Nat Genet 2001;29:342–4.
40. Wong LJ, Naviaux RK, Brunetti-Pierri N, Zhang Q, Schmitt ES, Truong C, et al. Molecular and clinical genetics of mitochondrial diseases due to POLG mutations. Hum Mutat 2008;29:E150–72.
41. El-Hattab AW, Li FY, Schmitt E, Zhang S, Craigen WJ, Wong LJ. MPV17-associated hepatocerebral mitochondrial DNA depletion syndrome: new patients and novel mutations. Mol Genet Metab 2010;99:300–8.
42. Naviaux RK, Nguyen KV. POLG mutations associated with Alpers' syndrome and mitochondrial DNA depletion. Ann Neurol 2004;55:706–12.
43. Scalais E, Francois B, Schlesser P, Stevens R, Nuttin C, Martin JJ, et al. Polymerase gamma deficiency (POLG): clinical course in a child with a two stage evolution from infantile myocerebrohepatopathy spectrum to an Alpers syndrome and neuropathological findings of Leigh's encephalopathy. Eur J Paediatr Neurol 2012 Feb 17. [Epub ahead of print].
44. Ostergaard E, Christensen E, Kristensen E, Mogensen B, Duno M, Shoubridge EA, Wibrand F. Deficiency of the alpha subunit of succinate-coenzyme A ligase causes fatal infantile lactic acidosis with mitochondrial DNA depletion. Am J Hum Genet 2007;81:383–7.
45. Carrozzo R, Dionisi-Vici C, Steuerwald U, Lucioli S, Deodato F, Di Giandomenico S, et al. SUCLA2 mutations are associated with mild methylmalonic aciduria, Leigh-like encephalomyopathy, dystonia and deafness. Brain 2007;130:862–74.
46. Bourdon A, Minai L, Serre V, Jais JP, Sarzi E, Aubert S, et al. Mutation of RRM2b, encoding p53-controlled ribonucleotide reductase (p53r2), causes severe mitochondrial DNA depletion. Nat Genet 2007;39:776–80.
47. Hirano M, Pavlakis SG. Mitochondrial myopathy, encephalopathy, lactic acidosis, and strokelike episodes (MELAS): current concepts. J Child Neurol 1994;9:4–13.
48. Sengers RC, Trijbels JM, Willems JL, Daniels O, Stadhouders AM. Congenital cataract and mitochondrial myopathy of skeletal and heart muscle associated with lactic acidosis after exercise. J Pediatr 1975;86:873–80.
49. Zhang S, Li FY, Bass HN, Pursley A, Schmitt ES, Brown BL, et al. Application of oligonucleotide array CGH to the simultaneous detection of a deletion in the nuclear TK2 gene and mtDNA depletion. Mol Genet Metab 2010;99:53–7.
50. Mandel H, Szargel R, Labay V, Elpeleg O, Saada A, Shalata A, et al. The deoxyguanosine kinase gene is mutated in individuals with depleted hepatocerebral mitochondrial DNA. Nat Genet 2001;29:337–41.
51. Sarzi E, Goffart S, Serre V, Chrétien D, Slama A, Munnich A, et al. Twinkle helicase (PEO1) gene mutation causes mitochondrial DNA depletion. Ann Neurol 2007;62:579–87.

52. Spinazzola A, Viscomi C, Fernandez-Vizarra E, Carrara F, D'Adamo P, Calvo S, et al. Mpv17 encodes an inner mitochondrial membrane protein and is mutated in infantile hepatic mitochondrial DNA depletion. Nat Genet 2006;38:570–5.
53. Elpeleg O, Miller C, Hershkovitz E, Bitner-Glindzicz M, Bondi-Rubinstein G, Rahman S, et al. Deficiency of the ADP-forming succinyl-CoA synthase activity is associated with encephalomyopathy and mitochondrial DNA depletion. Am J Hum Genet 2005;76:1081–6.
54. Nishino I, Spinazzola A, Hirano M. Thymidine phosphorylase gene mutations in MNGIE, a human mitochondrial disorder. Science 1999;283:689–92.
55. Mayr JA, Haack TB, Graf E, Zimmermann FA, Wieland T, Haberberger B, et al. Lack of the mitochondrial protein acylglycerol kinase causes Sengers syndrome. Am J Hum Genet 2012;90:314–20.
56. Oskoui M, Davidzon G, Pascual J, Erazo R, Gurgel-Giannetti J, Krishna S, et al. Clinical spectrum of mitochondrial DNA depletion due to mutations in the thymidine kinase 2 gene. Arch Neurol 2006;63:1122–6.

Chapter **15**

Newborn Screening

Uttam Garg, Bryce A. Heese, and Laurie D. Smith

Newborn screening is designed to identify infants with significant disease before they become symptomatic to begin early treatment and improve outcome. The concept of newborn screening began in the 1960s with phenylketonuria (PKU) and the vision and direction of Dr. Robert Guthrie. Dr. Guthrie developed a bacterial inhibition assay method to detect high concentrations of phenylalanine in patient samples collected on filter paper *(1)*. This method allowed for many samples to be screened simultaneously, a necessary component of population-based screening. The bacterial inhibition assay has since been replaced by other high-throughput screening methods. Dr. Guthrie is also credited for developing a useful sample collection method—the blood spot on a filter paper. The filter paper blood spot is almost universally used in newborn screening programs and can be used for several methods, such as analyte detection, electrophoresis, enzyme assays, and molecular-based tests *(2)*.

New York was the first state to implement newborn screening of PKU in the United States in the 1960s. Over the following decades, other states adopted newborn screening, and other disorders have slowly been incorporated *(2)*. The addition of new screening tests has varied and has traditionally been at the jurisdiction of each individual screening program. In 2003, the Secretary's Advisory Committee on Heritable Disorders in Newborns and Children was formed to provide guidance to the Secretary of the U.S. Department of Health and Human Services *(3)*. The committee is charged with evaluating conditions nominated for addition to the uniform screening panel and consequently making recommendations to the Secretary of the U.S. Department of Health and Human Services *(4)*. This committee has recommended that newborn screening programs adopt a uniform panel of 30 diseases that is based on the best available evidence *(3, 5)* (see Table 15-1). Although it is difficult to identify all countries that have implemented some form of expanded newborn screening for the inborn errors of metabolism, it is sufficient to say that screening is becoming more universally accepted worldwide.

It is important to note that population-based newborn screening should not be considered diagnostic. False-positive results frequently occur; thus, abnormal newborn screening results must be confirmed using proper clinical and laboratory testing. It is also important to remember that newborn screening does not identify all inherited metabolic disorders. Also, some patients can have false-negative results on newborn screening. Therefore, a patient with suspected metabolic disorders should be investigated despite normal newborn screening results.

SAMPLE COLLECTION

Sample collection and handling may vary among different laboratories; therefore, reference to local screening program guidelines is recommended. Typically, a blood sample from the heel is collected on a filter paper at 24–48 h of life. The infant's heel can be warmed to improve circulation and should be wiped clean using an alcohol wipe and allowed to dry. Blood is obtained from the medial or lateral aspects of the heel using a sterile lancet or incision device. The first drop of

Table 15-1 Secretary's Advisory Committee on Heritable Disorders in Newborns and Children Recommended Uniform Screening Panel

Organic acid disorders
    Propionic acidemia
    Methylmalonic acidemia (methylmalonyl-CoA mutase)
    Methylmalonic acidemia (cobalamin disorders)
    Isovaleric acidemia
    3-Methylcrotonyl-CoA carboxylase deficiency
    3-Hydroxy-3-methylglutaric aciduria
    Holocarboxylase synthase deficiency
    β-Ketothiolase deficiency
    Glutaric acidemia type I
Fatty acid oxidation disorders
    Carnitine uptake defect/carnitine transport defect
    Medium-chain acyl-CoA dehydrogenase deficiency
    Very long-chain acyl-CoA dehydrogenase deficiency
    Long-chain L-3 hydroxyacyl-CoA dehydrogenase deficiency
    Trifunctional protein deficiency
Amino acid disorders
    Argininosuccinic aciduria
    Citrullinemia, type I
    Maple syrup urine disease
    Homocystinuria
    Classic phenylketonuria
    Tyrosinemia, type I
Other inherited metabolic disorders
    Classic galactosemia
    Biotinidase deficiency
Endocrine disorders
    Congenital adrenal hyperplasia
    Primary congenital hypothyroidism
Hemoglobin disorders
    S,S disease (sickle cell anemia)
    S, β-thalassemia
    S,C disease
Other disorders
    Critical congenital heart disease
    Cystic fibrosis
    Hearing loss
    Severe combined immunodeficiencies

blood should be wiped with sterile gauze. The following drops of blood are allowed to touch the card and soak through, and this process is continued until all of the circles provided on the screening card are filled. The blood on the filter paper must be allowed to completely air dry before transporting to the screening laboratory at ambient temperature. Improper technique and excessive heat can compromise the integrity of the sample. A detailed procedure on sample collection is available (6).

Table 15-1 lists the disorders recommended for screening by the Advisory Committee on Heritable Disorders in Newborns and Children. This chapter is limited to newborn screening for inherited metabolic diseases. These disorders can broadly be divided into the disorders detectable by tandem mass spectrometry (MS/MS) or by other techniques such as spectrophotometry or fluorometry. Details of these disorders are discussed throughout the book in other chapters. In this chapter, initial markers used in the screening and follow-up markers used for confirmation are discussed (7–9).

CLASSICAL GALACTOSEMIA

Classical galactosemia is caused by a defect in the erythrocyte enzyme, galactose-1-phosphate uridyltransferase (GALT). Most programs screen for erythrocyte GALT activity, and some programs include measurement of total galactose and/or second-tier molecular testing for common mutations (including the Duarte variant). Because the screening method typically relies on enzyme activity, the sample can be sensitive to mishandling, particularly heat and humidity. Also, because the enzyme is found in erythrocytes, false-negative results can occur if the patient has received a recent blood cell transfusion. If a pretransfusion sample is not collected, another sample collected 30 days after the last transfusion is recommended for GALT testing. The false-positive rate is much higher when total galactose is used as a screening marker. This technique is being used less frequently with the advent of DNA analysis. If GALT activity is used as a screening marker, galactosemia due to galactokinase and galactose-1,4-epimerase deficiency is not detected. For further information regarding galactosemia, refer to Chapter 6, "Disorders of Carbohydrate Metabolism."

BIOTINIDASE DEFICIENCY

Biotinidase deficiency is typically detected on newborn screening using a colorimetric assay of biotinidase activity. Similar to galactosemia, this screen is based on the activity of intact enzyme within the blood spot and may be sensitive to sample mishandling, particularly heat and humidity *(10)*. This enzyme is found predominantly in the serum. False negatives can occur if the patient has received a recent blood transfusion. If a pretransfusion sample is not collected, as with galactosemia, collection of another sample 30 days after the last transfusion is recommended for biotinidase testing. For a discussion of biotinidase deficiency, refer to Chapter 3, "Organic Acid Disorders."

AMINO ACIDS, FATTY ACID OXIDATION, AND ORGANIC ACID DISORDERS

These disorders are screened through MS/MS. MS/MS has inarguably changed the face of newborn screening and has made the greatest contribution to newborn screening within the past decade. With MS/MS, a single assay can detect dozens of analytes on the basis of molecular mass and charge, thereby identifying many disorders of amino acids, fatty acid oxidation, and organic acids *(11, 12)*. Table 15-2 lists the screening and confirmatory markers for these disorders *(7, 8)*. Details of these disorders are discussed throughout the book. Newborn screening act sheets and confirmatory algorithms can be found on the American College of Medical Genetics and Genomics (ACMG) website *(13)*.

FUTURE OF NEWBORN SCREENING

Newborn screening will inarguably expand for inborn metabolic and other disorders. New markers and techniques are the driving force behind the expanding newborn screening. Newborn screening for lysosomal disorders is currently highly debated and under intense scrutiny *(14, 15)*. Although not yet adopted on the recommended uniform screening panel by the Secretary's Advisory Committee on Heritable Disorders in Newborns and Children, several programs have mandated newborn screening for selected lysosomal storage diseases. New York State was the first to implement screening for a lysosomal storage disorder, Krabbe disease, in 2006. Many programs will add other conditions, including Gaucher disease, Fabry disease, Neimann-Pick A & B disease, Pompe disease, Hunter syndrome, and/or Hurler syndrome *(16)*. Lysosomal storage diseases can be detected in the blood spot by enzyme

Table 15-2 Screening Markers for Commonly Screened Disorders by MS/MS and Confirmatory and Additional Follow-up Testing

Disorder	Group	Metabolic defect	Screening marker(s)/change	Confirmatory/additional testing/change	Comments
Argininemia	AA	Arginase 1 (liver)	↑ Arginine	↑ Plasma NH$_3$, ↑ arginine on PAAP	
Argininosuccinic acidemia (ASA)	AA	Argininosuccinate lyase (ASL)	↑ Citrulline, ↑ citrulline/arginine ratio	↑ Plasma NH$_3$, ↑ argininosuccinic acid on UAAP and PAAP	Because citrulline is elevated in ASA and citrullinemia, MS/MS cannot distinguish these two disorders.
Citrullinemia type 1/2	AA	Type 1: Argininosuccinate synthase (ASS); type 2—citrin	↑ Citrulline, ↑ citrulline/arginine ratio	Type 1: ↑ plasma NH$_3$, ↑ citrulline on PAAP. Type 2: ↑ plasma NH$_3$, ↑ citrulline on PAAP; ↔↑ bilirubin, alkaline phosphatase, and GGT	With citrulline as screening marker, MS/MS cannot distinguish between citrullinemia and ASA. Citrulline is also high in pyruvate carboxylase deficiency.
Homocystinuria	AA	Cystathionine-β-synthase	↑ Methionine, ↑ homocysteine (currently only performed in a few laboratories)	↑ Blood and urine homocyst(e)ine on PAAP and UAAP	Most laboratories use methionine as a screening marker. Homocystinuria due to MTHFR/cobalamin/folate deficiency is not detected by MS/MS because plasma methionine concentrations are not elevated.
Maple syrup urine disease (MSUD)	AA	Branched-chain α-ketoacid dehydrogenase	↑ Total "leucine, isoleucine, alloisoleucine," and ↑ valine	↑ Leucine, isoleucine, alloisoleucine, and valine on PAAP; positive DNPH test on urine; ↑ branched-chain α-keto and hydroxy acids on UOAP	MS/MS does not distinguish among leucine, isoleucine, and alloisoleucine. Hydroxyproline appears in the same peak as "leucines" on MS/MS.
Nonketotic hyperglycinemia	AA	Glycine cleavage system	↑ Glycine	↑ Glycine on PAAP and CSF amino acid profile, ↑ CSF/plasma glycine ratio (>0.04)	↑ CSF/plasma glycine ratio has much better predictive value.
Phenylketonuria	AA	Phenylalanine hydroxylase (>95%); BH$_4$ synthesis/regeneration defects (<5%)	↑ Phenylalanine, ↑ phenylalanine/tyrosine ratio	↑ Phenylalanine, ↑ phenylalanine/tyrosine ratio on PAAP; abnormal urinary and/or blood or CSF pterins in BH$_4$ synthesis/regeneration defects	↑ Phenylalanine/tyrosine ratio has better predictive value.

Disorder	Type	Enzyme/Gene	Marker	Additional findings	Comments
Tyrosinemia type 1	AA	Fumarylacetoacetate hydrolase (FAH)	↑ Tyrosine, ↑ succinylacetone (currently only performed in a few laboratories)	↑ Tyrosine and methionine on PAAP; ↑ succinylacetone and tyrosine metabolites on UOAP	Because succinylacetone is generally not detected by MS/MS, the different types of tyrosinemia are indistinguishable. Tyrosinemia type 1 can be missed because tyrosine concentrations may not be high.
Tyrosinemia type 2/ oculocutaneous tyrosinemia	AA	Tyrosine aminotransferase	↑ Tyrosine	↑ Tyrosine on PAAP; ↑ tyrosine metabolites without increased succinylacetone on UOAP	Plasma tyrosine concentration is generally higher in type 2 than type 1.
Carnitine acylcarnitine translocase (CACT) deficiency	FAO	Carnitine acylcarnitine translocase	↑ Long-chain (C16, C18) acylcarnitines, ↓ free carnitine	↑ Long-chain (C16, C18) acylcarnitines on PACP; ↓ free carnitine, ↑ CK, ↓ glucose, ↑ NH₃ on plasma	May be difficult to detect because MS/MS instruments are not optimized to measure low concentrations.
Carnitine palmitoyl transferase type 1 (CPT-1) deficiency	FAO	CPT-1	↓ Long-chain (C16, C18) acylcarnitines, ↑ free (C0) carnitine	↓ Long-chain (C16, C18) acylcarnitines on PACP; ↑ free carnitine, ↑ CK, ↓ glucose, ↑ NH₃ on plasma	
Carnitine palmitoyl transferase type 2 (CPT-2) deficiency	FAO	CPT-2	↑ Long-chain (C16, C18) acylcarnitines, ↓ free (C0) carnitine	↑ Long-chain (C16, C18) acylcarnitines on PACP; ↓ free carnitine, ↑ CK, ↓ glucose, ↑ NH₃ on plasma	Carnitine-acylcarnitine translocase deficiency is detected with same screening markers.
Carnitine uptake/ transporter defect	FAO	SLC22A5 (encodes the sodium ion-dependent carnitine transporter OCTN2)	↓ Free carnitine, ↓ C16, C18:1, C18 acylcarnitines	↓ C16, C18:1, C18 acylcarnitines on PACP; ↑ urine carnitine, ↓ free carnitine, ↑ CK, ↓ glucose, ↑ NH₃ on plasma, ↓ fibroblast carnitine uptake	May be difficult to detect because MS/MS instruments are not optimized to measure low concentrations.
3-Hydroxy long-chain acyl-CoA dehydrogenase (LCHAD/TFP) deficiency	FAO	LCHAD/TFP	↑ Long-chain 3-hydroxy (C16:1-OH, C16-OH, C18:1-OH, C18-OH) acylcarnitines	↑ Long-chain 3-hydroxy (C16:1-OH, C16-OH, C18:1-OH, C18-OH) acylcarnitines on PACP; ↑ 3-hydroxy-dicarboxylic acids on UOAP; ↑ CK, ↓ glucose, ↑ NH₃ on plasma	G1528C mutation is the most common.

(Continued)

223

Table 15-2 Screening Markers for Commonly Screened Disorders by MS/MS and Confirmatory and Additional Follow-up Testing (Continued)

Disorder	Group	Metabolic defect	Screening marker(s)/change	Confirmatory/additional testing/change	Comments
Medium-chain acyl-CoA dehydrogenase (MCAD) deficiency	FAO	Medium-chain acyl-CoA dehydrogenase	↑ Medium-chain (C6, C8, C10:1, C10) acylcarnitines	↑ Medium-chain (C6, C8, C10:1, C10) acylcarnitines PACP; ↑ dicarboxylic acids, hexanoylglycine, phenylpropionylglycine, and suberylglycine on UOAP; ↑ CK, ↓ glucose, ↑ NH₃ on plasma	MCAD deficiency is the most common disorder of FAO. Fifty percent of affected individuals are homozygous whereas 40% are compound heterozygous for the common A985G (K304E) mutation.
Multiple acyl-CoA dehydrogenase (MAD) deficiency or glutaric acidemia-type 2	FAO	Electron transfer flavoprotein (ETF) α/β subunits, ETF dehydrogenase, riboflavin-responsive MAD deficiency	↑ Multiple (C4–C18 saturated and unsaturated) acylcarnitines	↑ Multiple (C4–C18 saturated and unsaturated) acylcarnitines on PACP; ↑ glutaric, ethylmalonic, dicarboxylic acids, hexanoylglycine, phenylpropionylglycine, and suberylglycine on UOAP; ↑ CK, ↓ glucose, ↑ NH₃ on plasma	
Short-chain acyl-CoA dehydrogenase (SCAD) deficiency	FAO	Short-chain acyl-CoA dehydrogenase	↑ Butyrylcarnitine (C4)	↑ Butyrylcarnitine on PACP; ↑ ethylmalonic, methylsuccinic, butyrylglycine on UOAP	Elevated C4 acylcarnitine is also seen in isobutyryl CoA dehydrogenase deficiency, MAD deficiency, and ethylmalonic encephalopathy (caused by ETH1 mutations).
Very-long-chain acyl-CoA dehydrogenase (VLCAD) deficiency	FAO	Very-long-chain acyl-CoA dehydrogenase	↑ Long-chain (C14:2, C14:1, C14) acylcarnitines, ↓ free (C0) carnitine	↑ Long-chain (C14:2, C14:1, C14) acylcarnitines on PACP; ↑ CK, ↓ glucose, ↑ NH₃ on plasma; ↓ free (C0) carnitine	Liver enzymes may also be high.
Glutaric aciduria 1 (GA I)	OA	Glutaryl-CoA dehydrogenase	↑ Glutarylcarnitine (C5-dicarboxylic/C5DC)	↑ Glutaric acid, 3-hydroxygluratic acid, and glutaconic acid on UOAP; ↑ glutarylcarnitine (C5-dicarboxylic/C5DC) on PACP	3-Hydroxyglutaric acid may be difficult to detect on UOAP.

Condition	Type	Enzyme			Comment
3-Hydroxy-3-methylglutaric (HMG) aciduria	OA	3-Hydroxy-3-methylglutaryl-CoA lyase	↑ 3-Hydroxyisovalerylcarnitine (C5-OH), 3-methylglutarylcarnitine (C6DC)	↑ 3-Hydroxy-3-methylglutaric, 3-methylglutaconic, 3-methylglutaric, 3-hydroxyisovaleric on UOAP; ↑ 3-hydroxyisovalerylcarnitine (C5-OH), 3-methylglutarylcarnitine (C6DC) on PACP	3-Hydroxyisovalerylcarnitine is also high in 3-MCC, 3-methylglutaconyl-CoA hydratase, and multiple carboxylase deficiencies. 3-Hydroxyisovalerylcarnitine is indistinguishable from 2-methyl-3-hydroxybutyrylcarnitine.
Isovaleric acidemia	OA	Isovaleryl-CoA dehydrogenase	↑ Isovalerylcarnitine (C5)	↑ Isovalerylglycine, 3-hydroxyisovaleric acid on UOAP; ↑ isovalerylcarnitine (C5) on PACP	On MS/MS, isovalerylcarnitine is indistinguishable from 2-methylbutyrylcarnitine and pivaloylcarnitine derived from antibiotics containing Sulbactam pivoxil.
3-Ketothiolase deficiency	OA	3-Ketothiolase	↑ Tiglylcarnitine (C5:1), ↑ 3-hydroxy-2-methylbutyrylcarnitine (C5-OH)	↑ 2-Methyl-3-hydroxybutyrate, 2-methylacetoacetic, tiglylglycine on UOAP; ↑ tiglylcarnitine (C5:1), ↑ 3-hydroxy-2-methylbutyrylcarnitine (C5-OH). Ketones are also generally very high in blood/urine	On MS/MS, 3-hydroxy-2-methylbutyrylcarnitine is indistinguishable from 3-hydroxyisovalerylcarnitine.
3-Methylcrotonyl carboxylase (MCC) deficiency	OA	3-MCC	↑ 3-Hydroxyisovalerylcarnitine (C5-OH)	↑ 3-Hydroxyisovaleric, 3-methylcrotonylglycine on UOAP; ↑ 3-hydroxyisovalerylcarnitine (C5-OH) on PACP	See comment for 3-Hydroxy-3-methylglutaric (HMG) aciduria. 3-Methylcrotonylcarnitine may also be high.
2-Methylbutyryl CoA dehydrogenase deficiency	OA	2-Methylbutyryl CoA dehydrogenase	↑ 2-Methylbutyrylcarnitine (C5)	↑ 2-Methylbutyrylglycine	On MS/MS, 2-methylbutyrylcarnitine is indistinguishable from isovalerylcarnitine.
3-Methylglutanoyl CoA hydratase deficiency	OA	3-Methylglutanoyl CoA hydratase	↑ 3-Hydroxyisovalerylcarnitine (C5-OH)	↑ 3-Hydroxyisovaleric, 3-methylglutaconic, 3-methylglutaric on UOAP; ↑ 3-hydroxyisovalerylcarnitine (C5-OH) on PACP	See comment for 3-Hydroxy-3-methylglutaric (HMG) aciduria.

(Continued)

Table 15-2 Screening Markers for Commonly Screened Disorders by MS/MS and Confirmatory and Additional Follow-up Testing (Continued)

Disorder	Group	Metabolic defect	Screening marker(s)/change	Confirmatory/additional testing/change	Comments
Methylmalonic acidemia	OA	Methylmalonyl CoA mutase, cobalamin deficiency/defects (A, B, C, D, F)	↑ Propionylcarnitine (C3), ↑ methylmalonylcarnitine (C4-DC)	↑ Methylmalonic, 3-hydroxypropionic, methylcitrate, propionylglycine on UOAP; ↑ propionylcarnitine (C3), methylmalonylcarnitine (C4-DC) on PACP. Fibroblast complementation to classify cobalamin defect	Elevated C3 acylcarnitine also occurs in propionic acidemia and multiple carboxylase deficiency.
Multiple carboxylase deficiency	OA	Holocarboxylase synthetase	↑ Propionylcarnitine (C3), ↑ 3-hydroxyisovalerylcarnitine (C5-OH)	↑ 3-Hydroxy-isovaleric, 3-methylcrotonylglycine, methylcitric, 3-hydroxy-propionic, lactic, pyruvic, acetoacetic, 3-hydroxy-butyric on UOAP; ↑ propionylcarnitine (C3), ↑ 3-hydroxyisovalerylcarnitine (C5-OH) on PACP	Deficiency of holocarboxylase synthetase leads to functional deficiency of all carboxylases (pyruvate carboxylase, propionyl CoA carboxylase, MCC, acetyl-CoA carboxylase).
Propionic acidemia	OA	Propionyl-CoA carboxylase	↑ Propionylcarnitine (C3)	↑ 3-Hydroxypropionic, methylcitratic, propionylglycine on UOAP; ↑ propionylcarnitine (C3) on PACP	C3 is also high in methylmalonic acidemia, multiple carboxylase deficiency, and cobalamin deficiencies.

AA = amino acidemia, BH$_4$ = tetrahydrobiopterin, CK = creatine kinase, CSF = cerebrospinal fluid, DNPH = dinitrophenylhydrazine, FAO = fatty acid oxidation, GGT = γ-glutamyl transpeptidase, LCHAD/TFP = long-chain 3-hydroxy acyl-CoA dehydrogenase/trifunctional protein, MTHFR = methylenetetrahydrofolate reductase, NH$_3$ = ammonia, OA = organic acidemia, PAAP = plasma amino acid profile, PACP = plasma acylcarnitine profile, UAAP = urine amino acid profile, UOAP = urine organic acid profile.

assays using synthetic substrates *(16, 17)*. Detection methods include colorimetry, fluorometry, or MS/MS. Newborn screening for many other disorders such as disorders of steroid synthesis, bile acid synthesis, long-chain fatty acids, and creatine synthesis is also under discussion *(15)*. However, challenges in developing high-throughput, multiplex methods appropriate for mass population-based screening still exist.

REFERENCES

1. Guthrie R, Susi A. A simple phenylalanine method for detecting phenylketonuria in large populations of newborn infants. Pediatrics 1963;32:338–43.
2. Marsden D, Larson C, Levy HL. Newborn screening for metabolic disorders. J Pediatr 2006;148:577–84.
3. U.S. Department of Health and Human Services, Health Resources and Services Administration. Maternal and child health. Newborn screening. http://www.mchb.hrsa.gov/screening (Accessed April 2012).
4. Calonge N, Green NS, Rinaldo P, Lloyd-Puryear M, Dougherty D, Boyle C, et al. Committee report: Method for evaluating conditions nominated for population-based screening of newborns and children. Genet Med 2010;12:153–9.
5. National Newborn Screening & Genetics Resource Center. http://genes-r-us.uthscsa.edu/index.htm (Accessed April 2012).
6. Hannon WH, Whitley R, Davin B, Fernhoff P, Halonen T, Lavochkin M, et al. Blood collection on filter paper for newborn screening programs; Approved guideline, 5th ed. Document LA4-A5. Wayne, PA: Clinical and Laboratory Standards Institute, 2007.
7. Dietzen DJ, Rinaldo P, Whitley RJ, Rhead WJ, Hannon WH, Garg UC, et al. National Academy of Clinical Biochemistry laboratory medicine practice guidelines: follow-up testing for metabolic disease identified by expanded newborn screening using tandem mass spectrometry; executive summary. Clin Chem 2009;55:1615–26.
8. Garg U, Dasouki M. Expanded newborn screening of inherited metabolic disorders by tandem mass spectrometry: clinical and laboratory aspects. Clin Biochem 2006;39:315–32.
9. Pasquali M, Longo N. Newborn screening and inborn errors of metabolism. In: Burtis CA, Ashwood ER, Bruns DE, eds. Tietz Textbook of Clinical Chemistry and Molecular Diagnostics, 5th ed. St. Louis, MO: Elsevier, 2012:2045–82.
10. Cowan TM, Blitzer MG, Wolf B. Technical standards and guidelines for the diagnosis of biotinidase deficiency. Genet Med 2010;12:464–70.
11. Chace DH, Kalas TA. A biochemical perspective on the use of tandem mass spectrometry for newborn screening and clinical testing. Clin Biochem 2005;38:296–309.
12. Chace DH, Kalas TA, Naylor EW. The application of tandem mass spectrometry to neonatal screening for inherited disorders of intermediary metabolism. Annu Rev Genomics Hum Genet 2002;3:17–45.
13. American College of Medical Genetics and Genomics. http://www.acmg.net/AM/Template.cfm?Section=NBS _ACT_Sheets_and_Algorithms_Table&Template=/CM/HTMLDisplay.cfm&ContentID=5072 (Accessed April 2012).
14. Ross LF. Newborn screening for lysosomal storage diseases: an ethical and policy analysis. J Inherit Metab Dis 2011. [Epub ahead of print]
15. Bennett MJ, Rinaldo P, Wilcken B, Pass KA, Watson MS, Wanders RJ. Newborn screening for metabolic disorders: how are we doing, and where are we going? Clin Chem 2012;58:324–31.
16. Marsden D, Levy H. Newborn screening of lysosomal storage disorders. Clin Chem 2010;56:1071–9.
17. Zhang XK, Elbin CS, Turecek F, Scott R, Chuang WL, Keutzer JM, et al. Multiplex lysosomal enzyme activity assay on dried blood spots using tandem mass spectrometry. Methods Mol Biol 2010;603:339–50.

Chapter **16**

Other Inherited Metabolic Diseases

Uttam Garg and Laurie D. Smith

In addition to the inherited metabolic disorders discussed in this book, there are many more that are less commonly encountered, are not well understood, or do not fit neatly into any of the previous book chapters. The following table lists clinical and laboratory findings of many inherited metabolic disorders not discussed elsewhere *(1–6)*. Disorders such as the dyslipoproteinemias, steroid biogenesis disorders, porphyrias, bile metabolism disorders, and immunological disorders that are often not encountered or managed by clinical biochemical geneticists are not listed. Like many other disorders described in the book, the disorders listed in Table 16-1 have a wide spectrum and continuum of clinical findings.

Table 16-1 Clinical and Laboratory Findings in Various Inherited Metabolic Disorders Not Covered in the Book

Disorder	Genetics	Clinical findings	Laboratory findings
Alanine:glyoxylate aminotransfer-ase deficiency, primary hyper-oxaluria type 1	AGXT, 2q37.3	Accumulation of calcium oxalate in various tissues, especially the kidney, resulting in renal failure	Increased plasma and urine oxalate and glycolate. Reduced enzyme deficiency in liver biopsy
γ-Aminobutyric acid (GABA) transaminase deficiency	ABAT, 16p13.2	Convulsions, mental retardation, axial hypotonia, lethargy	Increased GABA in plasma, urine, and CSF. Vegabatrin treatment increases GABA
Aspartylglucosaminuria	AGA, 4q34.3	Central nervous system involvement, skeletal abnormalities, connective tissue lesions, and progressive mental retardation	Glycosylasparaginase deficiency in leukocytes and fibroblasts
Formiminotransferase deficiency/ formiminoglutamic aciduria	FTCD, 21q22.3	Variable. Cases of megaloblastic anemia and mental retardation have been re-ported	Increased formiminoglutamate. May cause false increase in C4 in newborn screening
α-Fucosidosis	FUCA1, 1p36.11	Angiokeratoma, progressive psychomotor retardation, neurologic signs, coarse facial features, and dysostosis multiplex	Deficient α-fucosidase in leukocytes or fibroblasts. Increased urinary excretion of fucose-rich oligosaccharides by TLC
Galactosialidosis, protective protein/cathepsin A deficiency, secondary β-galactosidase, and α-neuraminidase deficiency	CTSA, 20q13.12	Hurler like phenotype, dysostosis multiplex, kidney involvement, hepatosplenomegaly, intellectual disability	Enzyme deficiencies in leukocytes and fibroblasts
γ-Glutamylcysteine synthetase deficiency	GCLC, 6p12.1	Hemolytic anemia	Decreased erythrocyte glutathione and the enzyme, increased reticulocytes, decreased hemoglobin
Glutathione synthetase deficiency	GSS, 20q11.22	Hemolytic anemia	Decreased erythrocyte glutathione and the enzyme; increased reticulocytes, decreased hemoglobin, increased 5-oxoproline on urine organic acids profile
D-Glyceric acidemia	GLYCTK, 3p21.1	Highly variable. Some patients have an encephalopathic presentation, with severe mental retardation, seizures, and micro-cephaly. Others have mild speech delay or even have normal development	Increased urinary D-glyceric acid
Glyoxylate reductase deficiency, primary hyperoxaluria type 2	GRHPR, 9p13.2	Accumulation of calcium oxalate in various tissues, especially the kidney, resulting in renal failure	Urinary excretion of oxalate and commonly L-glycerate

Disorder	Gene, location	Clinical features	Laboratory findings
Hartnup disease	SLC6A19, 5p15.33	Variable. Cases with pellagra-like light-sensitive rash photodermatitis and cerebellar ataxia have been reported	Increased urinary neutral amino acids
Hawkinsinuria	HPD, 12q24.31	Autosomal-dominant disorder characterized by metabolic acidosis and failure to thrive in infancy. Symptoms improve in first year of life although patients continue to excrete the Hawkinsin and tyrosine metabolites in urine	Increased Hawkinsin (2-L-cystein-S-yl-1,4-dihydroxycyclohex-5-en-1-yl)-acetic acid and tyrosine metabolites (4-hydroxyphenylpyruvate, 4-hydroxyphenyllactate, 4-hydroxyphenylacetate) in urine
Histidinemia	HAL, 12q23.1	Variable, probably not related to the disorder	Increased histidine and decreased urocanic acid in blood and urine
Hydroxyproline oxidase deficiency	—	Benign condition not clearly associated with clinical manifestations	Increased hydroxyproline in plasma and urine
Hypophosphatasia	ALPL, 1p36.12	Highly variable. Different forms: perinatal, infantile, childhood, and adult depending on time of clinical manifestations. Defective mineralization of bone and/or teeth	Low activity of serum and bone alkaline phosphatase. Increased urinary phosphoethanolamine on amino acid profile
2-Ketoglutarate dehydrogenase complex deficiency	OGDH, 7p13	Variable. Cases of hypotonia, metabolic acidosis, hypoglycemia, and hyperlactatemia have been reported	Increased 2-ketoglutarate on urine organic acid profile
α-Mannosidosis type I and type II	MAN2B1, 19p13.2	Hurler-like phenotype, macrocephaly, dysostosis multiplex, hearing loss, hepatosplenomegaly, and intellectual disability	Deficient α-mannosidase in leukocytes or fibroblasts. Increased urinary excretion of mannose-rich oligosaccharides by TLC. Molecular analysis
β-Mannosidosis	MANBA, 4q22-q25	Mild Hurler-like phenotype, hearing loss	Deficient β-mannosidase in leukocytes or fibroblasts. Increased urinary excretion of mannose-rich oligosaccharides by TLC. Molecular analysis
Menkes, copper transport disorder	ATP7A, Xq21.1	Psychomotor retardation, convulsions, connective tissue abnormalities, hair abnormalities (kinky hair)	Low serum copper and ceruloplasmin concentrations, low liver copper
Mevalonate kinase deficiency	MVK, 12q24.11	Developmental delay, hepatosplenomegaly, lymphadenopathy, anemia, diarrhea, and malabsorption	Increased mevalonic acid on urine organic acid profile

(Continued)

Table 16-1 Clinical and Laboratory Findings in Various Inherited Metabolic Disorders Not Covered in the Book (Continued)

Disorder	Genetics	Clinical findings	Laboratory findings
α-NAGA deficiency type 2 (Kanzaki disease)	NAGA, 22q13.2	Neuroaxonal dystrophy, angiokeratoma corporis diffusum, and mild intellectual impairment	N-Acetyl-α-D-galactosaminidase deficiency in leukocytes and fibroblasts
N-Acetyl-α-D-galactosaminidase (NAGA) deficiency type 1 (Schindler disease)	NAGA, 22q13.2	Intellectual impairment	N-Acetyl-α-D-galactosaminidase deficiency in leukocytes and fibroblasts
Ornithine-5-aminotransferase deficiency	OAT, 10q26.13	Gyrate atrophy of choroid and retina. Blindness in adulthood	Increased blood and urinary ornithine; increased urinary arginine and lysine. Plasma creatine may be low
3-Phosphoglycerate dehydrogenase deficiency	PHGDH, 1p12	Microcephaly. Not well defined	Decreased plasma and CSF serine on amino acid profile
Prolidase deficiency	PEPD, 19q13.11	Chronic, slowly healing ulcerations, mainly on the legs and feet. The ulcers are often preceded by other dermatologic manifestations such as erythematous papular eruptions and telangiectasias with pruritus	Imidodipeptiduria and lack of or reduced prolidase activity in erythrocytes, leukocytes, or cultured fibroblasts
Proline oxidase deficiency/hyperprolinemia type 1	PRODH, 22q11.21. The PRODH gene falls within the region deleted in the 22q11 deletion syndrome, including DiGeorge syndrome and velocardiofacial syndrome	Benign condition not clearly associated with clinical manifestations	Increased urinary proline, hydroxyproline, and glycine
Δ¹-Pyrroline-5-carboxylate dehydrogenase deficiency/hyperprolinemia type 2	ALDH4A1, 1p36.13	Not well defined	Increased urine proline, hydroxyproline, glycine, and pyrroline-5-carboxylate
Δ¹-Pyrroline-5-carboxylate synthase deficiency	PYCS, 10q24.1	Bilateral cataract and joint and skin laxity	Increased blood ammonia. Decreased proline, ornithine, citrulline, and arginine
Renal glucosuria (SGLT2 defect)	SLC5A2, 16p11.2	Patients with familial renal glucosuria have decreased renal tubular resorption of glucose from the urine in the absence of hyperglycemia and any other signs of tubular dysfunction	Increased urinary glucose

Disorder	Gene, locus	Clinical features	Laboratory findings
Sarcosine dehydrogenase deficiency	SARDH, 9q34.2	Most likely benign disorder. Some reports have associated the disorder with mental retardation and neurologic problems	Increased sarcosine in plasma and urine
Sialidosis, α–neuraminidase deficiency type 1 and 2, mucolipidosis type 1	NEU1, 6p21.33	Type 1: Cherry-red spots, progressive myoclonus, progressive visual loss. Type 2: Coarse facies, dysostosis multiplex, hearing loss, ataxia, myoclonus, and seizures	Deficient α-neuraminidase in fibroblasts. Sialyl-acid-rich oligosaccharides in urine
Sialuria, N-acetylneuraminic aciduria	GNE, 9p13.3	Cardiomegaly, hepatosplenomegaly	Free sialic acid (N-acetylneuraminic acid) excretion in urine. Sialuria differs from the sialidoses that have deficient neuraminidase activity and increased sialyl acid-rich oligosaccharides in urine
Smith-Lemli-Opitz syndrome, 7-dehydrocholesterol (7-DHC) reductase deficiency	DHCR7, 11q13.4	Growth retardation, microcephaly, intellectual disability, malformations including distinctive facial features, cleft palate, cardiac defects, underdeveloped external genitalia in males, postaxial polydactyly, and 2-3 syndactyly of the toes	Increased plasma 7-DHC, hypocholesterolemia
Succinic semialdehyde dehydrogenase deficiency	ALDH5A1, 6p22.3	Mental retardation, ataxia	Increased γ–hydroxybutyric acid in urine, plasma, CSF. In GC-MS urea coelutes with γ–hydroxybutyric acid making identification challenging
Trimethylaminuria, fish odor syndrome	FMO3, 1q24.3	Fishy odor resembling that of rotten or decaying fish	Increased urinary triethylamine
Urocanase deficiency	UROC1, 3q21.3	Variable, probably not related to the disorder	Increased urocanic acid in urine
Wilson disease, hepatolenticular degeneration	ATP7B, 13q14.3	Hepatosplenomegaly, cirrhosis, Kayser-Fleischer-ring, hemolytic anemia, ascites, movement disorders	Low serum copper and ceruloplasmin concentrations, increased urinary copper excretion, increased hepatic copper

CSF = cerebrospinal fluid, GC-MS = gas chromatography/mass spectroscopy, TLC = thin-layer chromatography.

REFERENCES

1. Blau N, Duran M, Blaskovics ME, Gibson KM, Scriver CR, eds. Physician's Guide to the Laboratory Diagnosis of Metabolic Diseases, 2nd ed. Berlin: Springer, 2003.
2. GeneTests. http://www.genetests.org (Accessed February 2012).
3. Hoffmann GF, Zschocke J, Nyhan WL, eds. Inherited Metabolic Diseases: A Clinical Approach. Heidelberg, Germany: Springer, 2010.
4. Online Mendelian Inheritance in Man. http://www.ncbi.nlm.nih.gov/omim.
5. Saudubray J-M, van den Berghe G, Walter JH, eds. Inborn Metabolic Diseases: Diagnosis and Treatment, 5th ed. New York: Springer-Verlag, 2011.
6. Scriver CR, Sly WS, Childs B, Beaudet AL, Valle D, Kinzler KW, Vogelstein B. The Metabolic & Molecular Bases of Inherited Disease, 8th ed. New York: McGraw-Hill, 2001.

Index